Global Health Perspectives in Prediabetes and Diabetes Prevention

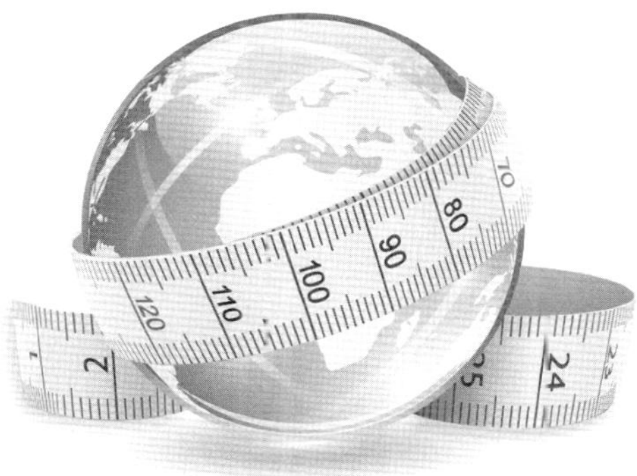

Global Health Perspectives in Prediabetes and Diabetes Prevention

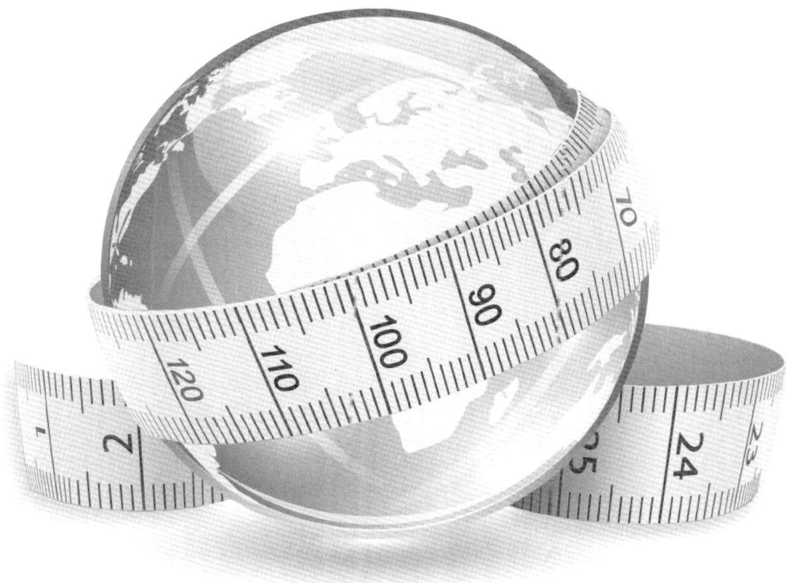

Editor

Michael Bergman, MD, FACP

NYU School of Medicine, USA

World Scientific

NEW JERSEY • LONDON • SINGAPORE • BEIJING • SHANGHAI • HONG KONG • TAIPEI • CHENNAI

Published by

World Scientific Publishing Co. Pte. Ltd.
5 Toh Tuck Link, Singapore 596224
USA office: 27 Warren Street, Suite 401-402, Hackensack, NJ 07601
UK office: 57 Shelton Street, Covent Garden, London WC2H 9HE

Library of Congress Cataloging-in-Publication Data
Global health perspectives in prediabetes and diabetes prevention / [edited by] Michael Bergman.
p. ; cm.
Includes bibliographical references and index.
ISBN 978-9814603300 (hardcover : alk. paper)
I. Bergman, Michael, editor.
[DNLM: 1. Diabetes Mellitus, Type 2--prevention & control. 2. Cross-Cultural Comparison.
3. Prediabetic State--prevention & control. 4. World Health. WK 810]
RA645.D5
362.1964'62--dc23

2014009132

British Library Cataloguing-in-Publication Data
A catalogue record for this book is available from the British Library.

In-house Editors: Darilyn Yap/Sandhya Devi

Typeset by Stallion Press
Email: enquiries@stallionpress.com

Printed in Singapore by FuIsland Offset Printing (S) Pte Ltd

Dedication

I am grateful to my wife Evelyn and our family for their love and support and encouraging my lifelong commitment to professional growth.

Contents

Preface

Michael Bergman

> "Prevention of disease is often difficult to put into practice. Among the obstacles: the success of prevention is invisible, lacks drama, often requires persistent behavior change, and may be long delayed … Prevention of disease will succeed over time insofar as it can be embedded in a culture of health."[1]

Type 2 diabetes imposes a substantial economic burden on healthcare systems. The International Diabetes Federation (IDF) estimates that in 2013, 382 million individuals representing more than 8% of adults globally have diabetes which is projected to increase by 55% to 592 million in 2035. These staggering figures result in health care expenditures estimated at $548 billion in 2013.[2]

An increase in global healthy life expectancy from 1990–2010 approximating four years has resulted principally through a reduction in child and adult mortality rather than in years lived with disability (YLD). Salomon *et al.* observed that "the failure to make substantial progress in reducing disability over the past 20 years should serve as a wake-up call to the global public health community… Most YLDs come from conditions for which we have not yet succeeded at effective, large-scale prevention."[3]

It is furthermore estimated that in 2010, 54% of worldwide disability-adjusted life-years (DALYs), a measure of overall disease burden representing the sum of years of life lost from premature death and years lived with disability, were due to non-communicable diseases (NCDs), an increase from 43% in 1990.[4] This includes a stark 69% increase in DALYs due to diabetes from 1990–2010 constituting the fourth leading contributing cause to global DALYs. Morbidity caused by diabetes including neuropathy, retinopathy, amputation, diabetic foot and chronic kidney diseases, is also substantial and increasing. Mortality related to NCDs increased from 57% to 65% in this same time period, 80% of which occurred in low- and middle-income countries which also have a high proportion of deaths in middle age. WHO, in an assessment of Global Burden of Disease, projects that by 2030 diabetes will represent the fourth leading cause of death in high-income countries, the sixth in middle-income countries and the ninth in low-income countries representing an increase in world ranking from eleventh place in 2002 to seventh in 2030.[5]

Despite recognition of the indisputable value of lifestyle modification in thwarting the insidious progression to diabetes, its global prevalence continues to increase. The vast majority of individuals with prediabetes remain undiagnosed and untreated. Efforts to identify markers for diagnosing dysglycemic states early on the lengthy continuum from normal glucose tolerance through prediabetes, prior to the emergence of diabetes, remains an area of considerable interest as current absolute diagnostic guidelines may ironically be delaying their timely detection.[6,7] In view of the global shift from communicable to chronic NCDs, the increasing prevalence of obesity, prediabetes and type 2 diabetes creates a considerable challenge to clinical and public health infrastructure. Therefore, the responsibilities of the medical and public health communities involve identifying new methods for screening and identifying those at risk as well availing high-risk individuals of treatment modalities.[8] In this context, inadequacies of current approaches to prediabetes and diabetes prevention with novel proposals for their remediation have recently been reviewed.[8,9]

Elliot P. Joslin already astutely recognized in 1921, coincidentally the same year insulin was discovered, that “It is well-known that diabetic patients come too late for treatment. If the disease is detected early, it is far more susceptible to diet…More energy must be exerted to discover this disease. One must hunt for it.”[10] Furthermore, he stated that “it is proper at the present time to devote attention not alone to treatment, but still more … to prevention. The results may not be quite so striking or as immediate, but they are sure to come and to be important … Real headway against the ravages of a disease begins with its prevention rather than with its treatment ..."[10] This text is an attestation to these very principles demonstrating the enormous global efforts being expended in the attempt to eradicate diabetes by implementing prevention programs in even the remotest communities. Although considerable progress is being made, clearly, much more needs to done. Effective coordination of governmental and non-governmental organizations, food and agricultural industries, regional and local health authorities, the practicing and academic medical communities is required with considerable investment of financial and other resources if the "diabesity" tsunami is to be thwarted. All sectors, government, industry, public health and clinical, therefore share a critical role in this process and by working together, ought to create the necessary synergies essential for making substantial forays in the prevention of type 2 diabetes.[8]

I am indebted to and grateful for the considerable efforts expended by all the notable authors who have taken from their valuable time to contribute to this authoritative and comprehensive text. We can all take immense satisfaction that this work represents a truly international cooperation and initiative appropriate for the global nature of this epidemic. I am especially grateful to Professors Peter Schwarz and Jaakko Tuomilehto, both renown for their substantial contributions to diabetes prevention, for their helpful suggestions regarding the contents and scope of this text. I am also grateful to the publisher, World Scientific Publishing, and editors for their support and acknowledging the fundamental importance of this text for global health efforts in diabetes prevention. It is hoped that its availability will further inform public health experts, policy makers and clinicians thereby stimulating and enhancing the global campaign to prevent diabetes leading to a reduction in associated morbidity, mortality, considerable economic burden and a dramatic improvement in the quality of life of citizenry throughout the world.

REFERENCES

1. Fineberg, HV. (2013) The paradox of disease prevention: celebrated in principle, resisted in practice. *JAMA* **310**: 85–90.
2. IDF Atlas (2013) 6th ed.

3. Salomon JA, Wang H, Freeman M, Vos T, Flaxman AD, Lopez AD, Murray CJL. (2012) Healthy life expectancy for 187 countries, 1990–2010: A systematic analysis for the Global Burden Disease Study 2010. *Lancet* **380**: 2144–2162.
4. Lim SS, Flazman AD, Danaei G *et al.* (2012) A comparable risk assessment of burden of disease and injury attributable to 67 risk factors and risk factor clusters in 21 regions, 1990–2010: A systematic analysis for the Global Burden of Disease Study 2010. *Lancet* **380**: 2224–22260.
5. Mathers CD, Loncar D. (2006) Projections of global mortality and burden of disease from 2002 to 2030. *PLoSMed* **3**: e442.
6. Bergman M, Dankner R, Roth J, Narayan KM. (2013) Are current diagnostic guidelines delaying early detection of dysglycemic states? Time for new approaches. Viewpoint. *Endocrine* **44**: 66–69.
7. Bergman M. (2010) Inadequacies of absolute threshold levels for diagnosing prediabetes. *Diabetes Metab Res Rev* **26**: 3–6.
8. Bergman M, Buysschaert M, Albright A, Schwarz P, Narayan KM, Yach D. (2012) Policy Perspective. Diabetes prevention: global health policy and perspectives from the ground. *Diabetes Manage* **2**: 309–321.
9. Bergman M. (2013) Inadequacies of current approaches to prediabetes and diabetes prevention. Viewpoint. *Endocrine* **44**: 623–633.
10. Joslin, EP. (1921) The prevention of diabetes mellitus. *JAMA* **76**: 79–84.

Chapter 1: Diagnosis and Definition

Martin Buysschaert, Vanessa Preumont,*[†]
Jose Luis Medina[‡] *and Michael Bergman*[§]

Diabetes mellitus is a metabolic disorder of multiple etiologies. Specifically, type 2 diabetes is characterized by chronic hyperglycemia together with disturbances of carbohydrate, fat, and protein metabolism. This condition results from defects of insulin secretion, insulin action, or both, as a consequence of a combination of genetic predisposition, unhealthy diet, physical inactivity, and increased weight.[1,2] Type 2 diabetes is a growing public health challenge globally with an estimated prevalence of the disease in 285 million people (corresponding to 6.4% of the world's adult population), which is expected to reach more than 550 million (7.8% of the population) by 2030, according to recent projections of the International Diabetes Federation (IDF). Of the total, 70% of these cases occur currently in low- and middle-income countries.[3,4] Long-term hyperglycemia in type 2 diabetes is associated with progressive damage of various organs, including eyes, kidneys, nerves, heart, and blood vessels, with premature mortality and has considerable economic impact.[2]

Prior to the development of type 2 diabetes, glucose levels can increase in a prediabetic state that may exist for many years before type 2 diabetes

*Corresponding author. Department of Endocrinology and Diabetology, Université Catholique de Louvain, University Clinic Saint-Luc, Brussels, Belgium. E-mail: martin.buysschaert@uclouvain.be

[†]Department of Endocrinology and Diabetology, University Clinic Saint-Luc, Brussels, Belgium. E-mail: vanessa.preumont@uclouvain.be

[‡]Medicine Department, Oporto Medical School, Oporto University, Sao Joao Hospital, San Joao, Portugal. Email: jlmedina40@gmail.com

[§]School of Medicine, Department of Medicine, Division of Endocrinology and Metabolism, New York. E-mail: michael.bergman@nyumc.org

comes to be diagnosed.[5,6] Dysglycemia is characterized by higher glucose levels than normal but lower than defined by conventionally established thresholds for diabetes. Globally, prediabetes should not be viewed as a clinical entity but rather a risk factor for diabetes development as well as for cardiovascular disease. This high-risk prediabetic state includes isolated impaired fasting glucose (IFG), isolated impaired glucose tolerance (IGT), or combined IFG/IGT.[7] The prevalence of IFG/IGT increases with age as indicated in the DECODE Study (IGT increased from 3.9% in 30 to 39-year-old men to 15.1% in the 70- to 79-year-old age group and from 4.5 in 30- to 39-year-old women to 16.9% in the 70- to 79-year-old age group).[8] It has been predicted that globally there will be 470 million people in 2030 with prediabetes.[4]

Diagnosis of prediabetes is mandatory since numerous clinical studies have confirmed that a substantial number of individuals with this disorder will later develop diabetes with an average annual risk approximating 5–10% compared with below 1% in normoglycemic subjects.[9–11] Furthermore, IFG/IGT is also associated with microvascular complications, neuropathy, and cardiovascular disease.[12–15] Kurihara *et al.* recently showed that coronary atherosclerosis and plaque vulnerability were more advanced in patients with prediabetes than those without diabetes and were comparable between individuals with prediabetes and diabetes.[16] Therefore, early recognition is crucial as lifestyle modification as well as medications have been shown to be effective, particularly in reducing progression to diabetes.[7,17–19]

Diagnosis of IFG/IGT is an evolving process as cutoff values have been revised several times in the past decades as new research data became available. Along this line, the aim of this chapter is to review the past and present definitions of prediabetes, including the place of HbA_{1c} as a diagnostic procedure.

1. THE PAST HISTORY OF "GLUCOSE INTOLERANCE"

Before 1979, a state of "borderline" diabetes had been recognized by the World Health Organization (WHO)'s First Expert Committee when there was uncertainty about the diagnosis of diabetes, but where blood glucose levels were above normal.[20]

The National Diabetes Data Group (NDDG), in 1979, confirmed that a raised blood glucose was the hallmark of diabetes but was also the first to introduce the concept of a prediabetic condition referred to as "glucose intolerance," defined as a metabolic (hyperglycemic) state intermediate between normal glucose homeostasis and diabetes.[21] The NDDG indicated that a 75 g load of glucose would be appropriate for diagnosis of both conditions when consumed in 300 mL water over 5 m (when at least 250 g carbohydrates were consumed for 3 days before the test). The fasting and 2-hr values diagnostic criteria for diabetes were largely established on the basis of predicting the development of retinopathy.[22] Briefly, diabetes was defined by a fasting plasma glucose (FPG) equal to or greater than 140 mg/dL (7.8 mmol/L) (on more than one occasion) or on a 2-hr value after a 75 g oral glucose tolerance test (OGTT) equal to or greater than 200 mg/dL (11.1 mmol/L) and at another time between 0 and 2 hr. Diabetes was also diagnosed in the presence of an "unequivocal" elevation of plasma glucose with classical signs and symptoms of hyperglycemia. In the NDDG report, "glucose intolerance" by itself was identified by the simultaneous presence of three criteria: a FPG level lower than 140 mg/dL (7.8 mmol/L), a glucose value between 140 and 199 mg/dL (7.8–11.0 mmol/L) 120 m after an OGTT, and at least one other glucose concentration equal to or exceeding 200 mg/dL (11.1 mmol/L) at 30, 60, and 90 m during OGTT (Table 1). These criteria were established in 1980 by the WHO, which stated, however, that glucose intolerance could be defined after OGTT by a single glucose level between 140 and 199 mg/dL (7.8–11.0 mmol/L) at 120 m if the FPG was below 140 mg/dL (7.8 mmol/L) (i.e., two criteria for "glucose intolerance" in the WHO vs. three in the NDDG).[23] In 1985, the WHO group adjusted their fasting and post-challenge values to precisely match the NDDG criteria.[24]

2. THE MODERN ERA OF "PREDIABETES"

2.1. Step 1

An International Expert Committee (IEC) convened by the American Diabetes Association (ADA) and IDF, in 1997, and the WHO, in 1998, re-examined the diagnostic criteria of (pre)diabetes in light of new

Table 1. Diagnostic criteria for prediabetes: historical synopsis.

NDDG (1979)[21]	Fasting	<140 (7.8)	
	OGTT 120′	140–199 (7.8–11.0)	Glucose
	OGTT 30, 60, 90′	1 value ≥ 200 (11.1)	Intolerance
WHO (1980)[23]	Fasting	<140 (7.8)	Glucose
	OGTT 120′	140–199 (7.8–11.0)	Intolerance
Expert Committee (1997)[25]	Fasting	110–125 (6.1–6.9)	IFG[a]
	OGTT 120′	140–199 (7.8–11.0)	IGT[b]
Expert Committee (2003)[30]	Fasting	100–125 (5.6–6.9)	IFG
	OGTT 120′	140–199 (7.8–11.0)[c]	IGT
WHO (2006)[32]	Fasting	110–125 (6.1–6.9)	IFG
	OGTT 120′	140–199 (7.8–11.0)[d]	IGT
Expert Committee (2009)[33]	Fasting	100–125 (5.6–6.9)[e]	IFG
ADA (2010/2013)[34,37]	OGTT 120′	140–199 (7.8–11.0)	IGT
	HbA_{1c} (%)	5.7–6.4[f]	IFG/IGT

Notes: Plasma glucose levels are expressed in mg/dL (mmol/L).
[a] IFG for impaired fasting glucose.
[b] IGT for impaired glucose tolerance.
[c] OGTT not recommended.
[d] OGTT recommended.
[e] 110–125 (6.1–6.9) for the WHO.
[f] WHO does not make any formal recommendation on the interpretation of HbA1c <6.5% in terms of prediabetes.

epidemiological data available since the *princeps* NDDG report.[25–27] One objective was to make the FPG and the 2-hr glucose value during OGTT equivalent for diagnosing diabetes: thus if one criterion was met, the other would likely be met as well. In this view, the IEC recommended that the FPG threshold for diagnosing diabetes be reduced from 140 to 126 mg/dL (7.8–7.0 mmol/L). The IEC linked the new levels with cross-sectional data showing that the risk of development of retinopathy already begins at approximately 126 mg/dL (7.0 mmol/L) in the fasting state in several cohorts, including Egyptians, Pima Indians, as well as a group of the Third National Health and Nutrition Survey (NHANES III).[25,28,29] The 2-hr glucose cutoff point for diagnosing diabetes after an OGTT remained unchanged as equal to or greater than 200 mg/dL (11.1 mmol/L), as well as based on the presence of clinical symptoms and measurement of a casual plasma glucose level equal to or greater than 200 mg/dL (11.1 mmol/L) (Table 1). It is of interest, however, that with the reduction of FPG threshold to 126 mg/dL (7.0 mmol/L), it was thought that it was no longer necessary to perform an OGTT in all individuals in order to diagnose those with diabetes.

As far as the prediabetic state was concerned, both the IEC and WHO introduced the concept of IFG as a fasting plasma glucose above normal but below the diabetes diagnostic level. Thus, IFG was defined by a plasma level between 110 and 125 mg/dL (6.1–6.9 mmol/L). The definition of IGT (previously "glucose intolerance") was kept unchanged with a 2-hr plasma glucose level during OGTT between 140 and 199 mg/dL (7.8–11.0 mmol/L). Collectively, both conditions, IFG and IGT, were referred in the new classification as prediabetes, even if they potentially represented different pathophysiological processes and identified different individuals. In other words, IFG and IGT sometimes diagnosed the same individuals, but often they did not coincide. Nonetheless, although IFG and IGT are potentially not interchangeable, ADA stated that FPG alone was the preferred test for diagnostic purposes and screening and that OGTT was unnecessary. This was not agreed to by the WHO, which continues to promote the use of the OGTT where necessary, in particular in individuals with IFG to exclude IGT or diabetes. In part, this rationale recognized that a considerable number of individuals diagnosed with diabetes by the 2-hr value have normal or IFG values when fasting.[26,27]

2.2. Step 2

Another change came about in 2003, when the Expert Committee group recommended lowering the threshold for IFG.[30] Thus, the original FPG range of 110–125 mg/dL (6.1–6.9 mmol/L) was lowered to 100–125 mg/dL (5.6–6.9 mmol/L), so that the population at risk of developing diabetes with IFG would be similar to that with IGT. The rationale for this decision was also based on data suggesting that individuals diagnosed using the lower glucose criteria for IFG were already at increased risk for developing type 2 diabetes. As expected, this change in the FPG cutoff point increased considerably the overall prevalence of IFG, approximately three- to fourfold. Although this decision seemed to be operationally adequate, some experts did not support this recommendation and the WHO still defines IFG with the previous FPG range of 110–125 mg/dL (6.1–6.9 mmol/L).[31,32]

2.3. Step 3

Conventionally, for decades, the diagnosis of (pre)diabetes was based on plasma glucose criteria. With the introduction of $HbA_{1c,}$ it was thought that this assay would prove useful for diagnosing (pre)diabetes as it requires neither fasting nor an OGTT. HbA_{1c} also reflects glycemic status over two to three months and therefore provides a measure of assurance that the individual may indeed be dysglycemic. However, there are several arguments against its use in particular that the HbA_{1c} was not sufficiently standardized and could be affected by several medical conditions. However, in 2009–2010, after an extensive review of biological and epidemiological evidence, an International Expert Committee representing the ADA, IDF, and the European Association for the Study of Diabetes (EASD) recommended that (pre)diabetes could be diagnosed, aside from glucose-based tests, by measuring HbA_{1c}.[33] The ADA adopted the criterion in 2010.[34] The rationale for this decision was based on the fact that most studies, including the recent DETECT 2, indicated that there was an increased risk for retinopathy when HbA_{1c} levels approximated 6.5%, which was similar to the risk of microangiopathy as had been shown for the corresponding FPG and 2-hr OGTT threshold.[35,36] Consequently, diabetes could be diagnosed by an HbA_{1c} level equal to or greater than 6.5%, with a $HbA_{1c} \geq 5.7–6.4\%$ identifying individuals that were at "increased risk" for diabetes. The Expert Committee suggested that a range of HbA_{1c} level of 6.0–6.5% represented the highest risk for the development of diabetes but that individuals with an HbA_{1c} lower than 6.0% were already of concern, especially in the presence of other risk factors. This statement was again confirmed by the ADA in 2013[37] (Table 2).

However, according to the Expert Committee and ADA, the diagnostic test of HbA_{1c} is valid only if performed using a method that is certified by the National Glycohemoglobin Standardization Program (NGSP) and standardized or traceable to the Diabetes Control and Complications Trial (DCCT) reference assay. Under these circumstances, HbA_{1c} has indeed superior attributes when compared with conventional blood glucose criteria. HbA_{1c} has also greater preanalytical stability and lower variability when

Table 2. Categories of increased risk for diabetes according to the ADA position statement 2013.[37]

FPG	100–125 mg/dL (5.6–6.9 mmol/L): → Impaired fasting glucose (IFG)
OR	
2-hr plasma glucose in the 75-g OGTT:	140–199 mg/dL (7.8–11.0 mmol/L) → Impaired glucose tolerance (IGT)
OR	
HbA_{1c}	5.7–6.4%: → IFG/IGT

compared with glucose-based tests.[38–40] The advantages of HbA_{1c} have, however, to be balanced with some caveats including limited availability, cost, interference of hemoglobinopathy variants as well as shortened erythrocyte life span, acute blood loss and/or transfusions, pregnancy (which lower HbA_{1c} values), and iron deficiency anemia, hypertriglyceridemia, uremia, and/or chronic alcohol consumption (which slightly increases the level). The latter conditions therefore require the exclusive use of glucose criteria.[38–40] It is also of interest to mention that HbA_{1c} levels tend to be higher (for the same glucose level) in African and Mexican Americans than in the Caucasian population.[41,42] However, Bower *et al.*, very recently, observed no clear ethnic differences in the association of HbA_{1c} with retinopathy.[43]

Nevertheless, it is now reasonable to consider, as stated by the ADA, HbA_{1c} as a valid test for identifying individuals with or at high risk for diabetes.[37] Whereas the use of HbA_{1c} for diagnosing prediabetes has been implemented by the ADA, the WHO is currently still considering this policy and has yet to make an official pronouncement.[44]

From a practical point of view, as with most diagnostic tests, a test result diagnostic of (pre)diabetes should be repeated to rule out laboratory error. It is preferable that the same test be repeated for confirmation. When two different tests are utilized, if both tests are abnormal, the diagnosis is clearly confirmed. If the results are discordant, the test whose result is above the diagnostic cutoff point should be repeated and the final diagnosis made on the basis of the confirmed test.[37]

2.4. Is HbA_{1c} [5.7–6.4%] the Gold Standard for Prediabetes?

2.4.1. *Pro*

Several studies using HbA_{1c} to predict the progression to diabetes have demonstrated a strong and continuous association between HbA_{1c} levels and the subsequent occurrence of diabetes. Zhang *et al.*, in 2010, reported in a review of 44,203 individuals with a follow-up averaging 5.6 years, that those with an HbA_{1c} between 5.5 and 6.0% had a substantially increased risk of diabetes with a 5-year incidence ranging from 9 to 25%. Moreover, an HbA_{1c} range of 6.0–6.5% was associated with a 5-year risk of developing diabetes between 25 to 50% and a relative risk 20 times higher compared with an HbA_{1c} of 5.0%.[45] Similarly, Bonora *et al.* also demonstrated that a "high normal" HbA_{1c} was an independent risk factor for developing diabetes during a 15-year follow-up. The hazard ratio was 12.50 for a baseline HbA_{1c} of 6.0–6.5% (vs. a range of 5.0–5.5% as a reference).[46] Bae *et al.*, in 2011, also indicated that an HbA_{1c} cutoff point of 5.7% was a suitable value for predicting future diabetes and that it was reasonable to consider the ADA recommended 5.7–6.4% as a category of increased risk of diabetes in a Korean population, similar to IFG and IGT.[47] Yang *et al.*, in a study of the Chinese population, indicated through receiver operating characteristic curves (ROC) that a cutoff point for HbA_{1c} of 5.9% for diagnosing prediabetes coincided with a sensitivity of 70% and a specificity of 87%.[48] Selvin *et al.*[15] also observed in black and white adults that the baseline HbA_{1c} was a stronger predictor of subsequent diabetes as well as of cardiovascular events than was the FPG. Other authors recently extended these observations for HbA_{1c} as a useful tool for diagnosing prediabetes as a main risk factor for later development of diabetes and/or cardiovascular disease.[49]

2.4.2. *Contra*

On the other hand, an HbA_{1c} level of 5.7–6.4% seems to identify a much smaller population of increased risk for diabetes than do IFG and IGT. Cowie *et al.* reported that participants in the 2003–2006 National Health and Nutrition Examination Survey, with an HbA_{1c} level between 6.0% and 6.4%, missed up to 90% of the individuals at increased risk for diabetes.[50] These data are in line with a report of Mann *et al.*, indicating that the prevalence of prediabetes among U.S. adults was 12.6% by the HbA_{1c} criterion and 28.2% by the FPG.[51] Zhou *et al.*,[52] in China, and Heianza *et al.*, in Japan,[53] clearly extended these observations and confirmed that blood glucose tests performed better than HbA_{1c}. Mohan *et al.*, in the context of racially discrepant results of HbA_{1c}, suggested that the cutoff point for diagnosing prediabetes could be different in non-Western than in Western populations with an optimal threshold of 5.6% in Asian Indians.[54] More recently, the strategy of using exclusively HbA_{1c} for detecting prediabetes has also been questioned by Olson *et al.*[55] and others[56–60] who considered that HbA_{1c} alone may overlook a large number of individuals with prediabetes and/or that concordance between tests is insufficient. It is also possible, as recently reported by Cosson *et al.*, that hemoglobin glycation could explain many of the discordant results between HbA_{1c} and OGTT.[61]

Alternatively, the use of HbA_{1c} may also lead to the reclassification of a considerable number of subjects without IFG to having prediabetes.[51,62] In view of these data, it was also considered that HbA_{1c} value of 5.7–6.4% detected in part different individuals with dysglycemia when compared with IFG and IGT.[63] Finally, it is also of interest to mention that the HbA_{1c} cutoff point in the obese pediatric population still has to be determined, as indicated by Kester *et al.*[64]

2.5. Is Prediabetes Really the First "Pathological" Threshold?

The scientific community continues to debate the status (and the definition) of prediabetes as a first pathological step in a (dys)glycemic continuum.

Accordingly, it is of interest to mention that the risk of diabetes clearly increases with incrementally higher FPG levels within the conventionally accepted normal range.[65,66] Thus, a FPG level of 90–94 mg/dL (5.0–5.2 mmol/L) conferred a 49% greater risk of developing diabetes when compared with a level lower than 85 mg/dl (4.7 mmol/L).[67]

Similarly, there is evidence that cardiovascular risk also increases continually with increasing FPG levels and that the progressive relationship between glucose levels and cardiovascular risk extends below the prediabetic threshold.[15,68,69] Thus, as indicated by Bergman, these "normoglycemic" subjects may already be at risk, in particular in the presence of other contributing factors.[70]

3. CURRENT STATUS OF PREDIABETES

Prediabetes is a risk factor for diabetes development as well as for cardiovascular disease. Diagnostic criteria for prediabetes have changed over time and still vary according to expert committees. Currently, screening procedures include three methods. Thus, persons with prediabetes are defined as having IFG (FPG: 100–125 mg/dL and 5.6–6.9 mmol/L) or IGT (2-hr values during the OGTT: 140–199 mg/dL and 7.8–11.0 mmol/L). It should be noted, however, that the WHO still defines the cutoff for IFG at 110 mg/dL (6.1 mmol/L) instead of 100 mg/dL (5.6 mmol/L). On the basis of a substantial number of studies, the ADA recommends that an HbA_{1c} range of 5.7–6.4% also may similarly identify individuals with prediabetes. However, the concordance between HbA_{1c} and either glucose-based test is not perfect due to lower sensitivity of HbA_{1c} at the designated cutoff points. Accordingly, the WHO estimates that there is currently insufficient evidence to make formal recommendations regarding the interpretation of HbA_{1c} levels below 6.5%.

It is also reasonable to postulate that the three tests could measure and identify different pathophysiological aspects of dysglycemia. Using HbA_{1c} alone could lead to reclassifying as normal the glucose status of large cohorts of individuals diagnosed with prediabetes with glucose-based tests. On the other hand, a substantial number of subjects without IFG may be reclassified as having prediabetes could also occur. Therefore, Bonora and Tuomilehto[71] suggested that using both FPG and HbA_{1c} could be a rational option for diagnosing prediabetes.

The debate concerning the relative merit of HbA_{1c} versus glucose measurements in diagnosing (pre)diabetes will only be resolved by further long-term research examining clinically relevant outcome parameters based on the different diagnostic criteria. Nonetheless, identification of prediabetes now permits early intervention and management in order to delay progression to diabetes and to prevent the development of chronic complications. It should be noted, however, that the evolution to diabetes may follow a continuum and could occur at blood glucose and HbA_{1c} values lower than those meeting current definitions of prediabetes. The final threshold for prompt diagnosis of prediabetes and implementation of treatment should also be determined by long-term prospective studies.

REFERENCES

1. Ferrannini E, Nannipieri M, Williams K *et al.* (2004) Mode of onset of type 2 diabetes from normal or impaired glucose tolerance. *Diabetes* **53**: 160–165.
2. Buysschaert M. (2011) Le diabète de type 2 et le syndrome métabolique. In: *Diabétologie Clinique,* 4e Edition, Novembre, pp. 19–32. De Boeck, Louvain-La-Neuve, Paris.
3. Shaw Je, Sicree RA, Zimmet PZ. (2010) Global estimates of the prevalence of diabetes for 2010 and 2030. *Diabetes Res Clin Pract* **87**: 4–14.
4. Bergman M, Buysschaert M, Schwarz PEH *et al.* (2012) Diabetes prevention: Global health policy and perspectives from the ground. *Diabetes Manage* **2**(4): 309–321.
5. Færch K, Borch-Johnsen K, Holst JJ *et al.* (2009) Pathophysiology and aetiology of impaired fasting glycemia and impaired glucose tolerance: Does it matter for prevention and treatment of type 2 diabetes? *Diabetologia* **52**: 1714–1723.
6. Tabák AG, Herder C, Rathmann W *et al.* (2012) Prediabetes: A high-risk state for diabetes development. *Lancet* **379**: 2279–2290.
7. Buysschaert M, Bergman M. (2013) Diagnosis of prediabetes and Diabetes Prevention. In: *Diabetes Prevention*. P. Schwarz, ed. Wiley-Blackwell. 232 pages. ISBN: 978-0-470-65465-1. P. 33–46.
8. DECODE Study Group. (2003) Age- and sex-specific prevalences of diabetes and impaired glucose regulation in 13 European cohorts. *Diabetes Care* **26**: 61–69.
9. Nathan M, Davidson MB, DeFronzo RA *et al.* (2007) Impraired fasting glucose and impaired glucose tolerance. *Diabetes Care* **30**: 753–759.
10. Gerstein H, Santaguida P, Raina P *et al.* Annual incidence and relative risk of diabetes in people with various categories of dysglycemia: A systematic

review and meta-analysis of prospective studies. *Diabetes Res Clin Pract* **78**: 305–312.

11. Aroda VR, Ratner R. (2008) Approach to the patient with prediabetes. *J Clin Endocrinol Metab* **93**(9): 3259–3265.
12. Diabetes Prevention Program Research Group. (2007) The prevalence of retinopathy in impaired glucose tolerance and recent-onset diabetes in the Diabetes Prevention Program. *Diabet Med* **24**: 137–144.
13. The Decode Study Group, on behalf of the European Diabetes Epidemiology Group. (2001) Glucose tolerance and cardiovascular mortality: Comparison of fasting and 2-hour diagnostic criteria. *Arch Intern Med* **161**: 397–404.
14. Gerstein HC, Islam S, Anand S *et al.* (2010) Dysglycemia and the risk of acute myocardial infarction in multiple ethnic groups: An analysis of 15,780 patients from the INTERHEART study. *Diabetologia* **53**: 2509–2517.
15. Selvin E, Steffes MW, Zhu H *et al.* (2010) Glycated hemoglobin, diabetes and cardiovascular risk in nondiabetic adults. *New Engl J Med* **362**: 800–811.
16. Kurihara O, Takano M, Yamamoto M *et al.* (2013) Impact of prediabetic status on coronary atherosclerosis. *Diabetes Care* **36**: 729–733.
17. Buysschaert M, Bergman M. (2011) Definition of prediabetes. *Med Clin N Am* **95**(2): 289–297.
18. Diabetes Prevention Program Research Group. (2002) Reduction in the incidence of type 2 diabetes with lifestyle intervention or metformin. *N Engl J Med* **346**: 393–403.
19. Perreault L, Pan Q, Mather KJ *et al.*, for the Diabetes Prevention Program Research Group. (2012) Effect of regression from prediabetes to normal glucose regulation on long-term reduction in diabetes risk: Results from the Diabetes Prevention Program Outcomes Study. *Lancet* **379**: 2243–2251.
20. World Health Organization (WHO) Expert Committee on Diabetes Mellitus. (1964) First Report. Technical Report Series 310. WHO, Geneva.
21. National Diabetes Data Group. (1979) Classification and diagnosis of diabetes mellitus and other categories of glucose intolerance. *Diabetes* **28**: 1039–1057.
22. Pettitt DJ, Knowler WC, Lisse JR *et al.* (1980) Development of retinopathy and proteinuria in relation to plasma-glucose concentrations in Pima Indians. *Lancet* **2**: 1050–1052.
23. World Health Organization (WHO) Expert Committee on Diabetes Mellitus. (1980) Second Report. Technical Report Series 646. WHO, Geneva.
24. World Health Organization (WHO). (1985) Diabetes mellitus: Report of a Study Group. Technical Report Series 727. WHO, Geneva.

25. The Expert Committee on the Diagnosis and Classification of Diabetes Mellitus. (1997) Report of the Expert Committee on the Diagnosis and Classification of Diabetes Mellitus. *Diabetes Care* **20**: 1183–1197.
26. Alberti KG, Zimmet PZ. (1998) Definition, diagnosis and classification of diabetes mellitus and its complications. Part 1: diagnosis and classification of diabetes mellitus provisional report of a WHO consultation. *Diabet Med* **15**(7): 539–553.
27. World Health Organization (WHO) Report of a WHO Consultation. (1999) Definition, diagnosis and classification of diabetes mellitus and its complications. Diagnosis and classification of diabetes mellitus WHO/NCD/NCS/99.2.WHO, Geneva.
28. Engelgau M, Thompson T, Herman WH *et al.* (1997) Comparison of fasting and 2-hour glucose and HbA_{1c} levels for diagnosing diabetes. Diagnostic criteria and performance revisited. *Diabetes Care* **20**: 785–791.
29. McLance D, Hanson R, Charles M *et al.* (1994) Comparison of tests for glycated hemoglobin and fasting and two hour plasma glucose concentrations as diagnostic methods for diabetes. *BMJ* **308**: 1323–1328.
30. The Expert Committee on the Diagnosis and Classification of Diabetes Mellitus. (2003) Follow-up report on the diagnosis of diabetes mellitus. *Diabetes Care* **26**: 3160–3167.
31. Davidson MB, Landsman PB, Alexander CM. (2003) Lowering the criterion for impaired fasting glucose will not provide clinical benefit. *Diabetes Care* **26**: 3329–3330.
32. World Health Organization (WHO) Consultation. (2006) Definition and diagnosis of diabetes mellitus and intermediate hyperglycaemia. WHO, Geneva.
33. The International Expert Committee. (2009) International Expert Committee Report on the role of the A_{1C} assay in the diagnosis of diabetes. *Diabetes Care* **32**: 1327–1334.
34. American Diabetes Association. (2010) Standards of medical care in diabetes — 2010. *Diabetes Care* **33**(Suppl. 1): S11–S61.
35. Sabanayagam L, Liew G, Tai ES *et al.* (2009) Relationship between glycated haemoglobin and microvascular complications: Is there a natural cut-off point for the diagnosis of diabetes? *Diabetologia* **52**: 1279–1289.
36. Colagiuri S, Lee CMY, Wong TY *et al.* for the DETECT-2 Collaboration Writing Group. (2011) Glycemic thresholds for diabetes-specific retinopathy. *Diabetes Care* **34**: 145–150.
37. American Diabetes Association. (2013) Standards of medical care in diabetes — 2013. *Diabetes Care* **36**(Suppl. 1): S11–S66.
38. Sacks DB. (2011) A_{1c} versus glucose testing: A comparison. *Diabetes Care* **34**: 518–523.

39. Sacks DB, Arnold M, Bakris GL *et al.* (2011) Position statement executive summary: Guidelines and recommendations for laboratory analysis in the diagnosis and management of diabetes mellitus. *Diabetes Care* **34**: 1419–1423.
40. Sacks DB. (2012) Measurement of hemoglobin A_{1c}. A new twist on the path to harmony. *Diabetes Care* **35**: 2674–2680.
41. Ziemer DC, Kolm P, Weintraub WS *et al.* (2010) Glucose-independent, Black-White differences in hemoglobin A_{1C} levels. *Ann Intern Med* **152**: 770–777.
42. Herman WH, Ma Y, Uwaifo G *et al.*, for the Diabetes Prevention Program. (2007) Differences in A_{1c} race and ethnicity among patients with impaired glucose tolerance in the diabetes prevention program. *Diabetes Care* **30**(10): 2453–2457.
43. Bower JK, Brancati FL, Selvin E. (2013) No ethnic differences in the association of glycated hemoglobin with retinopathy: the national health and nutrition examination survey 2005–2008. *Diabetes Care* **36**: 569–573.
44. WHO (2011) Use of glycated hemoglobin (HbA_{1c}) in the diagnosis of diabetes mellitus. *Diabetes Res Clin Pract* **93**(3): 299–309.
45. Zhang X, Gregg W, Williamson D *et al.* (2010) HbA_{1c} level and future risk of diabetes: A systematic review. *Diabetes Care* **33**: 1665–1673.
46. Bonora E, Kiechi S, Mayr A *et al.* (2011) High-normal HbA_{1c} is a strong predictor of type 2 diabetes in the general population. *Diabetes Care* **34**: 1038–1040.
47. Bae JC, Rhee EJ, Lee WY *et al.* (2011) Optimal range of HbA_{1c} for the prediction of the future diabetes: A 4-year longitudinal study. *Diabetes Res Clin Pract* **93**: 255–259.
48. Yang C, Liu Y, Li X *et al.* (2012) Utility of hemoglobin A_{1c} for the identification of individuals with diabetes and prediabetes in Chinese high risk population. *Scand J Clin Lab Invest* **72**(5): 403–409.
49. Silverman RA, Thakker U, Ellman T *et al.* (2011) Hemoglobin A_{1c} as a screen for previously undiagnosed prediabetes and diabetes in an acute-care setting. *Diabetes Care* **34**: 1908–1912.
50. Cowie CC, Rust KF, Byrd-Holt DD *et al.* (2010) Prevalence of diabetes and high risk for diabetes using A1C criteria in the U.S. population in 1988–2006. *Diabetes Care* **33**: 562–568.
51. Mann DM, Carson AP, Shimbo D *et al.* (2010) Impact of A_{1c} screening criterion on the diagnosis of pre-diabetes among U.S. adults. *Diabetes Care* **33**: 2190–2195.

52. Zhou X, Pang Z, Gao W, Wang S *et al.* (2010) Performance of an A_{1c} and fasting capillary blood glucose test for screening newly diagnosed diabetes and pre-diabetes defined by an oral glucose tolerance test in Qingdao, China. *Diabetes Care* **33**: 545–550.
53. Heianza Y, Hara S, Arase Y *et al.* (2011) HbA_{1c}: 5.7–6.4% and impaired fasting plasma glucose for diagnosis of prediabetes and risk of progression to diabetes in Japan (TOPICS 3): a longitudinal cohort study. *Lancet* **378**: 147–155.
54. Mohan V, Vijayachandrika V, Gokulakrishnan K *et al.* (2010) A_{1c} cut points to define various glucose intolerance groups in Asian Indians. *Diabetes Care* **33**: 515–519.
55. Olson DE, Rhee MK, Herrick K *et al.* (2010) Screening for diabetes and pre-diabetes with proposed A_{1c}-based diagnostic criteria. *Diabetes Care* **33**: 2184–2189.
56. Bersoux S, Cook CB, Wu Q *et al.* (2011) Hemoglobin A_{1c} testing alone does not sufficiently identify patients with prediabetes. *Am J Clin Pathol* **135**: 674–677.
57. Bhansali A, Walia R, Ravi Kumar P *et al.* (2012) Accuracy of glycated hemoglobin in screening for pre-diabetes in Asian Indians — A community survey: The Chandigarh Urban Diabetes Study (CUDS). *Diabet Med* **29**: 1385–1389.
58. Van't Riet E, Alssema M, Rijkelijkhuizen JM *et al.* (2010) Relationship between A_{1c} and glucose levels in the general Dutch population. The New Hoorn Study. *Diabetes Care* **33**: 61–66.
59. Du TT, Yin P, Zhang JH *et al.* Comparison of the performance of Hb_{1c} and fasting plasma glucose in identifying dysglycaemic status in Chinese high-risk subjects. *Clin Exp Pharmacol Physiol* 2013; **40**: 63–68.
60. Bianchi C, Miccoli R, Bonadonna R *et al.* (2012) Pathogenetic mechanisms and cardiovascular risk. Differences between HbA_{1c} and oral glucose tolerance test for the diagnosis of glucose tolerance. *Diabetes Care* **35**: 2607–2612.
61. Cosson E, Chiheb S, Cussac-Pillegand C *et al.* (2013) Haemoglobin glycation may partly explain the discordance between HbA_{1c} measurement and oral glucose tolerance test to diagnose dysglycemia in overweight/obese subjects. *Diabetes Metab* **39**: 118–125.
62. Bernal-Lopez MR, Santamaria-Fernandez S, Lopez-Carmona D *et al.* (2011) HbA_{1c} in adults without known diabetes from southern Europe. Impact of the new diagnostic criteria in clinical practice. *Diabet Med* **28**: 1319–1322.
63. Saukkonen T, Cederberg H, Jokelainen J *et al.* (2011) Limited overlap between intermediate hyperglycemia as defined by A_{1c} 5.7–6.4%, impaired

fasting glucose, and impaired glucose tolerance. *Diabetes Care* **34**: 2314–2316.

64. Kester LM, Hey H, Hannon TS. (2012) Using hemoglobin A_{1c} for prediabetes and diabetes diagnosis in adolescents: Can adult recommendations be upheld for pediatric use? *J Adolesc Health* **50**: 321–323.
65. Brambilla P, La Valle E, Falbo R *et al.* (2011) Normal fasting plasma glucose and risk of type 2 diabetes. *Diabetes Care* **34**: 1372–1374.
66. Pradhan AD, Rifai N, Buring JE *et al.* (2007) Hemoglobin A_{1c} predicts diabetes but not cardiovascular disease in nondiabetic women. *Am J Med* **120**: 720–727.
67. Nichols GA, Hillier TA, Brown JB. (2008) Normal fasting plasma glucose and risk of type 2 diabetes diagnosis. *Am J Med* **121**: 519–524.
68. Ning F, Tuomilehto J, Pyörälä K *et al.* for the DECODE Study Group (2010) Cardiovascular disease mortality in Europeans in relation to fasting and 2-h plasma glucose levels within a normoglycemic range. *Diabetes Care* **33**: 2211–2216.
69. Hoogwerf BJ, Spreche DL, Pearce GL *et al.* (2002) Blood glucose concentrations < or = 125 mg/dl and coronary heart disease risk. *Am J Cardiol* **89**: 556–559.
70. Bergman M. (2010) Inadequacies of absolute threshold levels for diagnosing prediabetes. *Diabetes Metab Res Rev* **26**(1): 3–6.
71. Bonora E, Tuomilehto J. (2011) The pros and cons of diagnosing diabetes with $H_{A1c.}$ *Diabetes Care* **34**: S184–S190.

Chapter 2: Epidemiology of Prediabetes

Crystal Man Ying Lee[†] *and Stephen Colagiuri*[†,*]

1. BACKGROUND

Several factors are contributing to the current diabetes epidemic including increased life expectancy of people with type 2 diabetes (T2D), earlier diagnosis, and younger age of onset. However, the largest single contributor is new cases of diabetes[1] and consequently, a key strategy to reducing the diabetes burden is to prevent people from developing diabetes. Community-based diabetes prevention programs are predicated on identifying individuals at high-risk of developing diabetes and implementing lifestyle modification programs to reduce the risk of progressing to diabetes. There are numerous studies demonstrating the success of this approach, which not only prevents the development of diabetes but may translate into a reduction in diabetes-related complications and chronic disability.[2]

Several risk factors place individuals at high-risk of diabetes, including obesity and family history of T2D. The term "prediabetes" is usually applied to individuals with a glycemia-related biochemical abnormality of fasting plasma glucose (FPG), 2-h post-glucose–load plasma glucose, or glycated hemoglobin (HbA_{1c}). Increasingly, risk assessment tools that combine a variety of risk factors for diabetes are being used to identify high-risk individuals rather than initially subjecting individuals to a blood test.

*Corresponding author. Email: stephen.colagiuri@sydney.edu.au

[†]Boden Institute of Obesity, Nutrition, Exercise and Eating Disorders, University of Sydney, Sydney, Australia

2. DEFINITIONS OF PREDIABETES

Risk states for future diabetes have been recognized for many years. One of the first definitions was proposed in 1965 by World Health Organization (WHO), which recommended the term "potential diabetes" but recognized that clinicians often referred to this as "prediabetes."[3] The term prediabetes has become popular to describe impaired glucose tolerance (IGT) and impaired fasting glucose (IFG) but has now been extended to include intermediate levels of HbA_{1c}.[4]

Despite the popularity of the term, the WHO 2006 report discouraged its use in order to avoid any stigma associated with the word "diabetes" and the fact that many people do not progress to diabetes as the term implies. Instead, it recommended that the term "intermediate hyperglycemia" be used to describe glycemic levels between normal glucose tolerance (NGT) and diabetes.[5]

2.1. Intermediate Hyperglycemia (IGT and IFG)

IGT and IFG were conceived to define categories of glycemia associated with an increased risk of developing diabetes.[6–9] Defining a lower limit for intermediate hyperglycemia is somewhat arbitrary, as the risk of diabetes with fasting and post-load plasma glucose follows a continuum, which extends into the levels considered normal. Therefore, guiding values are important for determining these somewhat arbitrary definitions.[5] For WHO, these values are population-based rather than premised primarily on an individual perspective and are rooted in scientific integrity with evidence of efficacy, feasibility, cost-effectiveness of interventions, sensitivity to local contexts, and on implications for health policymakers.[5]

IFG and IGT should not be viewed as clinical entities in their own right but rather as risk factors for diabetes as well as cardiovascular disease and are associated with obesity (especially abdominal or visceral obesity), dyslipidemia, and hypertension. IGT and IFG have become standardized ways of describing the prevalence of intermediate hyperglycemia and provide a sense of the projected diabetes burden.[10] The risk factors for prediabetes are similar to diabetes and include increasing age, family history of diabetes, abdominal obesity, and hypertension.[11]

A significant proportion of people with IGT and IFG revert to NGT. Data from Mauritius indicate that in people with IGT at baseline, 30% reverted to normal, 35% remained with IGT, 5% changed to IFG, and 30% developed diabetes over a 11-yr follow-up period.[12] As with all categories of glucose tolerance defined by measures of glycemia, reproducibility of prediabetes is moderate. One study that retested individuals within 6 weeks with an oral glucose tolerance test (OGTT) found that of individuals with IFG on the initial test, the proportion classified as IFG on both tests was 50–60%, with the majority being reclassified as normal and less than 10% having diabetes on repeat testing.[13] Reproducibility is even less for IGT. The proportion of people with IGT on the first OGTT and on retesting ranged from 33% to 48%, with 39% to 46% being reclassified as normal and 6–13% as having diabetes on repeat testing.[13]

Prediabetes is not only associated with an increased risk of developing diabetes, but is also associated with an increased risk of premature mortality and cardiovascular disease, although the risk is less than that of developing diabetes. The annualized relative risk for all-cause mortality was 1.5-fold higher in people with IGT compared with people with NGT and the relative risk of a fatal cardiovascular outcome was 1.7-fold higher for IGT and 1.2-fold higher with IFG.[13]

2.1.1. *Impaired glucose tolerance*

Numerous epidemiological studies from many countries have documented the prevalence of IGT. These are summarized in the latest International Diabetes Federation (IDF) Diabetes Atlas.[14] It is estimated that some 316 million people worldwide, or 6.9% in the age group 20–79 years, had IGT in 2013, the vast majority of whom live in low- and middle-income countries. By 2035, the number of people with IGT is projected to increase to 471 million, or 7.3% of the adult population. The prevalence of IGT varies by IDF region as shown in Table 1.

The prevalence of IGT increases with age as demonstrated in both the European DECODE and Asian DECODA studies.[15,16] For example, in European populations the prevalence of isolated IGT increased from 2.9% in 30- to 39-year-old men to 15.1% in 70- to 79-year-old men, and from 4.5% in 30- to 39-year-old women to 16.9% in 70- to 79-year-old women.[15]

Table 1. World estimates of IGT (adjusted to the world population) by IDF region.

Region	Prevalence (%)
Africa	8.3
Europe	8.1
Middle East and North Africa	7.5
North America and Caribbean	12.1
South and Central America	7.5
South East Asia	2.9
Western Pacific	6.6

The annualized relative risk of a person with IGT progressing to diabetes is increased six-fold compared with people with NGT.[13] This relative risk is 12-fold higher in those with both IFG and IGT. While risk is increased, absolute risk varies across studies ranging from 35.8 to 87.3/1,000 person-years.[15] Not surprising, those at the higher end of the glucose range for prediabetes have a higher incidence of developing diabetes. One study in Pima Indians reported a 5-yr cumulative incidence for new diabetes of 17% for those with a 2-h plasma glucose of 7.8–9.2 mmol/L (140–166 mg/dL) and 39% for those with a 2-h plasma glucose of 9.3–11.0 mmol/L (167–198 mg/dL).[16]

2.1.2. *Impaired fasting glucose*

Assessing and comparing the prevalence of IFG is complicated by the existence of two definitions — the WHO definition of FPG of 6.1–6.9 mmol/L (110–125 mg/dL)[5] and the American Diabetes Association (ADA) definition of 5.6–6.9 mmol/L (100–125 mg/dL).[19] Furthermore, when only FPG is measured, without also measuring a 2-h post-load plasma glucose, some defined as IFG will have IGT or even diabetes if a 2-h plasma glucose was measured. This is illustrated by the DECODE study, which showed that in those with a FPG of 6.1–6.9 mmol/L (110–125 mg/dL), 64.8% had isolated IFG, 28.6% had IGT, and 6.6%

actually had diabetes based on the 2-h plasma glucose.[15] Corresponding data from DECODA showed that in Asian individuals with a FPG level of 6.1–6.9 mmol/L (110–125 mg/dL) alone, 45.9% had isolated IFG, 35.2% had IGT and 18.9% had diabetes when the 2-h plasma glucose was measured.[16]

The impact of using different FPG levels to diagnose IFG is considerable. Use of the ADA criterion for IFG results in a two- to three-fold increase in IFG prevalence compared with WHO-defined IFG. The DETECT–2 study[20] compared the two definitions in population-based studies in Denmark, India, and the United States and reported an increase in prevalence of IFG from 11.8% to 37.6% in Denmark, from 10.6% to 37.6% in India and from 9.5% to 28.5% in the United States for WHO- and ADA-defined IFG criteria, respectively. This is further illustrated by two recent studies from China.[21,22] In the first, which used the WHO criterion, the prevalence of isolated IFG was 3.2% in men and 2.2% in women.[21] In the second study that used the ADA criterion, the overall prevalence of isolated IFG was 22.8% (23.7% in men and 21.7% women).[22] The total number of people with prediabetes in the first study was 148.2 million (76.1 million men and 72.1 million women) compared with 493.4 million (260.1 million men and 233.3 million women) in the second study. The public health implications of these findings are considerable.

The annualized relative risk of those with isolated IFG progressing to diabetes is 4.7-fold compared with those with NGT.[13] However, as in IGT, this risk varies according to plasma glucose level and is less at the lower end of the IFG range, especially with the ADA criterion, compared with those at the higher end of the IFG range.[23] Data from the Epidemiological Study on the Insulin Resistance Syndrome (DESIR) study reported diabetes incidence rates per 1,000 person-years for FPG categories of <5.6 mmol/L (101 mg/dL), 5.6–6.0 mmol/L (101–108 mg/dL), and 6.1–6.9 mmol/L (110–124 mg/dL) were, respectively, 1.8, 5.7, and 43.2 in men and 0.7, 6.2, and 54.7 in women.[24] In the Mauritius study, the 5-yr incidence of diabetes was on the order of 15% for a FPG between 5.5 and 5.7 mmol/L (99 and 103 mg/dL) compared with 30% for a FPG between 6.1 and 6.9 mmol/L (110 and 124 mg/dL).[12]

The observed differences in progression to diabetes have implications for diabetes prevention strategies.

2.2. Glycated Hemoglobin (HbA_{1c})

HbA_{1c} is now an accepted criterion option for diagnosing diabetes with a level ≥6.5% diagnostic of diabetes.[25] WHO concluded that there was currently insufficient evidence to make any formal recommendation on interpreting HbA_{1c} levels below 6.5%. An International Expert Committee did not recommend a level of HbA_{1c}, which could be used to diagnose states of intermediate hyperglycemia but recognized that levels of HbA_{1c} just below 6.5% may indicate increased risk of future diabetes and recommended that people with an HbA_{1c} between 6.0 and 6.5% were at a particularly high-risk and might be considered for prevention.[26] The ADA has recommended that individuals with HbA_{1c} level between 5.7 and 6.4% be categorized at an increased risk for diabetes and cardiovascular disease and should receive counseling about strategies to lower their risk.[25]

Based on the 2003–2006 US National Health and Nutrition Examination Survey (NHANES) data, 3.5% of those 20 years and older (7.4 million individuals) were at high-risk for diabetes defined by a HbA_{1c} between 6.0 and 6.4%. Prevalence increased significantly with age (3.7% in those aged 40–59 years and 7.1% in those aged 60–74 years) but did not differ by gender. Prevalence using the HbA_{1c} criterion was about one-tenth that using fasting or 2-h plasma glucose criteria (29.0% combined, 25.2% IFG, and 13.6% IGT).[27] Racial differences have been reported in the proportion of those 65 years and older being at high-risk for diabetes — 13.2% in non-Hispanic blacks, 7.7% in non-Hispanic whites, and 8.3% in Mexican Americans. These racial and ethnic differences may, in part, be explained by the well-established difference in the relationship between blood glucose and HbA_{1c} levels with black individuals having higher levels than white individuals across the glycemic spectrum, with the increasing degree of abnormal glucose tolerance.[28]

There are large differences in the proportion of those classified as having prediabetes by a HbA_{1c} level between 5.7 and 6.4% or with plasma glucose measurements. Using the 1999–2006 NHANES data, the prevalence of prediabetes was 12.6% with the HbA_{1c} criterion of 5.7–6.4% and

28.2% using the FPG criterion of 5.6–6.9 mmol/L (100–125 mg/dL), 7.7% having prediabetes according to both definitions. The use of HbA_{1c} criteria would reclassify 37.6 million Americans with IFG to not having prediabetes and 8.9 million without IFG to having prediabetes (46.5 million reclassified).[29] This discrepancy is also highlighted in the recently published study from China in which 38.2% had an isolated HbA_{1c} between 5.7 and 6.4% (27.5% in men and 38.9% in women)[22] compared with 22.8% with isolated IFG and 3.6% with isolated IGT, and 6.1% meeting all three criteria (fasting, 2-h glucose, and HbA_{1c}). These population differences may be real or reflect methodological difference with HbA_{1c} analysis.

HbA_{1c} predicts the development of diabetes. Pradhan *et al.*[29] measured HbA_{1c} at baseline in a cohort of 26,563 U.S. females aged ≥45 years without a known history of diabetes or vascular disease. During a median follow-up of 10.1 years, 1,238 cases of diabetes and 684 cardiovascular events occurred. After multivariate adjustment, HbA_{1c} was a strong predictor of diabetes but not cardiovascular disease. The adjusted relative risks for incident diabetes in HbA_{1c} categories of <5.0%, 5.0–5.4%, 5.5–5.9%, 6.0–6.4%, 6.5–6.9%, and ≥7.0% were 1.0, 2.9, 12.1, 29.3, 28.2, and 81.2, respectively.

Selvin *et al.*[31] analyzed data from the Atherosclerosis Risk in Communities (ARIC) cohort to assess the relationship of HbA_{1c} and incident diabetes, coronary heart disease, and stroke. The cumulative incidence over 15 years of diagnosed diabetes was 6%, 12%, 21%, 44%, and 79% among participants with an HbA_{1c} of <5.0%, 5.0 to < 5.5%, 5.5 to <6.0%, 6.0 to <6.5%, and ≥6.5%, respectively. HbA_{1c} at baseline was associated with newly diagnosed diabetes and cardiovascular outcomes. For HbA_{1c} values of <5.0%, 5.0 to <5.5%, 5.5 to <6.0%, 6.0 to <6.5%, and ≥6.5%, the multivariable-adjusted hazard ratios for diagnosed diabetes were 0.52, 1.00 (reference), 1.86, 4.48, and 16.47, respectively. For coronary heart disease, the hazard ratios were 0.96, 1.00 (reference), 1.23, 1.78, and 1.95, respectively. The hazard ratios for stroke were similar.

A systematic review[32] examined HbA_{1c} for identifying people at high-risk of diabetes. From 16 studies, which included 44,203 individuals, annualized diabetes incidence ranged from 0.1% with a HbA_{1c} level <5.0% to 54.1% with a HbA_{1c} level ≥6.1%. As with glucose measurements, risk of incident diabetes increased steeply with HbA_{1c} across the range from 5.0 to 6.5%, with a 25 to 50% incidence over 5 years for HbA_{1c} levels from 6.0 to 6.5% and 9 to 25% incidence over 5 years for HbA_{1c} levels from 5.5 to 6.0%.

2.3. Risk Assessment Tools

Risk assessment tools are increasingly used to identify individuals at high-risk of developing diabetes in community-based diabetes prevention programs. Although glycemic cut-points for intermediate hyperglycemia are operationally adequate, they may not be the most appropriate method for defining future risk of diabetes or cardiovascular disease. Consequently, the 2006 WHO report concluded that a risk score combining known risk factors, which includes a measure of glycemia, would seem a more logical approach to predicting risk of diabetes.[5] In addition, community screening for diabetes prevention programs requires simple methods for identifying high-risk individuals and using invasive blood tests, such as the OGTT, is not feasible at the population level. Although including fasting glucose or HbA_{1c} can increase the discriminatory power of a risk score, it defeats the purpose of developing a simple method to first identify high-risk individuals before conducting a more costly blood test for diagnosing dysglycemic states. Consequently, risk assessment tools have evolved to identify people at high-risk either alone or as the initial step in a two-step screening procedure in which the risk tool is used to identify people who require further testing.

The Finnish Diabetes Risk Score was one of the first risk scores developed to predict future risk of diabetes from easily obtainable clinical markers.[33] There are now more than 46 diabetes prediction risk scores developed for use in different populations.[34] Although most diabetes risk scores include similar risk factors such as age, body mass index, family history of diabetes, and known hypertension, applying a risk score that was developed from a specific population to an unrelated population generally results in poorer performance. Hence, the numerous population-specific diabetes risk tools emerged to predict the future risk of diabetes.

A systematic review of multivariate risk scores for predicting the development of diabetes examined aspects of their development, validation, and comparative performance.[34] Overall, risk tools showed good discriminatory ability in populations for whom they were developed but discriminatory performance was more heterogeneous and generally weaker in external populations. The accuracy of risk tools to estimate absolute risk remains unknown. The performance of risk tools is improved by including FPG but the usefulness of genetic profiling was limited.[35] Risk tools are now recommended in guidelines for diabetes prevention[36] and have been used in some prevention programs.[37–39]

Many low- and middle-income countries do not have data to develop their own risk scores. A current International Diabetes Federation initiative, the PREDICT-2 (risk prediction tools for identifying people at high-risk of developing type 2 diabetes) project, is attempting to establish and validate a methodology for adapting diabetes risk prediction scores for populations with locally available demographic data.[40] The aim of this project is to facilitate countries without longitudinal data to adapt an established diabetes prediction score using easily obtainable local diabetes risk factor variables. An IDF website is being established with currently available risk tools and the methodology to allow country adaption using local data.

3. CONCLUSIONS

Identifying those at increased risk of developing diabetes is critical to implementing diabetes prevention programs and reducing the global diabetes burden. The different methods for identifying individuals at high-risk of diabetes have advantages and disadvantages in their ability to accurately quantify risk and be applied practically. The number of individuals identified by each method will vary and a particular individual may be classified as being at high-risk by one method but not another. In general, all methods perform satisfactorily at a population level but many identified as being at increased risk may never develop diabetes. Offering these individuals a lifestyle modification program, though, is unlikely to be harmful compared with the derived potential benefit.

REFERENCES

1. Colagiuri S, Glumer C, Vistisen D, Borch-Johnsen K. (2005) For debate — there really is a diabetes epidemic. *Diabetologia* **48**: 1459–1463.
2. Gong Q, Gregg EW, Wang J, An Y, Zhang P, Yang W, Li H, Jiang Y, Shuai Y, Zhang B, Zhang J, Gerzoff RB, Roglic G, Hu Y, Li G, Bennett PH. (2011) Long-term effects of a randomised trial of a 6-year lifestyle intervention in impaired glucose tolerance on diabetes-related microvascular complications: The China Da Qing Diabetes Prevention Outcome Study. *Diabetologia* **54**: 300–307.
3. World Health Organization (1965) Diabetes Mellitus: Report of a WHO Expert Committee, World Health Organisation, Geneva (Tech. Rep. Ser., no. 310). http://www.who.int/diabetes/publications/Definition%20and%20diagnosis%20of%20diabetes_new.pdf
4. American Diabetes Association (2013) Diagnosis and classification of diabetes mellitus. *Diabetes Care* **36**: S67–S74
5. World Health Organization (2006) Definition and diagnosis of diabetes mellitus and intermediate hyperglycemia, World Health Organisation, Geneva. http://www.who.int/diabetes/publications/Definition%20and%20diagnosis%20of%20diabetes_new.pdf
6. National Diabetes Data Group (1979) Classification and diagnosis of diabetes mellitus and other categories of glucose intolerance. *Diabetes* **28**: 1039–1057.
7. World Health Organization (1980) Expert Committee on Diabetes Mellitus, World Health Organisation, Geneva (Tech. Rep. Ser., no. 646). http://www.who.int/diabetes/publications/Definition%20and%20diagnosis%20of%20diabetes_new.pdf
8. The Expert Committee on the Diagnosis and Classification of Diabetes Mellitus (1997) Report of the expert committee on the diagnosis and classification of diabetes mellitus. *Diabetes Care* **20**: 1183–1197.
9. World Health Organization (1999) Definition, Diagnosis and Classification of Diabetes Mellitus and its Complications: Report of a WHO Consultation. Part 1: Diagnosis and Classification of Diabetes Mellitus, World Health Organisation, Geneva.
10. Colagiuri S, Borch-Johnsen K, Wareham NJ. (2008) Back to the future — Do IGT and IFG have value as clinical entities? *Diabetes Res Clin Pract* **81**: 131–133.
11. Anjana RM, Pradeepa R, Deepa M, Datta M, Sudha V, Unnikrishnan R, Bhansali A, Joshi SR, Joshi PP, Yajnik CS, Dhandhania VK, Nath LM, Das

AK, Rao PV, Madhu SV, Shukla DK, Kaur T, Priya M, Nirmal E, Parvathi SJ, Subhashini S, Subashini R, Ali MK, Mohan V; ICMR–INDIAB Collaborative Study Group. (2011) Prevalence of diabetes and prediabetes (impaired fasting glucose and/or impaired glucose tolerance) in urban and rural India: Phase I results of the Indian Council of Medical Research-INdia DIABetes (ICMR-INDIAB) study. *Diabetologia* **54**: 3022–3027.

12. Soderberg S, Zimmet P, Tuomilehto J, *et al.* (2004) High incidence of type 2 diabetes and increasing conversion rates from impaired fasting glucose and impaired glucose tolerance to diabetes in Mauritius. *J Intern Med* **256**: 37–47.
13. McMaster University Evidence Based Practice Center. Diagnosis, prognosis and treatment of impaired glucose tolerance and impaired fasting glucose, Evidence Report 128, www.ahrq.gov.
14. Diabetes Atlas, 6th ed. (2013) Brussels, International Diabetes Federation. http://www.diabetesatlas.org/
15. DECODE Study Group (2003) Age- and sex-specific prevalences of diabetes and impaired glucose regulation in 13 European cohorts. *Diabetes Care* **26**: 61–69.
16. DECODA Study Group (2003) Age- and sex-specific prevalence of diabetes and impaired glucose regulation in 11 Asian cohorts. *Diabetes Care* **26**: 1770–1780.
17. Edelstein SL, Knowler WC, Bain RP, *et al.* (1997) Predictors of progression from impaired glucose tolerance to NIDDM: An analysis of six prospective studies. *Diabetes* **46**: 701–710.
18. Gabir MM, Hanson RL, Dabelea D, *et al.* (2000) The 1997 American Diabetes Association and 1999 World Health Organization criteria for hyperglycemia in the diagnosis and prediction of diabetes. *Diabetes Care* **23**: 1108–1112.
19. The Expert Committee on the Diagnosis and Classification of Diabetes Mellitus (2003) Follow-up Report on the Diagnosis of Diabetes Mellitus. *Diabetes Care* **26**: 3160–3167.
20. Borch-Johnsen K, Colagiuri S, Balkau B, *et al.* (2004) Creating a pandemic of prediabetes: The proposed new diagnostic criteria for impaired fasting glycaemia. *Diabetologia* **47**: 1396–1402.
21. Yang W, Lu J, Weng J, *et al.* for the China National Diabetes and Metabolic Disorders Study Group (2010) Prevalence of diabetes among men and women in China. *N Engl J Med* **362**: 1090–1101.
22. Xu Y. Wang L. He J. Bi Y. Li M. Wang T. Wang L. Jiang Y. Dai M. Lu J. Xu M. Li Y. Hu N. Li J. Mi S. Chen CS. Li G. Mu Y. Zhao J. Kong L. Chen J. Lai S. Wang W. Zhao W. Ning G. (2013) 2010 China Noncommunicable

Disease Surveillance Group. Prevalence and control of diabetes in China. *JAMA* **310**: 948–959.
23. Forouhi NG, Balkau B, Borch-Johnsen K, *et al.* (2006) The threshold for diagnosing impaired fasting glucose: A position statement by the European Diabetes Epidemiology Group. *Diabetologia* **49**: 822–827.
24. Balkau B, Hillier T, Vierron E, *et al.* (2005) Comment to: Borch-Johnsen K, Colagiuri S, Balkau B *et al.* (2004) Creating a pandemic of prediabetes: the proposed new diagnostic criteria for impaired fasting glycaemia. *Diabetologia* **47**: 1396–1402. *Diabetologia* **48**: 801–802.
25. Report of a World Health Organization Consultation (2011) Use of glycated haemoglobin (HbA_{1c}) in the diagnosis of diabetes mellitus. *Diabetes Res Clin Pract* **93**: 299–309.
26. International Expert Committee (2009) Report on the role of the A1C assay in the diagnosis of diabetes. *Diabetes Care* **32**: 1327–1334.
27. Cowie C, Rust K, Byrd-Holt D, *et al.* (2010) Prevalence of diabetes and high risk for diabetes using A1C criteria in the U.S. population in 1988–2006. *Diabetes Care* **33**: 562–568.
28. Ziemer DC, Kolm P, Weintraub WS, *et al.* (2010) Glucose-independent, black–white differences in hemoglobin A1c levels. A cross-sectional analysis of 2 studies. *Ann Intern Med* **152**: 770–777.
29. Mann DM, Carson AP, Shimbo D, Fonseca V, *et al.* (2010) Impact of A1C screening criterion on the diagnosis of pre-diabetes among U.S. adults. *Diabetes Care* **33**: 2190–2195.
30. Pradhan AD, Rifai N, Buring JE, Ridker PM. (2007) Hemoglobin A1c predicts diabetes but not cardiovascular disease in nondiabetic women. *Am J Med* **120**: 720–727.
31. Selvin E, Steffes MW, Zhu H *et al.* (2010) Glycated hemoglobin, diabetes, and cardiovascular risk in nondiabetic adults. *N Engl J Med* **362**: 800–811.
32. Zhang X, Gregg EW, Williamson DF, Barker LE, Thomas W, Bullard KW, Imperatore G, Williams DE, Albright AL. (2010) A1C level and future risk of diabetes: A systematic review. *Diabetes Care* **33**: 1665–1673.
33. Lindstrom J, Tuomilehto J. (2003) The Diabetes Risk Score: A practical tool to predict type 2 diabetes risk. *Diabetes Care* **26**: 725–731.
34. Buijsse B, Simmons RK, Griffin SJ, Schulze MB. (2011) Risk assessment tools for identifying individuals at risk of developing type 2 diabetes. *Epidemiol Rev* **33**: 46–62.
35. Bao W, Hu FB, Rong S, Rong Y, Bowers K, Schisterman EF, Liu L, Zhang C. (2013) Predicting risk of type 2 diabetes mellitus with genetic risk models on

the basis of established genome-wide association markers: A systematic review. *Am J Epidemiol* **178**: 1197–1207.

36. Lindstrom J, Neumann A, Sheppard KE, *et al.* (2010) Take action to prevent diabetes — the IMAGE toolkit for the prevention of type 2 diabetes in Europe. *Horm Metab Res* **42**: S37–S55.
37. Ackermann RT, Marrero DG. (2007) Adapting the Diabetes Prevention Program lifestyle intervention for delivery in the community: The YMCA model. *Diabetes Educ* **33**: 69–78.
38. Kilkkinen A, Heistaro S, Laatikainen T, *et al.* (2007) Prevention of type 2 diabetes in a primary health care setting. Interim results from the Greater Green Triangle (GGT) Diabetes Prevention Project. *Diabetes Res Clin Pract.* **76**: 460–462.
39. Saaristo T, Peltonen M, Keinänen-Kiukaanniemi S, *et al.* (2007) National type 2 diabetes prevention programme in Finland: FIN-D2D. *Int J Circumpolar Health* **66**: 101–112.
40. Lee CM, Colagiuri S. (2013) Risk scores for diabetes prediction: The International Diabetes Federation PREDICT-2 project. *Diabetes Res Clin Pract* **100**: 285–286.

Chapter 3: Pathophysiology of Prediabetes: Role of Lipotoxicity?

Amalia Gastaldelli and Ele Ferrannini†*

1. INTRODUCTION

Prediabetes is a condition of high-risk for diabetes defined by glycaemic measures intermediate between normal and diagnostic of diabetes.[1] By convention, prediabetes includes impaired fasting glucose (IFG) and impaired glucose tolerance (IGT). The latter is detected as a postprandial glucose level between 140 and 200 mg/dL (7.8 and 11.1 mmol/L) after a standard glucose load of 75 g oral glucose tolerance testing (OGTT). Both IFG and IGT are risk factors for type 2 diabetes, with risk greater with combined IFG and IGT. Several studies have indicated that despite normal fasting glucose levels, many subjects have IGT. With IFG defined by a fasting glucose between 100 and 126 mg/dL (5.6 and 7.0 mmol/L), individuals have a 20–30% chance of developing diabetes in the ensuing 5–10 years.[2,3] Furthermore, IFG and IGT are associated with a modestly increased risk of cardiovascular disease.[4,5] Plasma glucose concentration starts to increase when glucose appearance exceeds glucose disappearance, and continues to increase until these two rates are again equal. As a consequence, fasting hyperglycemia is closely correlated with reduced peripheral glucose clearance and increased endogenous glucose

*Corresponding author. Cardiometabolic Risk Laboratory, CNR Institute of Clinical Physiology, Pisa, Italy. Email: amalia@ifc.cnr.it

†Department of Clinical and Experimental Medicine, University of Pisa School of Medicine, Pisa, Italy. Email: ferranni@ifc.cnr.it

production (EGP).[6,7] On the other hand, postprandial hyperglycemia is due mainly to a reduction in β-cell function and peripheral insulin sensitivity.

As only fasting glycemia is routinely checked, most subjects with IGT and early type 2 diabetes are not diagnosed. The International Diabetes Federation (IDF) has estimated that approximately half of subjects with type 2 diabetes are unaware of their condition. The population-based US National Health and Nutrition Examination Survey (NHANES) reported that 35% of US adults older than 20 years and 50% of those older than 65 years had prediabetes in 2005–08 defined by fasting plasma glucose (FPG) or HbA_{1c} concentrations.[8] Application of these percentages to the entire US population in 2010 yielded an estimated 79 million adults with prediabetes.[8] Figure 1 shows the IGT prevalence in 2011 and the projection for 2030 according to IDF.[9] The number of subjects worldwide with IGT is expected to increase dramatically to upward of 400 million by 2030 with the greatest absolute rise in Asia and Western Pacific regions.[9]

The major problem of delaying the diagnosis of diabetes is the relentless progression of diabetic complications, both microvascular and macrovascular. Thus, it has been estimated that ~50% of patients with diabetes already have some manifestations of cardiovascular disease at the time of diagnosis.[10]

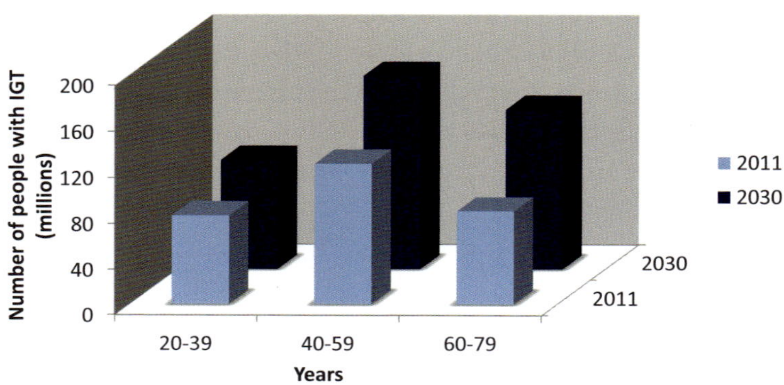

Fig. 1. Actual and projected prevalence of impaired glucose tolerance (IGT) in adults aged 20–79 years in 2011 and 2030. Data from Ref. [9].

In the present chapter, we will review current understanding of the pathophysiology of prediabetes and recent findings concerning new biomarkers for increased risk for type 2 diabetes.

2. β-CELL DYSFUNCTION AND INSULIN RESISTANCE

Impaired β-cell function and insulin resistance are the major determinants of altered glucose concentrations.[7] With regard to β-cell function, both basal insulin secretion rate (ISR) and total insulin output during the 2-hr following a standard oral glucose load increase progressively as glucose tolerance deteriorates,[11,12] consistently more in obese than lean subjects (Fig. 2). In those with diabetes with more severe fasting hyperglycemia, basal ISR tends decline to levels seen in those without diabetes and post-OGTT insulin output is reduced (Fig. 2). Thus, increased absolute insulin secretion rates are characteristic of prediabetes and predict progression to overt diabetes.[6,11,12]

Insulin resistance also plays an important role in determining glucose tolerance. Insulin resistance occurs in different organs (Fig. 3): in the liver,

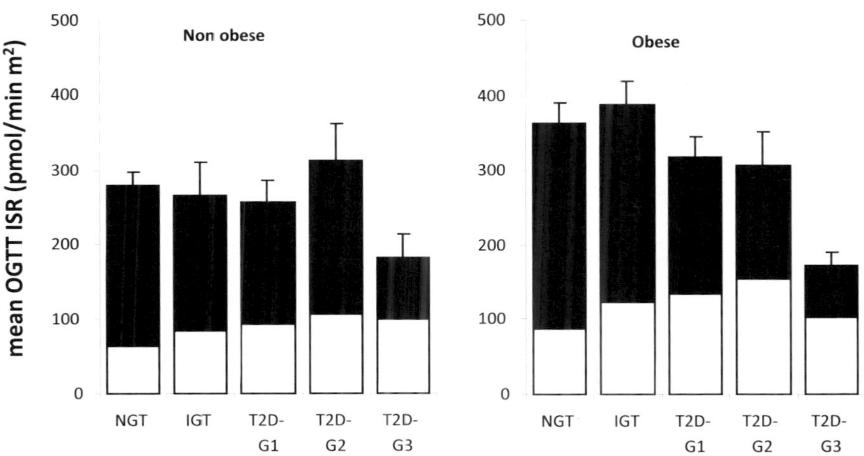

Fig. 2. Mean insulin secretion rates after OGTT in lean (left panel) and obese subjects (right panel), grouped according to glucose tolerance and fasting glycemia (G1 = FPG < 140 mg/dL; G2 = FPG from 140 to 180 mg/dL; G3 = FPG > 180 mg/dL). Empty bars represent fasting ISR, filled bar represents incremental secretion after OGTT. Reproduced with permission from Ref. [11].

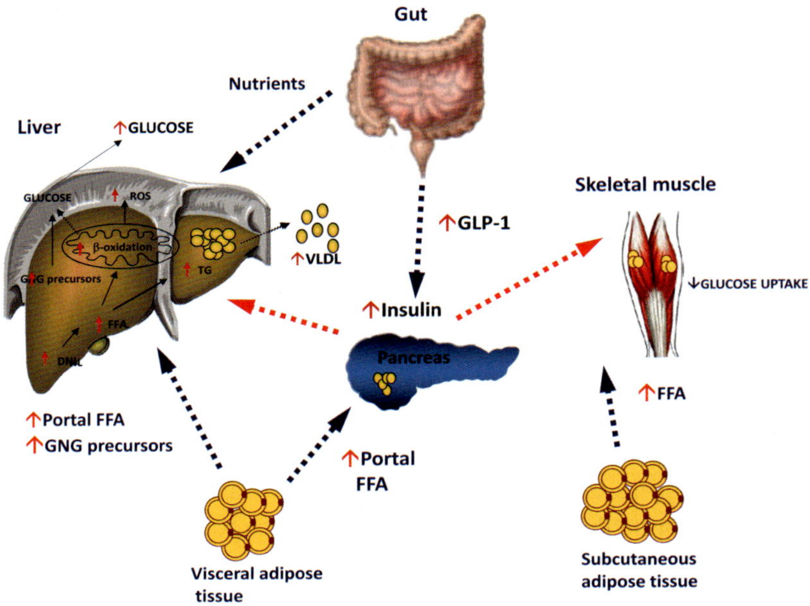

Fig. 3. Increased adipose tissue and visceral fat leads to ectopic fat accumulation in liver, muscle, and pancreas and to insulin resistance with the consequence of increased hepatic glucose, production, decreased muscle glucose uptake, and impaired suppression of lipolysis with the consequent of fatty acids overload to target tissues. Reproduced with permission from Ref. [11].

where, despite increased insulin levels, glucose production and in particular gluconeogenesis are elevated[13,14]; in skeletal muscle, where glucose uptake is impaired, but also in adipose tissue where rates of lipolysis are elevated despite increased insulin levels. Hepatic insulin resistance is the main determinant of fasting hyperglycemia while peripheral insulin sensitivity is mainly related to postprandial hyperglycemia.[11]

Both decreased hepatic and peripheral insulin sensitivity and decreased β-cell glucose sensitivity are responsible for increased mean OGTT glucose values (Fig. 4). β-cell glucose sensitivity is defined as the ability of the β-cell to quickly respond to changes in glucose concentrations by secreting more insulin. As long as the β-cell is able to secrete more insulin to overcome insulin resistance, glucose tolerance remains normal and as soon as the β-cell becomes dysfunctional, subjects progress to IGT and type 2 diabetes (Fig. 4).

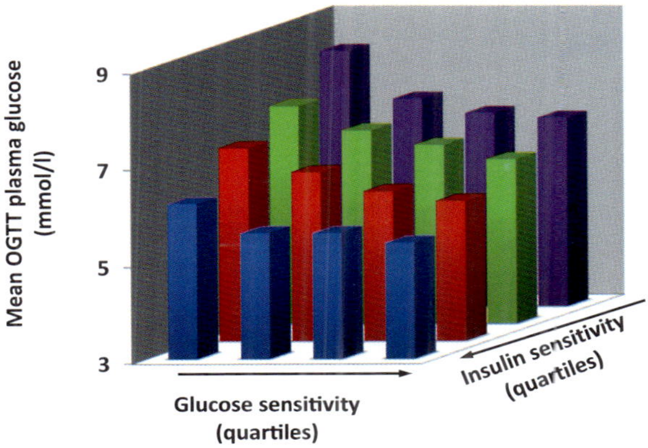

Fig. 4. Glucose concentration during OGTT is increased in subjects with decreased peripheral insulin sensitivity and decreased β-cell glucose sensitivity. Data from the Relationship between Insulin Sensitivity and Cardiovascular disease (RISC) study.

We have previously shown that subjects with IGT have already lost substantial β-cell function.[12,15] In addition, a reduced insulin secretion to insulin resistance ratio, an index of β-cell dysfunction, is one of the strongest predictors of type 2 diabetes in subjects with IGT.[16] Although the relative contributions of insulin resistance and β-cell glucose sensitivity to the development of type 2 diabetes may differ in various ethnic groups, the onset and pace of β-cell failure determine the rate of progression of hyperglycemia.[17] Genetic factors could also play an important role in this process. Subjects with a family history of diabetes (FHD) are genetically predisposed to type 2 diabetes; defects in insulin sensitivity and β-cell insulin secretion are accentuated along maternal inheritance.

Insulin is secreted in response to changes in glucose concentrations initially as a rapid response (first phase) followed by a slower second phase. β-cell rate sensitivity, which is an index of first-phase insulin response, is reduced as well as the second phase. In general, with most methods of glucose administration (e.g., oral glucose tolerance test, OGTT; mixed meal tolerance test, MTT; intravenous glucose tolerance test, IVGTT), the slope of the dose response of insulin secretion to glucose changes, i.e., β-cell glucose sensitivity, is less steep as subjects become glucose intolerant and then diabetic.[17] The β-cell responds proportionally to increases in glucose concentrations in order to maintain normal glucose levels.[17] As subjects become

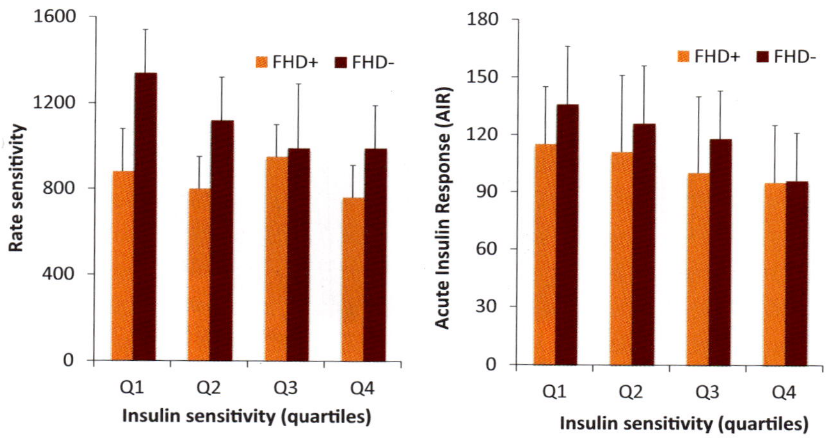

Fig. 5. Mean ± sd β-cell rate sensitivity (*left*) and acute insulin response, AIR1 (*right*) according to increasing quartiles of insulin sensitivity (M/I) in FHD^- (*red*) and FHD^+ (*orange*) subjects. Redrawn from Ref. [18].

glucose intolerant, the β-cell dynamic responses to glucose changes are lost concomitantly with insulin sensitivity. In subjects with FHD, β-cell dynamic responses to insulin resistance are lost regardless of whether the line of inheritance is maternal or paternal (as shown in the RISC study)[18] (Fig. 5).

Subjects with FHD but without type 2 diabetes have a normal response to the hyperglycemic clamp, i.e., both first- and second-phase insulin secretion are similar to that obtained in subjects without FHD. When the hyperglycemic clamp was repeated after prolonged lipid exposure, control subjects showed an increase in insulin secretion due to lipid-induced increase in insulin resistance while those with FHD showed an impaired insulin response manifested as a reduction in both first- and second-phase insulin secretion to 25% and 42% of that in control subjects[19] (Fig. 6). This is a clear indication that in subjects with FHD, lipotoxicity is an early defect that impairs not only peripheral glucose metabolism by increasing insulin resistance but also affects the dynamics of β-cell response.

3. ABDOMINAL OBESITY AND ECTOPIC FAT

Abdominal obesity, and in particular, visceral fat accumulation, is associated with an adverse metabolic risk profile and a greater risk of

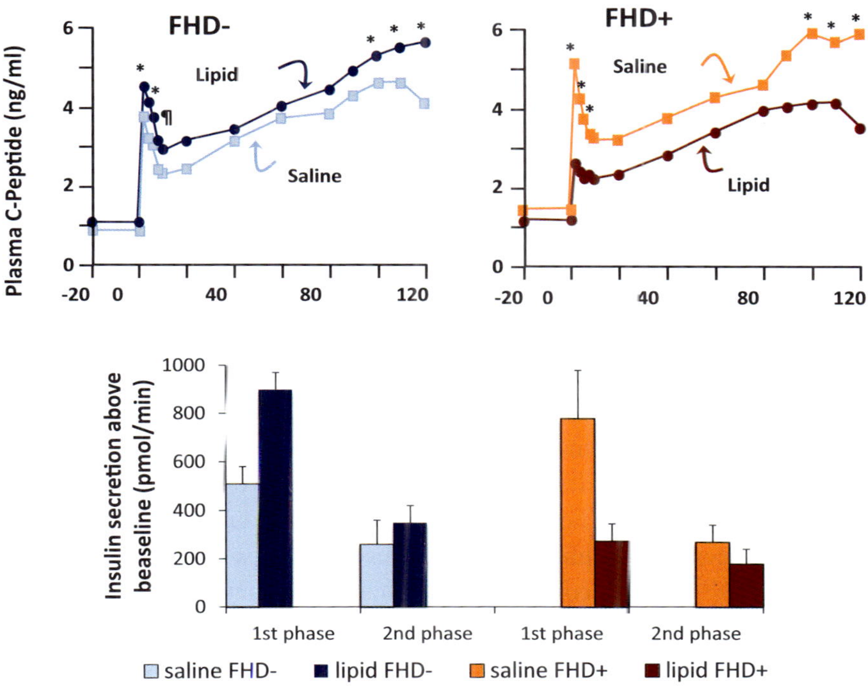

Fig. 6. Reduced β-cell response after lipid infusion in subjects with family history of diabetes but not in controls. Redrawn from Ref. [19].

developing type 2 diabetes.[20,21] The Paris Prospective Study was the first large prospective study to confirm the close relationship between adipose tissue insulin resistance (i.e., elevated plasma free fatty acids FFA, concentration) and the deterioration of glucose tolerance over time.[22] A recent analysis of the Dallas Heart Study, conducted in 512 obese participants, showed that incident prediabetes and type 2 diabetes were independently associated with insulin resistance and visceral fat [VAT, measured by magnetic resonance imaging (MRI)], but not general adiposity [i.e., body mass index (BMI), total fat, or subcutaneous fat].[23] In obese subjects with increased VAT and subcutaneous (SAT) adipose tissue, whole body lipolysis is increased compared to lean subjects.[24,25] When adipose tissue becomes dysfunctional, it also becomes resistant to the antilipolytic effect of insulin, thus not suppressing release of FFAs despite high levels of circulating insulin. It has been shown that visceral adipose tissue, in comparison to subcutaneous fat, is more sensitive to catecholamine-induced lipolysis and less sensitive to insulin.[25] Moreover, visceral fat releases FFA directly into the portal vein,[25,26] therefore explaining the close relationship between visceral, liver, and pancreatic fat.[27,28] This could explain also why VAT has a more direct impact not only on liver metabolism but also on liver histology and inflammation than fat from peripheral (subcutaneous) lipolysis.[29]

The liver takes up a large proportion of FFA entering the splanchnic bed through the portal vein with only a small fraction of FFA being taken up by nonhepatic splanchnic tissues.[30] The proportion of FFA delivered to the liver coming from VAT lipolysis increases as a function of visceral fat mass but more in women than men.[30] On average, approximately 20% of hepatic FFA delivery is from visceral fat[31] but in extreme viscerally obese women, postabsorptive hepatic FFA delivery from visceral fat may be up to 50%. Excess FFA delivery to the liver stimulates hepatic VLDL-TG production[32,33] and gluconeogenesis,[27] thus contributing to the altered metabolic profile and increasing the risk of type 2 diabetes.

While the "portal hypothesis" is appealing to explain the development of hepatic insulin resistance by visceral adipose tissue, this is unlikely the case for peripheral insulin resistance. In healthy obese individuals, the contribution of visceral fat to the overall FFA pool increases only modestly (from ~10% to only ~25%) compared to lean subjects,[31] suggesting that expansion of subcutaneous fat adipose tissue also plays an important role in the development of insulin resistance. It is also possible that the deleterious role of visceral fat is mediated not so much by FFA but primarily by the release of a number of adipocytokines (TNF-α, leptin, interleukins, etc.) that have been shown to promote insulin resistance,[34,35] thereby offering a unifying explanation for how a rather modest amount of adipose tissue (i.e., 10–15% of total body fat) may hold the potential to impair hepatic and peripheral (muscle) insulin action.

Visceral and ectopic fat accumulation probably are the consequences of dysfunctional subcutaneous adipose tissue. A recent study showed that overfeeding determines different patterns of fat accumulation. In particular, only subjects that showed defective SAT expression of lipid storage-related genes (DGAT2, SREBP1c, and CIDEA) exhibited the largest visceral depot accumulation.[36] The inability of SAT to metabolize circulating FFA could be one explanation for ectopic fat accumulation in other organs such as liver, pancreas, heart and skeletal muscle, leading to cell lipotoxicity with alteration of organ metabolism.[27,28,37,38]

Individuals with more visceral fat tend to also accumulate pancreatic fat.[28,39] It has been hypothesized that ectopic fat accumulation in the pancreas could impair insulin secretion and be a major risk factor for type 2 diabetes. A study conducted in subjects with IGT and/or IFG showed that the impairment in insulin secretion and β-cell function was associated with both visceral and intrapancreatic fat but not hepatic fat.[28] However, the relationship between pancreatic fat and decreased insulin secretion was stronger than with visceral fat. The close relationship between ectopic fat, insulin resistance, and insulin secretion was confirmed in a dietary intervention in subjects with type 2 diabetes that resulted in normalization of both β-cell function and hepatic insulin sensitivity associated with a decrease in both pancreatic and liver triglyceride stores.[37]

4. LIPOTOXICITY AND GLUCOTOXICITY

An emerging body of evidence indicates that triglyceride accumulation within ectopic tissues, such as liver, pancreas, heart, and skeletal muscle, leads to cell lipotoxicity[40, 41] with alteration of organ metabolism.[27,28,37,38] Initially triglyceride accumulation is probably not harmful for tissues, but can be seen as a protective mechanism against excessive lipid overflow and lipotoxicity. However, at a later stage, when adipose tissue becomes hypertrophic, infiltrated with macrophages and secreting proinflammatory adipokines, the intracellular lipid metabolism becomes impaired, thus increasing production of reactive oxygen species (ROS) and leading to tissue inflammation.[42] Therefore, only when adipose tissue becomes dysfunctional, it becomes responsible for metabolic alterations either systemically (through release of cytokines) or by altering specific organ functions through ectopic fat lipotoxicity.[42]

Lipotoxicity triggers multiple cellular processes including impaired insulin signaling,[43,44] oxidative stress,[45,46] alterations in local renin-angiotensin system,[47] enhanced adrenergic sensitivity of vascular smooth muscle cells,[48] and mitochondrial dysfunction.[40] The first alteration caused by lipotoxicity is the impairment of insulin signaling as FFA reduce basal and insulin-stimulated glucose uptake,[49] muscle ATP synthesis,[50] and nitric oxide

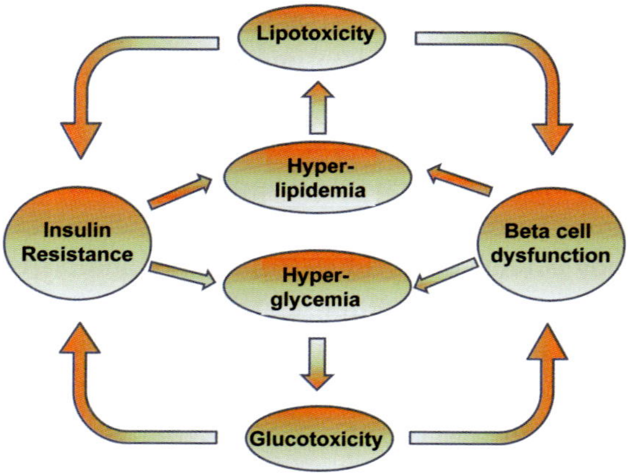

Fig. 7. Both lipotoxicity and glucotoxicity contribute to insulin resistance and β-cell dysfunction, thus determining hyperglycemia.

production,[44] and impair insulin-stimulated activation of phosphoinositol-3 kinase (PI3K), pyruvate dehydrogenase kinase, isozyme 1, RAC-alpha serine/threonine-protein kinase (also known as proto-oncogene c-Akt), and endothelial nitric oxide synthase (eNOS).[44] Moreover, FFA exposure increases cellular levels of diacylglycerols, ceramide, and long-chain fatty acyl-coenzyme A (CoA), lipid metabolites that activate transcription factors such as nuclear factor-κB (NF-κB), involved in inflammatory processes.[51] Long-chain acyl-CoA esters directly stimulate the opening of ATP-sensitive potassium channels leading to K^+ efflux, shortened action potentials, reduced Ca^{2+} influx, and decreased contractile force.[52] Mitochondrial dysfunction increases oxidative stress and uncouples oxidative phosphorylation.

Glucotoxicity and lipotoxicity are closely interrelated and both contribute to the deterioration of insulin resistance and β-cell function (Fig. 7).

5. MARKERS OF PROGRESSION FROM IGT TO TYPE 2 DIABETES

Several diabetes prediction models have been developed on the basis of indices available to family physicians (e.g., age, BMI, waist circumference, hypertension, family history of diabetes in first degree relatives), but so far none has been universally accepted.[53] In particular, given that ethnic origin is strongly related to diabetes risk, recalibration of prediction algorithms might be necessary when models are applied to different populations.[53]

Glycemic measures (fasting or 2-hr plasma glucose levels and HbA_{1c}) are more useful when used as continuous instead of categorical variables[54,55] since categorization could exclude borderline subjects as increased glycemia usually occurs as a a continuous process. The hypertriglyceridemic waist model phenotype (i.e., waist circumference >90 cm in men or >85 cm in women), in conjunction with a plasma triglyceride concentration of >177 mg/dL (>2.0 mmol/L) has also been proposed as a model of cardiometabolic risk.[56] Again, the use of a score based on continuous variables — such as the fatty liver index (FLI), which includes both TG and waist — could be more efficient in estimating risk. FLI has been associated not only with increased liver fat but also with impaired glucose and lipid metabolism and insulin resistance.[57]

β-cell dysfunction and postprandial hyperglycemia are robust predictors for development of type 2 diabetes in subjects with IFG/IGT[7] although these measurements are currently used only in a clinical research setting. A recent analysis of the Actos Now for the prevention of diabetes (ACTNOW) study has indicated that several metabolic factors — namely, increased fasting plasma glucose, 2-hr plasma glucose, G_{0-120} during an OGTT, HbA1c, adipocyte insulin resistance index, fasting plasma insulin, and mean insulin concentration during an OGTT, as well as family history of diabetes and presence of metabolic syndrome — are associated with an increased risk of diabetes in IGT subjects.[16] At baseline, higher insulin secretion (as the ratio of mean insulin to mean glucose in the OGTT) was associated with decreased risk of diabetes. Better β-cell function (insulin secretion/insulin resistance or disposition index) was the variable most closely associated with reduced risk of diabetes (with an odds ratio of 0.11, $p < 0.0001$).

Recent advances in *omics* technology have also allowed the identification of new predictors of abnormalities in glucose tolerance. Metabolomic screening of fasting plasma from nondiabetic subjects identified α-hydroxybutyrate (α-HB) and linoleoyl-glycerophosphocholine (L-GPC) as joint markers of insulin resistance (IR) and β-cell dysfunction.[58,59] The two markers have been tested in two observational cohorts, comprising

1,261 participants without diabetes from the RISC study and 2,580 from the Botnia Prospective Study, with 3-year and 9.5-year follow-up data, respectively. In both cohorts, α-HB was a positive correlate and L-GPC a negative correlate of insulin sensitivity with α-HB reciprocally related to indices of β-cell function derived from the OGTT. Both markers were predictors of dysglycemia (RISC) or type 2 diabetes (Botnia) independent of familial diabetes, sex, age, BMI, and fasting glucose.[58]

6. CONCLUSIONS

Diabetes mellitus is one of the major clinical problems worldwide. New methods of early detection based on high throughput screening, molecular targeting, and nanotechnology are currently being investigated given the importance of early identification of the disease and the possibility of intervention to stop its epidemic spread.

REFERENCES

1. Tabak AG, Herder C, Rathmann W, Brunner EJ, Kivimaki M. (2012) Prediabetes: A high-risk state for diabetes development. *Lancet* **379**: 2279–2290.
2. Tirosh A, Shai I, Tekes-Manova D, Israeli E, Pereg D, Shochat T, Kochba I, Rudich A. (2005) Normal fasting plasma glucose levels and type 2 diabetes in young men. *N Engl J Med* **353**: 1454–1462.
3. Meigs JB, Muller DC, Nathan DM, Blake DR, Andres R. (2003) The natural history of progression from normal glucose tolerance to type 2 diabetes in the Baltimore Longitudinal Study of Aging. *Diabetes* **52**: 1475–1484.
4. Meigs JB, Nathan DM, D'Agostino RB, Sr, Wilson PW. (2002) Fasting and postchallenge glycemia and cardiovascular disease risk: The Framingham Offspring Study. *Diabetes Care* **25**: 1845–1850.
5. Levitan EB, Song Y, Ford ES, Liu S. (2004) Is nondiabetic hyperglycemia a risk factor for cardiovascular disease? A meta-analysis of prospective studies. *Arch Intern Med* **164**: 2147–2155.
6. DeFronzo RA. (2009) Banting Lecture. From the triumvirate to the ominous octet: A new paradigm for the treatment of type 2 diabetes mellitus. *Diabetes* **58**: 773–795.
7. Ferrannini E, Gastaldelli A, Iozzo P. (2011) Pathophysiology of prediabetes. *Med Clin North Am* **95**: 327–339, vii–viii.

8. Centers for Disease Control and Prevention C, Department of Health and Human Services U. (2011) National Diabetes Fact Sheet: National estimates and general information on diabetes and prediabetes in the United States. Centers for Disease Control and Prevention, Atlanta, GA.
9. International Diabetes Federation (2011) IDF Diabetes Atlas, 5th edn. Brussels, Belgium: International Diabetes Federation.
10. Turner R, Cull C, Holman R. (1996) United Kingdom Prospective Diabetes Study 17: The effect of improved metabolic control on complications of NIDDM. *Ann Intern Med* **124**: 136–145.
11. Gastaldelli A. (2011) Role of beta-cell dysfunction, ectopic fat accumulation and insulin resistance in the pathogenesis of type 2 diabetes mellitus. *Diabetes Res Clin Pract* **93**: S60–S65.
12. Ferrannini E, Gastaldelli A, Miyazaki Y, Matsuda M, Mari A, DeFronzo RA. (2005) Beta-Cell function in subjects spanning the range from normal glucose tolerance to overt diabetes: A new analysis. *J Clin Endocrinol Metabol* **90**: 493–500.
13. Gastaldelli A, Baldi S, Pettiti M, Toschi E, Camastra S, Natali A, Landau BR, Ferrannini E. (2000) Influence of obesity and type 2 diabetes on gluconeogenesis and glucose output in humans: A quantitative study. *Diabetes* **49**: 1367–1373.
14. Gastaldelli A, Miyazaki Y, Pettiti M, Buzzigoli E, Mahankali S, Ferrannini E, DeFronzo RA. (2004) Separate contribution of diabetes, total fat mass, and fat topography to glucose production, gluconeogenesis, and glycogenolysis. *J Clin Endocrinol Metabol* **89**: 3914–3921.
15. Gastaldelli A, Ferrannini E, Miyazaki Y, Matsuda M, DeFronzo RA. (2004) Beta-cell dysfunction and glucose intolerance: Results from the San Antonio metabolism (SAM) study. *Diabetologia* **47**: 31–39.
16. DeFronzo RA, Tripathy D, Schwenke DC, Banerji M, Bray GA, Buchanan TA, Clement SC, Henry RR, Kitabchi AE, Mudaliar S *et al.* (2013) Prediction of diabetes based on baseline metabolic characteristics in individuals at high risk. *Diabetes Care* **36**: 3607–3612.
17. Ferrannini E, Gastaldelli A, Matsuda M, Miyazaki Y, Pettiti M, Glass L, DeFronzo RA. (2003) Influence of ethnicity and familial diabetes on glucose tolerance and insulin action: A physiological analysis. *J Clin Endocrinol Metabol* **88**: 3251–3257.
18. Natali A, Muscelli E, Mari A, Balkau B, Walker M, Tura A, Anderwald C, Golay A, Ferrannini E. (2010) Insulin sensitivity and beta-cell function in the offspring of type 2 diabetic patients: Impact of line of inheritance. *J Clin Endocrinol Metabol* **95**: 4703–4711.

19. Kashyap S, Belfort R, Gastaldelli A, Pratipanawatr T, Berria R, Pratipanawatr W, Bajaj M, Mandarino L, DeFronzo R, Cusi K. (2003) A sustained increase in plasma free fatty acids impairs insulin secretion in nondiabetic subjects genetically predisposed to develop type 2 diabetes. *Diabetes* **52**: 2461–2474.
20. Fox CS, Massaro JM, Hoffmann U, Pou KM, Maurovich-Horvat P, Liu CY, Vasan RS, Murabito JM, Meigs JB, Cupples LA *et al.* (2007) Abdominal visceral and subcutaneous adipose tissue compartments: Association with metabolic risk factors in the Framingham Heart Study. *Circulation* **116**: 39–48.
21. Gastaldelli A. (2008) Abdominal fat: Does it predict the development of type 2 diabetes? *Am J Clin Nutr* **87**: 1118–1119.
22. Charles M, Eschwege E, Thibult N, Claude J-R, Warnet J-M, Rosselin G, Girard J, Balkau B. (1997) The role of non-esterified fatty acids in the deterioration of glucose tolerance in Caucasian subjects: Results of the Paris Prospective Study. *Diabetologia* **40**: 1101–1106.
23. Neeland IJ, Turer AT, Ayers CR, Powell-Wiley TM, Vega GL, Farzaneh-Far R, Grundy SM, Khera A, McGuire DK, de Lemos JA. (2012) Dysfunctional adiposity and the risk of prediabetes and type 2 diabetes in obese adults. *JAMA* **308**: 1150–1159.
24. Albu JB, Curi M, Shur M, Murphy L, Matthews DE, Pi-Sunyer FX. (1999) Systemic resistance to the antilipolytic effect of insulin in black and white women with visceral obesity. *American J Physiol* **277**: E551–E560.
25. Wajchenberg BL. (2000) Subcutaneous and visceral adipose tissue: Their relation to the metabolic syndrome. *Endocr Rev* **21**: 697–738.
26. Ferrannini E, Sironi AM, Iozzo P, Gastaldelli A. (2008) Intra-abdominal adiposity, abdominal obesity, and cardiometabolic risk. *Eur Heart J Suppl* **10**: B4–B10.
27. Gastaldelli A, Cusi K, Pettiti M, Hardies J, Miyazaki Y, Berria R, Buzzigoli E, Sironi AM, Cersosimo E, Ferrannini E *et al.* (2007) Relationship between hepatic/visceral fat and hepatic insulin resistance in nondiabetic and type 2 diabetic subjects. *Gastroenterology* **133**: 496–506.
28. Heni M, Machann J, Staiger H, Schwenzer NF, Peter A, Schick F, Claussen CD, Stefan N, Haring HU, Fritsche A. (2010) Pancreatic fat is negatively associated with insulin secretion in individuals with impaired fasting glucose and/or impaired glucose tolerance: A nuclear magnetic resonance study. *Diabetes Metab Res Rev* **26**: 200–205.
29. van der Poorten D, Milner KL, Hui J, Hodge A, Trenell MI, Kench JG, London R, Peduto T, Chisholm DJ, George J. (2008) Visceral fat: A key mediator of steatohepatitis in metabolic liver disease. *Hepatology* **48**: 449–457.

30. Ebbert JO, Jensen MD. (2013) Fat depots, free fatty acids, and dyslipidemia. *Nutrients* **5**: 498–508.
31. Nielsen S, Guo Z, Johnson C, Hensrud D, Jensen M. (2004) Splanchnic lipolysis in human obesity. *J Clin Invest* **113**: 1582–1588.
32. Adiels M, Taskinen MR, Packard C, Caslake MJ, Soro-Paavonen A, Westerbacka J, Vehkavaara S, Hakkinen A, Olofsson SO, Yki-Jarvinen H *et al.* (2006) Overproduction of large VLDL particles is driven by increased liver fat content in man. *Diabetologia* **49**: 755–765.
33. Fabbrini E, Mohammed BS, Magkos F, Korenblat KM, Patterson BW, Klein S. (2008) Alterations in adipose tissue and hepatic lipid kinetics in obese men and women with nonalcoholic fatty liver disease. *Gastroenterology* **134**: 424–431.
34. Shoelson S, Lee J, Goldfine A. (2006) Inflammation and insulin resistance. *J Clin Investig* **116**: 1793–1801.
35. Fontana L, Eagon J, Trujillo M, Scherer P, Klein S. (2007) Visceral fat adipokine secretion is associatd with systemic inflammation in obese humans. *Diabetes* **56**: 1010–1013.
36. Alligier M, Gabert L, Meugnier E, Lambert-Porcheron S, Chanseaume E, Pilleul F, Debard C, Sauvinet V, Morio B, Vidal-Puig A *et al.* (2013) Visceral fat accumulation during lipid overfeeding is related to subcutaneous adipose tissue characteristics in healthy men. *J Clin Endocrinol Metab* **98**: 802–810.
37. Lim EL, Hollingsworth KG, Aribisala BS, Chen MJ, Mathers JC, Taylor R. (2011) Reversal of type 2 diabetes: Normalisation of beta cell function in association with decreased pancreas and liver triacylglycerol. *Diabetologia* **54**: 2506–2514.
38. Szendroedi J, Phielix E, Roden M. (2012) The role of mitochondria in insulin resistance and type 2 diabetes mellitus. *Nat Rev Endocrinol* **8**: 92–103.
39. Le KA, Ventura EE, Fisher JQ, Davis JN, Weigensberg MJ, Punyanitya M, Hu HH, Nayak KS, Goran MI. (2011) Ethnic differences in pancreatic fat accumulation and its relationship with other fat depots and inflammatory markers. *Diabetes Care* **34**: 485–490.
40. DeFronzo RA. (2010) Insulin resistance, lipotoxicity, type 2 diabetes and atherosclerosis: The missing links. The Claude Bernard Lecture 2009. *Diabetologia* **53**: 1270–1287.
41. Arner P. (2002) Insulin resistance in type 2 diabetes: Role of fatty acids. *Diabetes Metabol Res Rev* **18**: S5–S9.
42. Morelli M, Gaggini M, Daniele G, Marraccini P, Sicari R, Gastaldelli A. (2013) Ectopic fat: The true culprit linking obesity and cardiovascular disease? *Thromb Haemost* **110**: 651–660.

43. Belfort R, Mandarino L, Kashyap S, Wirfel K, Pratipanawatr T, Berria R, Defronzo RA, Cusi K. (2005) Dose–response effect of elevated plasma free fatty acid on insulin signaling. *Diabetes* **54**: 1640–1648.
44. Wang XL, Zhang L, Youker K, Zhang MX, Wang J, LeMaire SA, Coselli JS, Shen YH. (2006) Free fatty acids inhibit insulin signaling-stimulated endothelial nitric oxide synthase activation through upregulating PTEN or inhibiting Akt kinase. *Diabetes* **55**: 2301–2310.
45. Chinen I, Shimabukuro M, Yamakawa K, Higa N, Matsuzaki T, Noguchi K, Ueda S, Sakanashi M, Takasu N. (2007) Vascular lipotoxicity: Endothelial dysfunction via fatty-acid-induced reactive oxygen species overproduction in obese Zucker diabetic fatty rats. *Endocrinology* **148**: 160–165.
46. Inoguchi T, Li P, Umeda F, Yu HY, Kakimoto M, Imamura M, Aoki T, Etoh T, Hashimoto T, Naruse M *et al.* (2000) High glucose level and free fatty acid stimulate reactive oxygen species production through protein kinase C--dependent activation of NAD(P)H oxidase in cultured vascular cells. *Diabetes* **49**: 1939–1945.
47. Watanabe S, Tagawa T, Yamakawa K, Shimabukuro M, Ueda S. (2005) Inhibition of the renin-angiotensin system prevents free fatty acid-induced acute endothelial dysfunction in humans. *Arterioscl, Thromb Vasc Biol* **25**: 2376–2380.
48. Egan BM, Hennes MM, Stepniakowski KT, O'Shaughnessy IM, Kissebah AH, Goodfriend TL. (1996) Obesity hypertension is related more to insulin's fatty acid than glucose action. *Hypertension* **27**: 723–728.
49. Boden G, Lebed B, Schatz M, Homko C, Lemieux S. (2001) Effects of acute changes of plasma free fatty acids on intramyocellular fat content and insulin resistance in healthy subjects. *Diabetes* **50**: 1612–1617.
50. Brehm A, Krssak M, Schmid AI, Nowotny P, Waldhausl W, Roden M. (2006) Increased lipid availability impairs insulin-stimulated ATP synthesis in human skeletal muscle. *Diabetes* **55**: 136–140.
51. Itani SI, Ruderman NB, Schmieder F, Boden G. (2002) Lipid-induced insulin resistance in human muscle is associated with changes in diacylglycerol, protein kinase C, and IkappaB-alpha. *Diabetes* **51**: 2005–2011.
52. Liu GX, Hanley PJ, Ray J, Daut J. (2001) Long-chain acyl-coenzyme A esters and fatty acids directly link metabolism to K(ATP) channels in the heart. *Circ Res* **88**: 918–924.
53. Noble D, Mathur R, Dent T, Meads C, Greenhalgh T. (2011) Risk models and scores for type 2 diabetes: Systematic review. *BMJ* **343**: d7163.
54. Rathmann W, Kowall B, Heier M, Herder C, Holle R, Thorand B, Strassburger K, Peters A, Wichmann HE, Giani G *et al.* (2010) Prediction

models for incident type 2 diabetes mellitusin the older population: KORA S4/F4 cohort study. *Diabet Med* **27**: 1116–1123.

55. Wilson PW, Meigs JB, Sullivan L, Fox CS, Nathan DM, D'Agostino RB, Sr. (2007) Prediction of incident diabetes mellitus in middle-aged adults: The Framingham Offspring Study. *Arch Intern Med* **167**: 1068–1074.
56. He S, Zheng Y, Shu Y, He J, Wang Y, Chen X. (2013) Hypertriglyceridemic waist might be an alternative to metabolic syndrome for predicting future diabetes mellitus. *PLoS One* **8**: e73292.
57. Gastaldelli A, Kozakova M, Hojlund K, Flyvbjerg A, Favuzzi A, Mitrakou A, Balkau B. (2009) Fatty liver is associated with insulin resistance, risk of coronary heart disease, and early atherosclerosis in a large European population. *Hepatology* **49**: 1537–1544.
58. Ferrannini E, Natali A, Camastra S, Nannipieri M, Mari A, Adam KP, Milburn MV, Kastenmuller G, Adamski J, Tuomi T *et al.* (2013) Early metabolic markers of the development of dysglycemia and type 2 diabetes and their physiological significance. *Diabetes* **62**: 1730–1737.
59. Gall WE, Beebe K, Lawton KA, Adam KP, Mitchell MW, Nakhle PJ, Ryals JA, Milburn MV, Nannipieri M, Camastra S *et al.* (2010) Alpha-hydroxybutyrate is an early biomarker of insulin resistance and glucose intolerance in a nondiabetic population. *PLoS One* **5**: e10883.

Chapter 4: Primary Prevention Trials in Type 2 Diabetes

Ambady Ramachandran,,† Chamukuttan Snehalatha,† Samith A. Shetty† and Arun Nanditha†*

1. INTRODUCTION

1.1. Burden of Type 2 Diabetes

Type 2 diabetes (T2DM) constitutes more than 95% of all diabetic population and is a major public health burden in the 21st century. T2DM has a long, asymptomatic, latent, prediabetic stage, which is associated with insulin resistance and other cardiometabolic risk factors. The global prevalence of impaired glucose tolerance (IGT) is 6.9% (316 million), which foretells an impending future increase in the number of people affected with diabetes.[1] It has been shown that people with IGT have two- to seven-fold higher risk of progression to T2DM than people with normal glucose tolerance (NGT).

The recent epidemic can be attributed mainly to the rise in environmental risk factors as genetic factors do not change in a short period. In many developing countries, especially in South East Asia (SEA), diabetes develops earlier than in the white population, and the rising rate of obesity occurs even among children and youth which accelerates the metabolic decompensation to diabetes, at an early age.[2]

Diabetes-related morbidity and mortality cause a severe public health burden. The International Diabetes Federation (IDF) estimates show that

* Corresponding author. Email: ramachandran@vsnl.com

†India Diabetes Research Foundation and Dr. A. Ramachandran's Diabetes Hospitals Chennai, India.

the annual health expenditure due to diabetes in 2013 has been more than $548 billion.[1]

Landmark long-term studies such as the Diabetes Control and Complications Trial in Type 1 diabetes (DCCT)/Epidemiology of Diabetes Interventions and Complications Study (EDIC)[3] and the UK Prospective Diabetes Study (UKPDS)[4] have unequivocally proven that tight control of glycemia instituted early in the course of diabetes produces a "legacy effect" (metabolic memory) that reduces the risk of vascular complications.[4]

It is well-known that the toxic effect of dysglycemia at the cellular level begins well before diabetes is diagnosed.[5] Therefore, it is imperative that appropriate strategies are developed and instituted to identify people at risk of diabetes and to prevent the deterioration of pancreatic β-cell secretion and insulin sensitivity, which ultimately leads to diabetes. Prevention of diabetes reduces human suffering, alleviates the economic burden resulting from the disease, and also prevents the morbidity and mortality from diabetes-related complications such as cardiovascular diseases (CVD). There is consensus that early detection, treatment, and prevention of diabetes are imperative for the well-being of society, the healthcare system, and to improve the economic scenario in any country.[6]

This chapter gives a description of systematic, randomized, prospective clinical trials of primary prevention of T2DM with a minimum follow-up of 2 years. Reviews, monograms, and original publications of the studies have been referenced. Emphasis is placed on studies using lifestyle modification (LSM)/behavioral strategies since they have been proven to be effective, safe, more economical, and sustainable than pharmacological interventions.

2. PRIMARY PREVENTION OF DIABETES

2.1. Risk Factors

Risk factors associated with T2DM are (a) nonmodifiable, such as genetic factors, demographic determinants (age, family history of diabetes, and ethnicity) and (b) modifiable, which include behavioral changes and adverse intrauterine environment and lifestyle-related factors.[6] Obesity and physical inactivity are the major modifiable factors, the prevalences of which are high and rising phenomenally in developing countries.

Genome-wide association studies have shown modest effect of certain loci with T2DM in different ethnic populations. But they do not add to the predictive power for clinical diabetes beyond the traditional risk factors.[7] Epigenetic effects — heritable changes to DNA structure that do not involve changes in the DNA sequence — occurring during gestation appear to influence adiposity and related phenotypes in offspring. In high-risk populations such as the South Asian populations, the predisposition for T2DM appears to be associated with genetic, epigenetic, and unhealthy lifestyle factors.[8]

2.2. Types of Intervention

Primary prevention is defined as the prevention of a disease by controlling modifiable risk factors through population prevention programs.

Primordial prevention strategies instituted in potential mothers during the preconception stage and during pregnancy mainly involving adequate nutrition have been advocated especially in middle- and low-income populations. Such strategies are difficult to implement and no valid results on such studies are available.[8]

3. INTERVENTION STRATEGIES

3.1. Lifestyle Modification (LSM)

There is unequivocal evidence from studies conducted in subjects of varied ethnicity, in men and women, in overweight or lean subjects showing that LSM involving healthy diet, enhanced physical activity, and improved behavior is effective in preventing T2DM.[6,8–16]

The principles of LSM are sustained physical activity of 30 to 40 minutes on all or a minimum of 5 days a week and restricted calorie intake, with reduction of refined carbohydrate and fat content and inclusion of food fiber. Reduction of weight in obese/overweight persons by intensive practice of LSM has shown beneficial effects. Cessation of tobacco use and unhealthy use of alcohol are also advised. LSM has been recommended as the safe and preferred mode for a prevention strategy.

Table 1 shows the most successful randomized, controlled primary prevention studies in diabetes using LSM.

Table 1. Landmark diabetes prevention trials using lifestyle modification.

Study[ref]	Ethnic group/ selection criterion	Number of patients by treatment group	Mean BMI (kg/m^2) and age (years)	Duration (Years)	Lifestyle goals	Behavioral intervention	Weight loss at 1 year (kg) intervention vs. control	Diabetes cumulative incidence (%)	Relative risk reduction (%)
Da Qing study (1997)[10]	Asian (Chinese)/ IGT	Control: 133 Diet: 130 Exercise: 141 Diet + Exercise: 126	BMI: 26.0 Age: 45.0	Mean 6.0	Weight loss and maintenance of healthy diet and/or exercise	NR	NR	Control: 67.7 Diet: 43.8 Exercise: 41.1 Diet+ exercise: 46	31.0 46.0 42.0
DPS (2001)[11]	Finnish/IGT	Control: 257 Intervention: 265	BMI: 31.1 Age: 55.0	Mean 3.2	5% weight loss, calorie restriction: low fat, high-fiber diet + 30 min exercise per day	Food records; goal setting	4.2 vs 0.8 ($p<0.0001$)	Control: 23 Intervention: 11	58
DPP (2002)[12]	Multi ethnic/ IGT	Control: 1082 Intervention: 1079	BMI: 34.0 Age: 50.6	Median 2.8	7% weight loss + 150 min exercise per week	Culturally sensitive materials and motivational strategies	5.6 vs 0.1 ($p<0.0001$)	Control: 11 Intervention: 4.8	58

(Continued)

Table 1. *(Continued)*

Study[ref]	Ethnic group/ selection criterion	Number of patients by treatment group	Mean BMI (kg/m^2) and age (years)	Duration (Years)	Lifestyle goals	Behavioral intervention	Weight loss at 1 year (kg) intervention vs. control	Diabetes cumulative incidence (%)	Relative risk reduction (%)
IDPP-1 (2006)[13]	Asian Indian/ IGT	Control: 136 Intervention: 133	BMI: 25.8 Age: 45.9	Median 2.6	Weight maintenance by restricting refined carbohydrates and fat + 30 min exercise per day	Motivational strategies	NS	Control: 55 Intervention: 39.3	28.5
Japanese (2005)[a,14]	Asian (Japanese)/ IGT/Men	Control: 102 Intervention: 356	BMI: 23.5 Age: 51.5	Mean 4.0	Reduction in BMI to ≤22 kg/m^2 by 30–40 min exercise per day	Goal setting; Repeated motivation at 2–3 monthly interval	2.2 vs. 0.39 ($p<0.0001$)	Control: 9.3 Intervention: 3	67.4
Japanese (2011)[15]	Asian (Japanese)/ IFG/Obese	Control: 311 Intervention: 330	BMI: 27.0 Age: 49	Mean 3.0	5% weight loss, calorie restriction, low fat consumption, pedometer steps 70,000/ week	Motivational strategies	2.5 vs 1.1 ($p<0.0001$)	Control: 16.6 Intervention: 12.2	26.5

(Continued)

Table 1. *(Continued)*

Study[ref]	Ethnic group/ selection criterion	Number of patients by treatment group	Mean BMI (kg/m^2) and age (years)	Duration (Years)	Lifestyle goals	Behavioral intervention	Weight loss at 1 year (kg) intervention vs. control	Diabetes cumulative incidence (%)	Relative risk reduction (%)
JDPP (2011)[16]	Asian (Japanese)/ IGT	Control: 152 Intervention: 152	BMI: 24.5 Age: 51	Mean 3.0	5% weight loss in overweight / obese subjects to increase energy expenditure due to leisure time physical activity by 700 kcal / week	Educational settings; existing primary healthcare setup	1.5 vs 0.7 ($p = 0.023$)	Control: 14.8 Intervention: 8.2	Effect significant ($p = 0.027$) only if BMI > 22.5 Kg/m^2

Abbreviations: BMI — body mass index (kg/m^2); DPP — Diabetes Prevention Programme; JDPP — Japanese Diabetes Prevention Program.
[a]In this study, the oral glucose tolerance test used 100 g glucose and modified criteria for recruitment.

3.2. The China Da Qing Study[10]

The Da Qing Diabetes Prevention Study in China was one of the earliest multicentre, randomized, controlled clinical trials conducted in 577 subjects with IGT. There were four arms in this study: (1) regulated diet, (2) increased physical activity, (3) diet regulation and improved physical activity, and (4) no intervention (control).

The intervention groups were counseled individually by physicians on lifestyle parameters. The initial analysis at 6 years showed that all three interventions were equally effective in reducing the incidence of diabetes versus the control group. More importantly, a 20-year follow-up completed in 2006 showed that the combined intervention group had a 43% lower incidence of diabetes than the control group (Table 2).[17] The extended study showed that the benefits were evident up to 14 years after the active intervention ceased. Onset of diabetes was delayed by an average of 3.6 years.

At this point in time no significant difference was seen between the intervention and control groups in the rate of first CVD events (0.98; 95% CI, 0.71–1.37), CVD mortality (0.83; 95% CI, 0.48–1.10), and all-cause

Table 2. Long-term effectiveness of diabetes prevention studies.

Study[ref]	Intervention (*n*)	Duration (years)	Risk reduction	Extended follow-up (years)	Risk reduction vs. control (%, 95% CI)
Da Qing study,[17] China	Control: 133	6	31	20	43 (19–59)
	Diet: 130		46		
	Exercise: 141		42		
	Diet+ exercise: 126				
DPS,[19] Finland	Control: 257	3.2	58	7	43.0 (24–57)
	LSM: 265			13	38.6 (21.1–52.2)
DPP,[20] US	Placebo: 1082	2.8	58	10	LSM: 34 (24–42)
	LSM: 1079				
	Metformin: 1073		31		Metformin: 18 (7–28)

Notes: NR — not reported; NS — not significant.
Abbreviations: DPS — Diabetes Prevention Study, Finland; DPP — Diabetes Prevention Programme; LSM — lifestyle modification.

mortality (0.96; 95% CI, 0.65–1.41). There was limited statistical power to detect differences for these relatively rare outcomes. A statistically significant reduction in severe diabetic retinopathy was noted. In April 2014, the results of the prolonged 23 years follow-up of the study were published in *The Lancet Diabetes & Endocrinology* by Li *et al.* The breakthrough finding of the study was that lifestyle intervention could reduce cardiovascular and all cause mortality in people with prediabetes. Of the original 577 persons with IGT, 542(94%) had complete data for mortality and 568(99%) contributed data for the analysis. As the incidence of diabetes in the 6-year and in the 20-year intervention periods was similar in all the intervention groups, they were combined in this analysis. Cumulative incidence of cardiovascular disease mortality was 11.9% (95% CI 8.8–15.0) in the intervention group ($n=439$) versus 19.6% (12.9–26.3) in the control group ($n=138$) [hazard ratio (HR) 0.59, 95% CI 0.36–0.96; $p=0.033$]. All cause mortality was 28.1% (95% CI 23.9–32.4) versus 38.4% (30.3–46.5; HR 0.71, 95% CI 0.51–0.99; $p=0.049$). Incidence of diabetes was 72.6% (68.4–76.8) versus 89.9% (84.9–94.9; HR 0.55, 95% CI 0.40–0.76; $p=0.001$). A post-hoc analysis showed that the effect of intervention resulted in much lower mortality rate among women than in men. Lack of the beneficial effect of the intervention in men was largely attributed to higher rates of smoking and higher age than among women. The reduction in diabetes incidence was similar in men and women.

The analysis also showed that the reduction in mortality associated with the intervention was mediated by its effect in delaying the onset of diabetes. The difference between the intervention and control groups started to emerge 12 years after the study began. A non-significant 17% difference in cardiovascular mortality was noted at 20-year follow-up. Only after 23 years, could statistical significance be observed.

The study was the first to show that lifestyle intervention in people with IGT can not only reduce the incidence of diabetes but can also reduce mortality.[18]

3.3. The Finnish Diabetes Prevention Study (DPS)[11]

The DPS, a study in Finland, randomized 522 overweight individuals (mean BMI, 31.1 kg/m^2) with IGT from five centers into two groups: (a) the control group, which received advice on general healthy lifestyle at the baseline visit and (b) the intervention group, which received continued individualized advice and behavioral support. The goals of the intervention were body weight reduction of 5% or more; total fat intake of less than 30% of energy, with saturated fat intake of less than 5%; fiber intake of 15 g/1000 cal; and moderate exercise of at least 30 minutes per day. Intensive training including one-on-one consultation, instructions via phone calls, and voluntary group discussions were given at frequent intervals. At the end of the 3-year follow-up, a 58% risk reduction was noted (Table 1). Remarkably, none among those who achieved all the lifestyle goals developed T2DM.

After an active intervention period of a median of 4 years, 366 participants (200 in the intensive group and 166 in the control group) free of diabetes were further studied until the end of 2009 with a total follow-up of 9 years and a time span of 13 years from baseline.[19] The interim follow-up at 7 years showed a 43% risk reduction with the intervention versus control (Table 2). At the 13-year follow-up, the absolute risk reduction was 19.4% and the relative risk reduction was 38.6%.[19]

3.4. The Diabetes Prevention Program (DPP)[12]/The DPP Outcome Study (DPPOS)[20]

The DPP was the largest primary prevention trial in diabetes conducted in a multiethnic population in the United States involving 3234 obese/overweight men and women with IGT. Originally four groups were studied: placebo control group, intensive LSM group, metformin group, and troglitazone group. Due to the adverse effect of troglitazone, this was withdrawn within a year of starting the study. The LSM group was personally trained by case managers on healthy, low calorie, low fat diet, and physical activity of moderate intensity with the goals of weight loss (≥ 7.0%) and increased physical activity. The metformin group received 850 mg twice daily. Individualized and culturally appropriate training sessions were conducted. The initial analysis at a mean of 2.8 years of follow-up showed a 58% relative risk reduction in the LSM group and a 31% risk reduction in the metformin group. Most of the effect was explained by the reduction in body weight[12] (Table 1).

All active participants of the original trial were eligible for continued follow-up for 10 years. After unblinding the treatment assignments, placebo was stopped. All participants including the original LSM group and those who had developed diabetes were offered a group-administered lifestyle curriculum. Participants in the metformin group received 850 mg of the same, twice daily, in an unblinded fashion. A total of 88% ($n = 2766$) enrolled for an additional median follow-up period of 5.7 years. During the extended follow-up, the LSM group partially regained weight and moderate weight loss was maintained with metformin. Diabetes incidence in 10 years since DPP randomization was reduced by 34% in the LSM group and 18% in the metformin group when compared with placebo.[20]

The three studies described above have shown that prevention or delay in onset of diabetes with LSM can be sustained for at least 10 years. It is not known whether the sustained reduction in diabetes incidence results from permanent lifestyle changes or whether it is the legacy effect of improved glycaemia in the initial periods of the trial.

4. STUDIES IN ASIAN POPULATIONS

4.1. The Indian Diabetes Prevention Programs (IDPP)[13]

South Asian populations have a high predisposition to develop type 2 diabetes, hence, primary prevention of the disease is of utmost importance in these countries. China and India, two large Asian countries undergoing rapid urbanization and economic transition, have the first and second rankings among countries with the largest number of individuals with diabetes. The Asian population has several peculiar demographic and metabolic characteristics that lead to the development of diabetes at a young age, at lower BMI levels, and also have high insulin resistance despite having lean or ideal body weights. Studies in China,[10] India,[13] and in Japan[14] showed that prevention of T2DM with LSM was feasible even among lean populations with high familial predisposition to develop diabetes (Table 1).

The Indian Diabetes Prevention Programme-1 (IDPP-1)[13] was designed to test the feasibility and the effectiveness of prevention strategies in Asian Indian populations who were younger, leaner, and highly insulin resistant when compared with European populations.

IDPP-1[13] was a community-based randomized controlled study in 531 participants with IGT diagnosed with two glucose tolerance tests (421 men, 110 women). They were younger (45.9 ± 5.7 years) and had lower BMI (25.8 ± 3.5 kg/m^2) than the participants in Western studies; the characteristics were similar to the Chinese cohort in the Da Qing Study.[10] The study groups were (1) control with standard advice, (2) LSM of moderate intensity, (3) treatment with metformin (250 mg twice daily), and (4) a combination of LSM and metformin therapy. In a median follow-up of 2.6 years, the rate of conversion to diabetes was high in the control group (18.3 persons/year). However all three interventions resulted in equal relative risk reductions approximating 29%. There was no additional benefit of combining LSM with metformin. More importantly, beneficial changes in glycemia and in basic pathophysiology, i.e., improvement in insulin sensitivity and maintenance of β-cell secretion, occurred without significant weight reduction (Table 1).

Another three-year study (IDPP-2)[21] of 407 participants with IGT showed that there was no additional benefit of adding pioglitazone to LSM. The cumulative incidence of diabetes in the placebo (31.6%) and pioglitazone (29.8%) groups were similar (adjusted hazards ratio of 1.084, $p=0.0665$). Normoglycaemia was achieved in 32.3% and 40.9% of participants in the placebo and pioglitazone groups, respectively.

The most probable explanation for the lack of additional benefit of adding an insulin sensitizer to LSM in the Indian population was that the maximum possible benefit could be produced with LSM alone.

4.2. Japanese Diabetes Prevention Studies

Three long-term diabetes prevention trials in Japan with varied study designs were reported (Table 1). In the 4-year study by Kosaka *et al.*[14] published in 2005, men with IGT, identified during hospital health screening were randomized to control and LSM groups (1:4 ratio). The subjects in the control and in the intervention groups were advised to maintain BMI of <24.0 kg/m^2 and of <22.0 kg/m^2, respectively by diet and exercise. In the intervention groups, detailed instructions on lifestyle were repeated every 3–4 months during hospital visits. Diabetes was diagnosed when two or more fasting glucose values exceeded 140 mg/dL (7.7 mmol/L).

In a mean period of 4 years, weight loss was higher and a relative risk reduction of 67.4% was observed with intervention.

Another study by the Japan Diabetes Prevention Program (JDPP)[16] Research Group demonstrated the feasibility of conducting the prevention program using existing resources in a primary health care setting. The cumulative incidence of diabetes was lower in the intervention group, 8.2% in the intervention vs 14.8% in the control group ($p=0.097$). However, due to the small number of individuals studied, the difference between the groups did not reach statistical significance (Log Rank Test; $p = 0.097$). A subanalysis of subjects with BMI ≥ 22.5 kg/m^2 showed a significant decrease in the cumulative incidence with intervention ($p=0.027$), suggesting that the effects of intervention differed for lean men versus those with ideal body weight. The impact of lifestyle in prevention in individuals with varying BMI needs to be studied further.

Subjects with impaired fasting glucose (IFG) were recruited in another Japanese trial, which showed a relative risk reduction of 26.5% with LSM when compared with the control group.[15] The baseline BMI of the participants in this study was higher (mean 27.0 kg/m^2) than in other cohorts in the Asian studies.

In a meta-analysis of published diabetes prevention trials, Gillies *et al.*[9] reported pooled hazard ratios of 0.51 (95% CI, 0.44–0.60) for lifestyle interventions vs. standard advice, and 0.70 (0.62–0.79) for oral diabetes drugs vs. control. These corresponded to estimated number needed to treat (NNT) to prevent one case of diabetes of 6.4 with the lifestyle intervention and 10.8 for oral diabetes drugs, during follow-up ranging from 3 to 6 years. This showed that the effectiveness of LSM as a prevention strategy for diabetes was better than that for oral drugs.

4.3. Malmo Feasibility Study[22]

A study in Malmo, Sweden, was the first study to show the feasibility of using LSM even in men with normoglycemia (NGT). In this nonrandomized study, a significant reduction in the incidence of diabetes was shown even in people with NGT who practiced LSM for a period of 6 years. Further, a 12-year follow-up indicated that LSM prevented mortality in people with IGT, [6.5 and 14% per 1,000 person-years, respectively in LSM and standard care groups ($p=0.009$)].[23]

5. RECENT DEVELOPMENTS

5.1. Efficacy of Mobile Phone Messaging in Prevention of Diabetes[24]

The efficacy of LSM as a preventive strategy has been proven in the research setting. Research is now being focused on translating the finding into a "real-world" setting, using pragmatic, scalable, and economical adaptations. In India, the authors in collaboration with researchers in the Imperial College, London, UK conducted a 2-year prospective trial in 537 men with IGT, which assessed whether mobile phone messaging that encouraged lifestyle change could reduce incident type 2 diabetes, which concluded in November 2012 (NCT00819455).[24]

At the end of a 2-year study period, the cumulative incidence of T2DM was lower in those who received frequent messages promoting lifestyle changes (18%) than in controls (27%) who were provided standard care. (Hazard ratio 0.64, 95% CI 0.45–0.92, $p = 0.015$). The number needed to treat to prevent one case of diabetes was 11.0 (95% CI 6–55). The messages were acceptable to the participants and were effective.

The results are the first to show benefit from a targeted mobile phone intervention in the prevention of type 2 diabetes. This strategy showed similar preventive effectiveness as that noted by a direct contact method in the IDPP-1 study. Mobile phones are used worldwide by individuals at all socioeconomic levels. The cost of short messaging service (SMS) is low and the messages can be individualized. Having proven its efficacy as a communication tool in preventive endeavors in diabetes in a developing country, a similar strategy can be used in other countries as well.

6. STUDIES USING PHARMACOLOGICAL AGENTS

Table 3 shows the major prospective trials that tested the preventive potential of several antidiabetic agents.

6.1. Metformin

The DPP study[12] in the United States and the IDPP-1[13] in India were the major studies that showed the efficacy of metformin in reducing the incidence of diabetes in subjects with IGT. The benefit of metformin for prevention of diabetes has been tested in other small studies. An analysis of 31 trials with 4,570 participants followed up for 8,267 person-years showed a reduction in the incidence of diabetes by 40% with an absolute risk reduction of 6%.[34] Beneficial changes were also seen in body weight, lipid profile, and insulin resistance.

6.2. Alpha Glucosidase Inhibitors

The effectiveness of acarbose was demonstrated in a multiethnic population with IGT in the Study to Prevent NIDDM (STOP NIDDM)[25] study. A relative risk reduction of 25% was seen in a mean period of 3.3 years.

A large Japanese study tested the use of voglibose in a 3-year prospective study and the relative risk reduction was nearly 60%.[26]

6.3. Thiazolidinediones (TZD)

Troglitazone, rosiglitazone, and pioglitazone have been shown to be effective oral agents in reducing the incidence of T2DM in subjects with IGT of multiethnic origin in different trials (Table 3). Ethnic variations seemed to be present in the action of pioglitazone. In the Asian Indian study IDPP-2,[21] addition of pioglitazone did not enhance the effectiveness of LSM. The relative risk reductions with glitazones have been high, varying from 50% to 75% in all the other trials, which had used these drugs in individuals with high risk for T2DM.

6.4. The CAnadian Normoglycemia Outcomes Evaluation Trial[31]

The CAnadian Normoglycemia Outcomes Evaluation (CANOE) trial in 207 patients with IGT randomized to receive a combination of 2 mg rosiglitazone and 500 mg metformin twice daily or matching placebo for a median period of 3.9 years showed that the combination was highly effective in preventing T2DM (Table 3).

6.5. Studies Using Other Drugs

The antiobesity agent orlistat was compared with placebo in the XENical in the prevention of Diabetes in Obese Subjects (XENDOS) study for its

Table 3. Studies of prevention of diabetes using pharmacological agents.

Study (year)^ref	Population	Patients in each group (*n*)	Medication (mg)	Subject at risk	Duration (Years)	Cumulative incidence in control (%)	Relative risk reduction % (95% CI)	Adverse events
Metformin								
DPP (2002)[12]	Multiethnic	Active: 1073; Placebo: 1082	Metformin: 850/ twice daily	IGT; BMI: 34.0	2.8	28.9	31 (17–43)	Gastrointestinal problems
IDPP-1 (2006)[13]	Asian Indian	Active: 133; Placebo: 136	Metformin: 250/ twice daily	IGT; BMI: 25.8	2.5	55	26.4 (19.1–35.1)	Hypoglycemia; Gastrointestinal problems
Alpha-Glucosidase inhibitors								
STOP-NIDDM (2002)[25]	Multi ethnic	Active:714; placebo: 715	Acarbose: 100/ thrice daily	IGT; BMI: 30.0	3.3	42	25 (10–37)	Gastrointestinal side effects
Voglibose (2009)[26]	Japanese	Active: 897; Placebo: 887	Voglibose: 0.2/ thrice daily	IGT; BMI: 25.8	3	12	59.5 (43.3–81.8)	Gastrointestinal side effects
Glitazones								
TRIPOD (2002)[27]	Hispanic woman	Active: 133; Placebo: 136	Troglitazone (400)	Previous GDM; BMI: 30 Kg/m^2	2.5	30	50 (28–89)	Liver toxicity

(Continued)

Table 3. *(Continued)*

Study (year)[ref]	Population	Patients in each group (*n*)	Medication (mg)	Subject at risk	Duration (Years)	Cumulative incidence in control (%)	Relative risk reduction % (95% CI)	Adverse events
DPP (2005)[28]	Multi ethnic	Active: 585; Placebo: 582	Troglitazone: 400/once daily	IGT; BMI: 34.0	0.9	12	75 (NR)	Liver toxicity
DREAM (2006)[29]	Multiethnic	Active: 2365; Placebo: 2634	Rosiglitazone: 8/once daily	IGT, IFG; BMI: 30.9	3	25	62 (35–46)	Liver toxicity
IDPP-2 (2009)[21]	Asian Indian	Active: 204; Placebo:203	Lifestyle modification+ Pioglitazone: 30/once daily	IGT; BMI: 25.9	3	31.6	NS	—
ACT NOW (2011)[30]	Multiethnic	Active: 308; Placebo: 299	Pioglitazone: 45/once daily	IGT, BMI: 34.5	2.4	7.6	72 (51–84)	Weight gain and edema
Combination drugs								
CANOE (2011)[31]	Multiethnic	Active: 103; Placebo: 104	Rosiglitazone (4) and metformin (1000)	IGT; BMI: 32	3.9	39	66 (41–80)	Increase in diarrhoea

(Continued)

Table 3. (*Continued*)

Study (year)^ref	Population	Patients in each group (*n*)	Medication (mg)	Subject at risk	Duration (Years)	Cumulative incidence in control (%)	Relative risk reduction % (95% CI)	Adverse events
Other agents								
XENDOS (2004)[32]	Multiethnic	Active: 1640; Placebo: 1637	Orlistat: 120/ once daily	BMI: 37.3; normal (69%); IGT (21%)	4	14.2	37.3 (13.7–54.5)	Gastrointestinal events
NAVIG-ATOR (2010)[33]	Multinational	Active: 4631; Placebo: 4675	Nateglinide: 60 mg thrice daily; Valsartan: upto 160/ daily	IGT; BMI: 30.5	5	36 36.8	NS 14 (8–20)	Hypoglycaemia Hypotension-related side effects

Abbreviations: DPP — Diabetes Prevention Programme; IDPP-1 & 2 — Indian Diabetes Prevention Programme-1 and 2; STOP-NIDDM — study to prevent noninsulin-dependent diabetes; TRIPOD, Troglitazone in prevention of diabetes; DREAM — Diabetes Reduction Assessment with ramipril and rosiglitazone medication; ACT NOW — Actos Now for prevention of diabetes; CANOE — CAnadian Normoglycemia Outcomes Evaluation; XENDOS — Xenical in the prevention of diabetes in obese subjects; NAVIGATOR — Nateglinide And Valsartan in Impaired Glucose Tolerance Outcomes; IGT — Impaired glucose tolerance; GDM — gestational diabetes; BMI — body mass index; NS — not significant; NR — not reported.

potential to reduce the incidence of diabetes.[32] Although significant weight reduction was seen with the drug, the results were not conclusive because of the high attrition rate of 57%.

6.6. Antihypertensive Agents

Diabetes incidence was not a prespecified primary end point in any of the studies using antihypertensive drugs given to patients at risk of developing T2DM. A review of 24 studies showed that diabetes incidence was unchanged or increased by thiazide diuretics and β-blockers and unchanged or decreased by angiotensin-converting enzyme inhibitors, calcium channel blockers, and angiotensin receptor blockers. In the Diabetes Reduction Assessment with Ramipril and Rosiglitazone Medication (DREAM) trial,[29] ramipril was found to be ineffective in preventing diabetes (hazard ratio 0.9). No additive effect was seen in patients randomized to receive ramipril plus rosiglitazone.

6.7. Safety of Pharmacological Agents

Metformin has been shown to be a safe and effective pharmacological agent for prevention of diabetes. Other drugs tested in different prevention studies have shown varied adverse events and therefore do not have acceptable safety profiles for long-term use. Moreover, the use of drugs requires constant monitoring by healthcare professionals and is more costly than LSM.

In addition to beneficial changes in glucose metabolism, preventive strategies also reduce other cardiometabolic risk factors such as hypertension, dyslipidaemia, and inflammatory markers. The DPP study[12] showed beneficial effects on blood pressure, and blood lipids, while the DPS study reported improvement in blood pressure lipids, and plasminogen activator inhibitor-1.[35] In the IDPP-1, beneficial changes were seen in the lipid profile.[36]

7. MECHANISM OF ACTION OF INTERVENTION

Obesity, elevated levels of fasting or 2-hr glucose, insulin resistance, and β-cell secretory defects are found to be highly predictive of conversion to diabetes.

The pivotal role of β-cell dysfunction in the conversion of IGT to diabetes has been demonstrated in several long-term prospective studies in prediabetes. The DPP, the DPS, and the IDPP-1 studies showed that preservation of β-cell function facilitated by improved insulin sensitivity decreased the conversion of IGT to diabetes and also promoted the reversal to normoglycaemia in some cases.[37] Deterioration in insulin resistance and β-cell function resulted in diabetes.

In the DPP[12] and DPS[11] studies, the beneficial biochemical mechanisms were associated with reduction in body weight. In the Asian studies, the beneficial changes were seen with LSM or with use of metformin irrespective of weight reduction.

It has been demonstrated that the impact of LSM on the incidence of T2DM could overcome the influence of genetic and familial risk. An analysis of the DPS cohort, with a mean follow-up of 6.2 years, showed that the effect of intervention on the incidence of diabetes was similar in subjects with or without a family history and 19 known genetic risk loci.[38] The DPP and IDPP-1 studies had also shown that the impact of familial risk could be overcome by LSM.

The effectiveness of preventive intervention is lower in the Asian than in the white populations and this might be associated with the higher conversion rate from prediabetes to diabetes in Asians. The benefit of preventive intervention might be lower in persons with IFG than in those with isolated IGT. This could be related to the differences in the pathophysiology of these groups. The result of IDPP-2[21] was at variance with that of the ACT-NOW study,[30] which showed a significant relative risk reduction in incident diabetes with pioglitazone therapy in participants with IGT (Table 3). An ethnicity-related difference in the action of pioglitazone in nondiabetic persons may have been responsible for the divergent observation.

7.1. Cost-Effectiveness of Prevention Programs

Only a few studies, such as the DPP,[39] and the IDPP-1[40] examined the cost and cost-effectiveness of prevention programs. From the health care perspective, the cost to prevent one case of diabetes in the DPP study was $15,700 with intensive lifestyle and with metformin it was $31,000. In the

IDPP-1 study, the cost of LSM was \$1,052 to prevent one case of diabetes and \$1,095 with metformin. The estimates from the IDPP-1 study suggested that nonpharmacological interventions for the prevention of type 2 diabetes in a developing country were cheaper and more cost-effective, similar to the observations made in the DPP study. The latter observation should encourage other developing countries to take similar preventive endeavors in diabetes management. However, it is a limitation that data on long-term cost-effectiveness and indirect cost estimates are not available from the Indian or Chinese studies.

8. NATIONAL PROGRAMS

National programs translating the findings of the research studies to the population level are urgently needed, especially among developing countries where diabetes is reaching pandemic levels. Many developing nations in Europe, the United States, and the United Kingdom, Canada, and Australia have included primary prevention of diabetes in their health care agendas. Such programs conducted over a decade in Finland have provided valuable information on strategies that can be emulated by other countries. The Development Program for the Prevention and Care of Diabetes (DEHKO 2000–2010) was Finland's national diabetes program coordinated by the Finnish Diabetes Association.[41] It aimed to prevent type 2 diabetes and diabetes-related complications, to improve the quality of diabetes care and to support self-care of individuals with diabetes. Currently, the One Life project is a continuation of the mission promoted by a multisectorial approach. At the beginning of 2012, the Finnish Brain Association, the Finnish Diabetes Association, and the Finnish Heart Association with their respective health promotion projects have joined forces in One Life.[42]

The European public health research project IMAGE has developed a toolkit for prevention of type 2 diabetes, which provides practical information on preventive interventions.[43]

India has implemented its plan of action on prevention strategies for noncommunicable diseases including diabetes. Guidelines have now been laid down by the Indian Council of Medical Research (ICMR),[44] Government of India, for providing minimum standards of care, prevention, survey of disease prevalence, and training health resource personnel. The Ministry of Health and Family Welfare of the Government of India has launched the pilot phase of the National Program for Prevention and Control of Diabetes, Cardiovascular Diseases, and Stroke.[45]

National diabetes programs have been initiated in Bangladesh, India, Pakistan, and Sri Lanka. Nepal is developing strategies to implement similar national programs as well.

9. CONCLUSIONS

The success of LSM interventions in subjects at high-risk for diabetes, performed in varied ethnic populations in different parts of the world, proves the efficacy and feasibility of this strategy in significantly reducing the incidence of T2DM. Three of these studies have also shown that the beneficial effects are sustained for over 10 years.

Several barriers exist for implementation of prevention programs at population levels, particularly in developing countries. The major ones are economic problems related to unavailability of sufficient resources, socio-cultural problems due to social taboos, beliefs and poor health-seeking behavior, and lack of knowledge and skills. Each country has to evolve nationally relevant programs for addressing the aforementioned issues.

Translating the research findings to the less-than-optimal real-world environment is a huge challenge. With the assistance of the National Institutes of Health (NIH), USA and BRiDGES (Bringing, Research in Diabetes to Global Environments Systems), initiated by the International Diabetes Federation (IDF) and World Diabetes Foundation (WDF), translational research endeavors for diabetes prevention have been initiated in developing countries, some of which are described in other chapters.

Primary prevention is essential, especially in resource-constrained countries. A multisectorial effort involving governmental and nongovernmental cooperation and coordination is needed. Health education of the public, training of health care providers, and national coordination of prevention efforts are of paramount importance.

REFERENCES

1. IDF Diabetes Atlas, 6th ed. International Diabetes Federation, 2013. www.idf.org/diabetesatlas
2. Ramachandran A, Ma RC, Snehalatha C. (2010) Diabetes in Asia. *Lancet* **375**: 408–418.
3. Nathan DM, Cleary PA, Backlund JY, *et al.* (2005) Intensive diabetes treatment and cardiovascular disease in patients with type 1 diabetes; Diabetes Control and Complications Trial/Epidemiology of Diabetes Interventions and Complications (DCCT/EDIC) Study Research Group. *N Engl J Med* **353**: 2643–2653.
4. Holman RR, Paul SK, Bethel MA, *et al.* (2008) 10-year follow-up of intensive glucose control in type 2 diabetes. *N Engl J Med* **359**: 1577–1589.
5. Gerstein HC, Pais P, Pogue J, *et al.* (1999) Relationship of glucose and insulin levels to the risk of myocardial infarction: a case control study. *J Am Coll Cardiol* **33**: 612–619.
6. Alberti KGMM, Zimmet P, Shaw J. (2007) International Diabetes Federation: a consensus on Type 2 diabetes prevention. *Diabetic Med* **24**: 451–463.
7. Hu FB. (2011) Globalization of diabetes: the role of diet, lifestyle, and genes. *Diabetes Care* **34**: 1249–1257.
8. Ramachandran A, Snehalatha A, Samith Shetty A, Nanditha A. (2013) Primary prevention of type 2 diabetes in South Asians-challenges and the way forward. *Diabet Med* **30**: 26–34.
9. Gillies CL, Abrams KR, Lambert PC, *et al.* (2007) Pharmacological and lifestyle interventions to prevent or delay type 2 diabetes in people with impaired glucose tolerance: systematic review and meta-analysis. *BMJ* **334**: 299.
10. Pan X, Li G, Hu Y, *et al.* (1997) Effects of diet and exercise in preventing NIDDM in people with impaired glucose tolerance: The Da Qing IGT and diabetes study. *Diabetes Care* **20**: 537–544.
11. Tuomilehto J, Lindstrom J, Eriksson JG, *et al.* The Finnish Diabetes Prevention Study group. (2001) Prevention of type 2 diabetes mellitus by changes in lifestyle among subjects with impaired glucose tolerance. *N Engl J Med* **344**: 1343–1350.
12. Knowler WC, Barrett-Conner E, Fowler SE, *et al.* The Diabetes Prevention Program Research Group. (2002) Reduction in the incidence of type 2 diabetes with lifestyle intervention or metformin. *N Engl J Med* **346**: 393–403.
13. Ramachandran A, Snehalatha C, Mary S, *et al.* (2006) The Indian Diabetes Prevention Programme shows that lifestyle modification and metformin

prevent type 2 diabetes in Asian Indian subjects with impaired glucose tolerance (IDPP-1). *Diabetologia* **49**: 289–297.

14. Kosaka K, Noda M, Kuzuya T. (2005) Prevention of type 2 diabetes by lifestyle intervention: a Japanese trial in IGT males. *Diab Res Clin Pract* **67**: 152–162.
15. Saito T, Watanabe M, Nishida J, *et al.* Zensharen Study for Prevention of Lifestyle Diseases Group. (2011) Lifestyle modification and prevention of type 2 diabetes in overweight Japanese with impaired fasting glucose levels: a randomized controlled trial. *Arch Intern Med* **171**: 1352–1360.
16. Sakane N, Sato J, Tsushita K, Tsujii S, *et al.* Japan Diabetes Prevention Program (JDPP) Research Group. (2011) Prevention of type 2 diabetes in a primary healthcare setting: three-year results of lifestyle intervention in Japanese subjects with impaired glucose tolerance. *BMC Public Health* **11**: 40.
17. Li G, Zhang P, Wang J, *et al.* (2008) The long-term effect of lifestyle interventions to prevent diabetes in the China Da Qing Diabetes Prevention Study: A 20-year follow-up study. *Lancet* **371**: 1783–1789.
18. Li G, Zhang P, Wang J, *et al.* (2014) Cardiovascular mortality, all-cause mortality, and diabetes incidence after lifestyle intervention for people with impaired glucose tolerance in the Da Qing Diabetes Prevention Study: a 23-year follow-up study. *Lancet Diabetes Endocrinol* http://dx.doi.org/10.1016/S2213–8587(14)70057–9. [Epub a head of print]
19. Lindstrom J, Peltonen M, Eriksson JE, *et al.* for the Finnish Diabetes Prevention Study (DPS) (2012) Improved lifestyle and decreased diabetes risk over 13 years: Ling-term follow-up of the randomized Finnish Diabetes Prevention Study (DPS). *Diabetologia* **56**: 284–293.
20. Knowler WC, Fowler SE, Hamman RF, *et al.* (2009) 10-Year follow-up of diabetes incidence and weight loss in the Diabetes Prevention Program Outcomes Study. *Lancet* **374**: 1677–1686.
21. Ramachandran A, Snehalatha C, Mary S, *et al.* (2009) Pioglitazone does not enhance effectiveness of lifestyle modification in preventing conversion of impaired glucose tolerance to diabetes in Asian Indians: Results of Indian Diabetes Prevention Programme-2 (IDPP-2). *Diabetologia* **52**: 1019 –1026.
22. Eriksson KF, Lindgard F. (1991) Prevention of type 2 non-insulin-dependent) diabetes mellitus by diet and physical exercise. The 6-year Malmö feasibility study. *Diabetologia* **34**: 891–898.
23. Eriksson KF, Lindgärd F. (1998) No excess 12-year mortality in men with impaired glucose tolerance who participated in the Malmö Preventive Trial with diet and exercise. *Diabetologia* **41**: 1010–1016.

24. Ramachandran A, Snehalatha C, Ram J, *et al.* (2013) Effectiveness of mobile phone messaging in prevention of type 2 diabetes by lifestyle modification in men in India: A prospective, parallel-group, randomized controlled trial. *Lancet Diabetes Endocrinol* **1**: 191–198.
25. Chiasson J, Homis R, Hanefeld M, *et al.* for The STOP-NIDDM Trial Research Group. (2002) Acarbose for prevention of type 2 diabetes mellitus: the STOP-NIDDM randomized trial. *Lancet* **359**: 2072–2077.
26. Kawamori R, Tajima N, Iwamoto Y, *et al.* on behalf of the Voglibose Ph-3 Study Group. (2009) Voglibose for prevention of type 2 diabetes mellitus: a randomised, double-blind trial in Japanese individuals with impaired glucose tolerance. *Lancet* **373**: 1607–1614.
27. Buchanan TA, Xiang AH, Peters RK, *et al.* (2002) Preservation of pancreatic beta-cell function and prevention of type 2 diabetes by pharmacological treatment of insulin resistance in high-risk hispanic women. *Diabetes* **51**: 2796–2803.
28. Knowler WC, Hamman RF, Edetstein SL, *et al.* (2005) Research Group Prevention of type 2 diabetes with troglitazone in the Diabetes Prevention Program. *Diabetes* **54**: 1150–1156.
29. Gerstein HC, Yusuf S, Bosch J, *et al.* DREAM (Diabetes Reduction Assessment with Ramipril and Rosiglitazone Medication) Trial Investigators. (2006) Effect of Rosiglitazone on the frequency of diabetes inpatients with impaired glucose tolerance or impaired fasting glucose: A randomized controlled trial. *Lancet* **368**: 1096–1105
30. DeFronzo RA, Tripathy D, Schwenke DCM, *et al.* (2011) Pioglitazone for diabetes prevention in impaired glucose tolerance. *N Engl J Med* **364**: 1104–1115
31. Zinman B, Harris SB, Neuman J, *et al.* (2010) Low-dose combination therapy with rosiglitazone and metformin to prevent type 2 diabetes mellitus (CANOE trial): a double-blind randomized controlled study. *Lancet* **376**: 103–111.
32. Torgerson JS, Hauptman J, Boldrin MN, *et al.* (2004) Xenical in the prevention of diabetes in obese subjects (XENDOS) study: a randomized study of orlistat as an adjunct to lifestyle changes for the prevention of type 2 diabetes in obese patients. *Diabetes Care* **27**: 155–161.
33. The NAVIGATOR study group. (2010) Effect of nateglinide on the incidence of diabetes and cardiovascular events. *N Engl J Med* **362**: 1463–1476.
34. Sally S. (2008) Meta-analysis: Metformin treatment in persons at risk for diabetes mellitus. *Am J Med* **121**: 149–157.

35. Goldberg RB, Temprosa M, Haffner S, *et al.* (2009) Effect of progression from impaired glucose tolerance to diabetes on cardiovascular risk factors and its amelioration by lifestyle and metformin intervention: the Diabetes Prevention Program randomized trial by the Diabetes Prevention Program Research Group. *Diabetes Care* **32**: 726–732.
36. Snehalatha C, Mary S, Vasant V, *et al.* (2008) Beneficial Effects of Preventive Strategies of Primary Prevention of Diabetes on Cardiovascular Risk Factors — Results of the Indian Diabetes Prevention Programme (IDPP). *Diab Compl Vas Res* **5**: 25–29.
37. Ramachadran A, Snehalatha C. (2011) Diabetes Prevention Programs. *Med Clin N Am* **95**: 353–372
38. Uusitupa MI[1], Stancáková A, Peltonen M, *et al.* (2011) Impact of positive family history and genetic risk variants on the incidence of diabetes: the Finnish Diabetes Prevention Study. *Diabetes Care* **34**: 418–423.
39. The Diabetes Prevention Program Research Group. (2003) Within-trial cost-effectiveness of lifestyle intervention or metformin for the primary prevention of type 2 diabetes. *Diabetes Care* **26**: 2518–2523.
40. Ramachandran A, Snehalatha C, Yamuna A, *et al.* (2007) Cost-effectiveness of the interventions in the primary prevention of diabetes among Asian Indians: Within-trial results of the Indian Diabetes Prevention Programme (IDPP). *Diabetes Care* **30**: 2548–2552.
41. Saaristo T, Moilanen L, Korpi-Hyövälti E, *et al.* (2010) Lifestyle intervention for prevention of type 2 diabetes in primary health care: One-year follow-up of the Finnish National Diabetes Prevention Program (FIN-D2D). *Diabetes Care* **33**: 2146–2151.
42. Finnish Diabetes Association. One life projects — promoting vascular health. www.diabetes.fi/en/finnish diabetes association/one life project, accessed September 17, 2013.
43. Schwarz PE, Reddy P, Greaves C, Dunbar J, Schwarz J (Eds.) (2010) *Diabetes Prevention in Practice*, TUMAINI Institute for Prevention Management, Dresden, Germany.
44. Shah B, Menon G. Burden of non-communicable disease in India. New Delhi, India: Indian Council of Medical Research; 2005.
45. A new initiative for a healthy nation National programme for prevention and control of diabetes, cardiovascular and stroke (NPDCS). Available at: http://mohfw.nic.in/for%20websitediabetes.htm. Accessed March 11, 2008.

Chapter 5: Treatment of Prediabetes

Muhammad A. Abdul-Ghani,[*,†] *Mustafa Kanat,*[‡]
and Ralph A. DeFronzo[†]

1. INTRODUCTION

Impaired glucose tolerance (IGT), 2-hr plasma glucose between 140–199 mg/dL (7.8–11.0 mmol/L), was introduced in 1979 as an intermediate stage in the transition from normal glucose tolerance (NGT) to overt type 2 diabetes mellitus (T2DM).[1] Individuals with IGT are at increased future risk to develop T2DM.[2] In 1997, the American Diabetes Association (ADA) revised its criteria for the diagnosis of T2DM and high-risk individuals and created a new category, impaired fasting glucose (IFG), fasting plasma glucose (FPG) between 100–125 mg/dL (5.6–6.9 mmol/L)[3], which was meant to represent, analogous to IGT, a transitional state of glucose tolerance from NGT to T2DM based upon the FPG concentration. Although individuals with IFG are at increased risk for future T2DM,[2] epidemiologic and clinical studies have demonstrated that IFG and IGT represent distinct entities of glucose intolerance.[4] Because individuals with IGT and IFG are at increased risk for future T2DM, these glucose intolerant states are referred to as "prediabetes" (reviewed in Ref. [4]). It is estimated that ~70 million Americans have prediabetes (IGT and/or IFG). Because of the impact of T2DM on public health in terms of disease prevalence (~7% of US population),[5] increased morbidity and mortality, and health care expenditure (annual cost estimated at S174 billion in 2007),

*Corresponding author. Email: abdulghani@uthscsa.edu
†Diabetes Division, University of Texas Health Science Center at San Antonio, San Antonio, TX, USA.
‡Department of Internal Medicine, Istanbul Medipol University, Istanbul.

preventing the conversion of IGT and/or IFG to T2DM represents a promising strategy to restrain the ongoing epidemic of diabetes and to decrease its impact on health care expenditure.

The Diabetes Control and Complications Trial,[6] the United Kingdom Prospective Diabetes Study (UKPDS),[7,8] and the Kumamoto Study[9] have documented that hyperglycemia is the major risk factor for microvascular and, to lesser extent, macrovascular[10,11] complications. Recent clinical trials have provided evidence that tight glycemic control is less effective in preventing diabetes vascular complications in subjects with long-standing, poorly controlled T2DM than in individuals with new-onset diabetes.[12,13] Consequently, in newly diagnosed T2DM, emphasis has been placed on achieving as close to normoglycemic control as possible without untoward side effects.[14] Because most of the morbidity and mortality in T2DM arises from long-term complications, early detection and effective intervention would be expected to have enormous beneficial human, social, medical, and economic impact. Thus, initiation of treatment in IGT individuals with interventions that reverse specific pathophysiological defects present in the prediabetic state[4,15–18] provides a promising strategy to prevent the development of hyperglycemia and its associated vascular complications.

2. PATHOGENESIS OF T2DM

Current evidence supports a two-step development of T2DM[15–24] (Fig. 1). Insulin resistance is the earliest metabolic abnormality detected in subjects destined to develop T2DM. In response to insulin resistance, the β-cells augment their secretion of insulin to compensate for the insulin resistance and normoglycemia is maintained. Thus, hyperinsulinemia is a characteristic feature of the underlying insulin resistance. When β-cells fail to compensate for insulin resistance, glucose tolerance deteriorates. Initially, this is manifested as IGT and subsequently as overt T2DM.[15,17,20,22–25] Although plasma insulin levels are elevated in IGT individuals, β-cell function is severely impaired.[22,23,25] Thus, it is important to distinguish between insulin secretion and β-cell health, i.e., β-cell function (see subsequent section on "Impaired β-Cell Function").

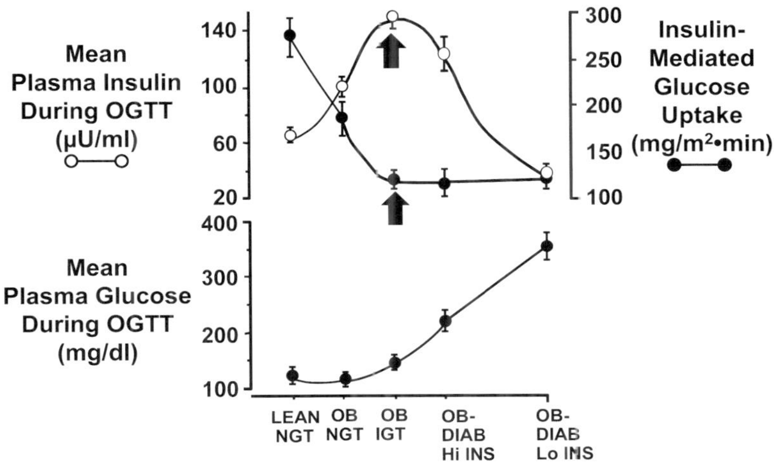

Fig. 1. Natural history of type 2 diabetes mellitus. The plasma insulin response (*open circles*) depicts the classic Starling's curve of the pancreas. *Closed circles* = insulin-mediated glucose uptake (*top panel*). DIAB = diabetes; Hi INS = high insulin secretion; IGT = impaired glucose tolerance; Lo INS = low insulin secretion; NGT = normal glucose tolerance; OB = obese; OGTT = oral glucose tolerance test.

2.1. Insulin Resistance

Insulin resistance is a core defect in both prediabetes and T2DM,[4,20,22,23,26–29] and involves liver,[20,22,23,30] muscle,[20,22,23,28,31,32] and adipose tissue.[23] Insulin resistance precedes the development of glucose intolerance and overt T2DM.[15–20,22,23,28,33] NGT offspring of two diabetic parents[15,34,35] and people with IGT[15–20,22–24,33,36] are markedly resistant to insulin[15,34,35] and manifest compensatory hyperinsulinemia. Much evidence supports a genetic component of the insulin resistance,[20] which is aggravated by environmental factors, e.g., weight gain and physical inactivity. Not surprisingly, interventions that ameliorate insulin resistance and reduce the insulin secretory demand on the β-cells have been shown to effectively prevent/delay IGT progression to T2DM.[37–40]

2.2. Impaired β-Cell Function

Although insulin resistance is a cardinal feature of IGT, ultimately, β-cell failure is responsible for the development of IGT and its progression to

T2DM.[15–17,20,22,23,33,41] It follows that interventions that halt/preserve β-cell function provide a promising strategy to prevent the development of T2DM. Low plasma insulin response during the OGTT predicts IGT progression to T2DM in all ethnic groups, and the impairment in first phase insulin secretion (0–10 m time period following an intravenous glucose challenge) is a strong predictor of progression to diabetes.[22,33,36,42,43] When the FPG exceeds 90 mg/dL (5.0 mmol/L), first phase insulin secretion begins to deteriorate, and, when the FPG exceeds 110 mg/dL (6.1 mmol/L), first phase insulin secretion is almost completely lost.[22,23,44,45]

As discussed earlier, it is important to distinguish between insulin secretion and β-cell function. The β-cells respond to an increment in glucose (ΔG) with an increment in insulin (ΔI), and this response is modulated by the severity of insulin resistance.[46] Therefore, the "gold standard" for β-cell function is the insulin secretion/insulin resistance (disposition) index (ΔI/ΔG ÷ IR). Simply measuring the plasma insulin response may provide misleading information about β-cell health.[15–17,23] Both genetic[20,23] and acquired factors (glucotoxicity,[47] lipotoxicity,[48] incretin deficiency/resistance[49–51]) play a major role in the demise in β-cell function. Although subjects with IGT have a four- to six-fold increase in the risk for T2DM compared to NGT individuals,[2] many NGT subjects are at increased future risk for T2DM.[2,52] In prospective epidemiologic studies, ~40% of subjects who developed T2DM at follow-up had NGT at baseline.[2] β-cell dysfunction is the best predictor of the 2-hr PG during the OGTT in NGT individuals,[43,52] as well as the best predictor of NGT progression to IGT and subsequently to T2DM.[15–17,23,24,52] Individuals in the upper tertile of NGT have a 50% decline in β-cell function, while subjects in the upper tertile of IGT manifest a 70–80% decline[15–17] (Fig. 2). Because individuals in the upper tertile of IGT are maximally/near maximally insulin resistant and have lost 70–80% of β-cell function, even a small further decline in insulin secretion will result in a marked increase in fasting/postprandial blood glucose levels. Once overt T2DM is present, β-cell function declines progressively with time[15,17,20,23,24,33,41,53] despite commonly employed interventions (metformin, sulfonylureas, insulin)[7,8,53] to control glycemia (reviewed in Ref. [23]). Multiple factors including genetic predisposition, insulin resistance causing increased insulin secretory demand, glucotoxicity, lipotoxicity, impaired incretin release/action, amylin accumulation, and decreased β-cell mass, all play a causative role in the progressive β-cell

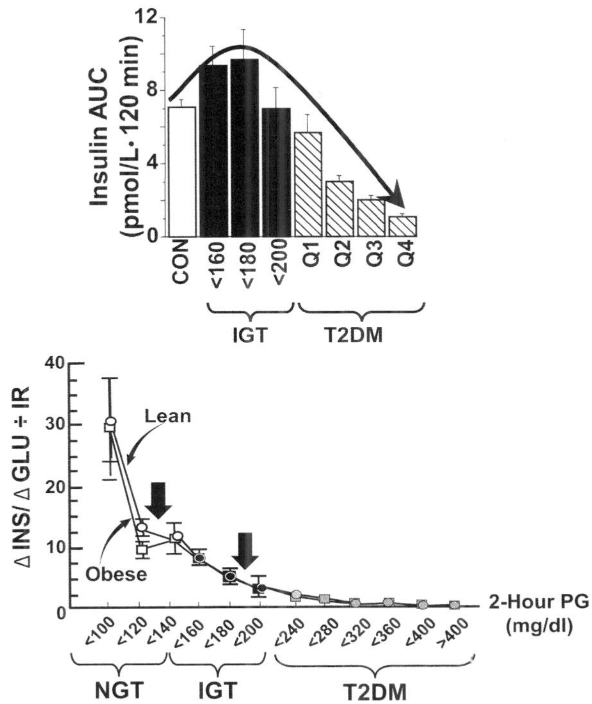

Fig. 2. Insulin secretion/insulin resistance (disposition) index (defined as change in insulin/change in glucose ÷ insulin resistance [ΔINS/ΔGLU ÷ IR]) in individuals with normal glucose tolerance (NGT), impaired glucose tolerance (IGT), and type 2 diabetes mellitus (T2DM) as a function of the 2-hour plasma glucose (PG) concentration in lean (*closed circles*) and obese (*open circles*) subjects. The inset depicts the incremental are under the plasma insulin concentration curve during the OGTT in control, IGT and T2DM individuals showing the classic Starling's curve of the pancreas.

dysfunction (reviewed in Refs. [20], [23] and [41]). Therefore, interventions designed to retard/prevent β-cell failure are of paramount importance in preventing the progression of IGT to T2DM.

3. INSULIN RESISTANCE AND β-CELL FUNCTION IN IFG AND IGT

Individuals with IGT and IFG, and especially those with combined IGT/IFG,[2,40,43,54,55] are at high-risk for T2DM.[21,56–58] Although both IGT and IFG

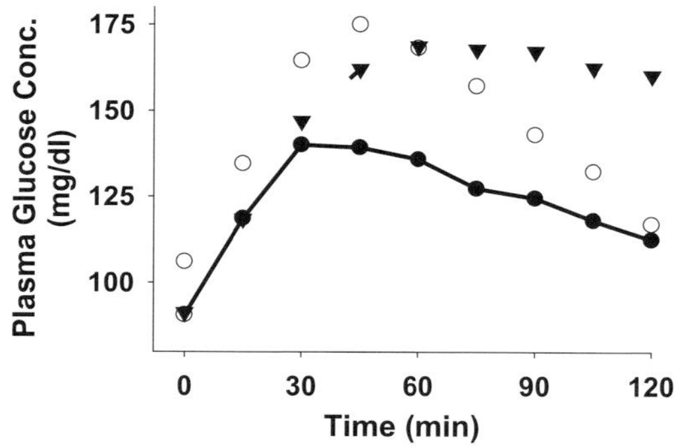

Fig. 3. Plasma glucose concentration during the OGTT in normal glucose tolerant (NGT) (*close circles*) individuals and in subjects with impaired glucose tolerance (IGT) (*closed triangles*) and impaired fasting glucose (IFG) (*open circles*).

are precursors of T2DM, they have distinct pathophysiological etiologies and different implications for future development of atherosclerotic cardiovascular disease. IFG individuals have moderate hepatic insulin resistance and impaired early insulin response (0–30 m) during the OGTT.[16,17,29,31,59] As such, they are characterized by elevated FPG and an excessive early rise (0–60 m) in PG during OGTT[60] (Fig. 3). However, because the late plasma insulin response (60–120 m) is intact and muscle insulin sensitivity is normal/near-normal, the 2-hr PG returns to its starting FPG level.[61,62] In contrast, IGT individuals have moderate–severe muscle insulin resistance and impaired early (0–30 m) and late (60–120 m) plasma insulin responses during the OGTT.[16,17,61,62] Thus, although the FPG is not elevated, there is a progressive, sustained rise in PG during the OGTT and the 2-hr PG remains well above the FPG level. Impaired first phase insulin secretion is characteristic of both IGT and IFG. However, they are distinguished by intact second phase insulin secretion in IFG and the tissues (liver in IFG vs muscle in IGT) responsible for insulin resistance. IGT and IFG also have different implications for atherosclerotic cardiovascular disease. IGT is associated with the metabolic syndrome and is a strong predictor of cardiovascular disease, whereas IFG is a much weaker predictor of atherosclerotic cardiovascular disease.[63]

4. INTERVENTION TO PREVENT THE PROGRESSION OF IGT TO T2DM

IGT and IFG represent early steps in the progression of NGT to T2DM.[20,22–24,33] Because impaired β-cell function and insulin resistance are characteristic of both IGT and IFG, it follows that interventions that preserve/augment β-cell function and ameliorate insulin resistance represent effective approaches to prevent the progression of IGT to diabetes.

4.1. Reversal of Insulin Resistance: Weight Loss

Obesity represents the single most important risk factor for the progression of IGT to diabetes[26,27,34,64] and is primarily responsible for the epidemic increase in T2DM over the last 20 years. Weight gain, together with physical inactivity, cause insulin resistance and place an increased insulin secretory demand on the β-cells. Weight loss, whether achieved via lifestyle modification or pharmacologic intervention, enhances insulin sensitivity, reduces the workload on the β-cells, and improves glucose tolerance in IGT individuals. Four lifestyle intervention studies have demonstrated that a regimen that decreases body weight by employing diet/exercise is very effective in reducing IGT progression to T2DM by improving insulin sensitivity and augmenting β-cell function.[37,58,65–67] A 5% reduction in body weight, which resulted in a ~30% improvement in whole body insulin sensitivity,[66] decreased the conversion rate of IGT to T2DM by 56%.[37]

Although lifestyle intervention is effective in decreasing the progression of IGT to T2DM, the maintenance of weight loss/physical activity is difficult to sustain over long periods,[68] as demonstrated in the DPP, in which the lost weight was largely regained when the DPP ended[69] (Fig. 4). Drug-induced weight loss also is effective in decreasing the progression rate of IGT to T2DM. In the XENDOS study, orlistat caused a 2.8 kg greater weight loss compared to lifestyle intervention (5.8 vs 3.0 kg) and was associated with a 37% decrease in the progression of IGT to T2DM.[70] However, similar to lifestyle intervention, weight loss induced by pharmacologic therapy is followed by weight regain when drug therapy is replaced by placebo, despite continued dietary intervention.[71] Thus,

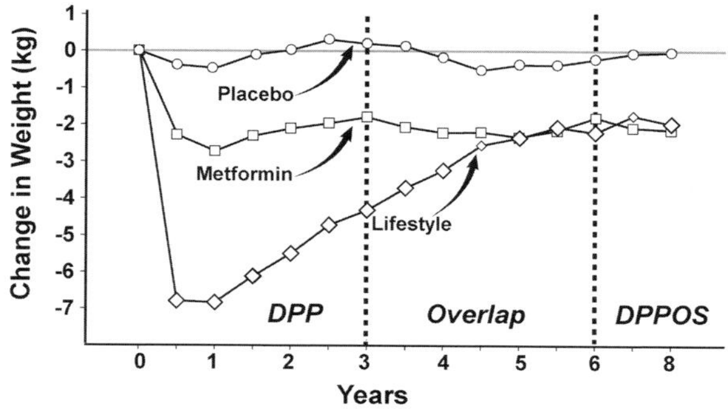

Fig. 4. Change in body weight during the DPP, during the overlap period, and during the DPP Outcomes Study (DPPOS) (reproduced from Eriksson and Lindgärde[58]).

weight regain is characteristic of most weight loss programs, irrespective of the type of intervention (lifestyle or pharmacologic), and follow-up studies have demonstrated that the conversion rate of IGT to T2DM after the cessation of weight loss intervention is similar to the control group.[72] This indicates lack of "legacy" effect of weight loss on prevention of progression of IGT to T2DM. Moreover, attempts to translate DPP results to "real world" clinical practice and achieve a 5% weight loss have proven difficult. In a community study in Finland,[73] 10,149 high-risk individuals were enrolled in a diabetes prevention program designed to achieve 5–7% body weight loss. Only one third of participants successfully reduced their body weight by more than 2.5%. Moreover, weight loss, even when achieved, is effective in decreasing the incidence of diabetes by only 50–60%.[37] Therefore, 40–50% of IGT subjects still progress to T2DM despite successful weight loss, indicating that lifestyle intervention alone is insufficient to prevent diabetes in a large percentage of individuals. In contrast to behavioral modification (diet plus exercise), pharmacological therapy uniformly reduces IGT/IFG conversion to T2DM.

4.2. Reversal of Insulin Resistance: Pharmacologic Intervention

Because improving insulin sensitivity with lifestyle intervention is difficult to achieve, pharmacologic agents have been employed as an alternative approach to enhance insulin action and decrease the conversion of IGT to T2DM. Clinical trials have shown that pharmacologic agents that improve insulin sensitivity in liver, muscle, and adipocytes are highly effective in preventing the progression of IGT to T2DM (Table 1).

4.2.1. *Metformin*

Metformin reduces the FPG concentration and hemoglobin A_{1c} (HbA_{1c}) in T2DM[74–76] by inhibiting hepatic glucose production[75,76] and, to a lesser extent, by improving insulin sensitivity.[76] Metformin does not stimulate insulin secretion[74–76] or preserve β-cell function,[76 77] and, after an initial decline, HbA_{1c} rises progressively as demonstrated in the UKPDS, ADOPT, and other studies.[7,78] In the DPP, metformin 1,700 mg/day reduced IGT conversion to T2DM by 31%[37] in association with improved insulin sensitivity[66] and decreased the incidence of metabolic syndrome. Metformin also reduced IGT conversion to T2DM in the Indian DPP.[79] In young (<65 years), obese (BMI>35) subjects with impaired fasting glucose, metformin was as effective as weight loss in decreasing the progression of IGT to T2DM.[37] Because metformin is generic and has an excellent long-term safety record, an ADA Consensus Conference recommended that high-risk individuals ($HbA_{1c} \geq 6.0\%$; body mass index ≥ 30 kg/m^2; age ≤ 60 yr) with IGT or IFG be treated with metformin.[80] However, metformin,[6,8,76] like sulfonylureas,[6,7] does not prevent the progressive β-cell failure that is characteristic of T2DM (reviewed in Ref. [23]), and HbA1c rises progressively after an initial good response.

4.2.2. *Thiazolidinediones (TZDs)*

Clinical studies have demonstrated that TZDs, working via the peroxisome proliferator activator receptor-γ (PPARγ), improve both core defects of IGT. They are powerful insulin sensitizers in muscle, liver, and adipocytes,[81–83] and they exert a potent effect to enhance/preserve β-cell function.[84]

Much evidence supports the hypothesis that TZDs improve muscle insulin sensitivity by reducing plasma-free fatty acid levels/intramyocellular lipid content, and redistributing fat from visceral to subcutaneous adipose depots.[48,81–83] A direct insulin-sensitizing effect mediated via the PPARγ receptor[81–83] in muscle and adipocytes also has been demonstrated. All three TZDs troglitazone,[85] pioglitazone,[86] and rosiglitazone,[87] similarly

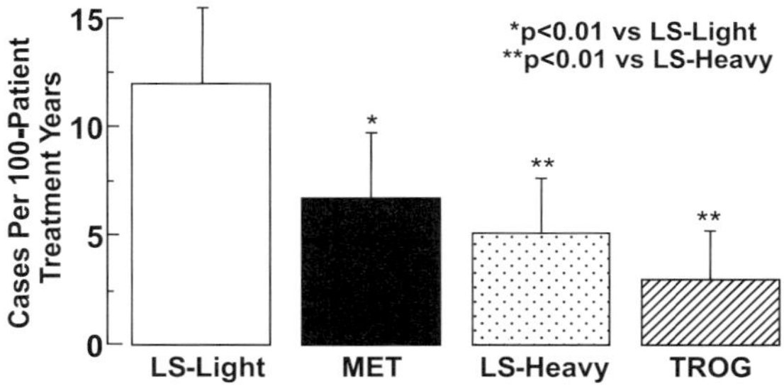

Fig. 5. Effect of lifestyle intervention, metformin, and troglitazone on the conversion rate of IGT to type 2 diabetes in the first 1.5 years of the DPP (i.e., before the discontinuation of troglitazone from the DPP). LS, lifestyle; MET, metformin; TROG, troglitazone.

improve insulin sensitivity and glycemic control in T2DM. In IGT individuals[38,88,89] and women with a history of gestational diabetes,[90] troglitazone enhances insulin sensitivity, improves glucose tolerance, and decreases the progression of IGT to T2DM. In the DPP, troglitazone reduced IGT conversion to diabetes by 23% after 3 years, although the drug was discontinued after 10 months.[38] When IGT subjects actively were taking troglitazone (initial 1.5 years), the diabetes incidence (3.0 cases/100 person-treatment years) was markedly reduced compared with placebo (12.0), metformin(6.7), and lifestyle intervention (5.1) groups ($p < 0.001$; $p = 0.02$; and $p = 0.18$), respectively (Fig. 5). In DREAM, rosiglitazone reduced IGT conversion to T2DM by 62%,[39] and the improvement in the insulin secretion/insulin resistance index was the best predictor of diabetes prevention. In women with history of gestational diabetes mellitus, both troglitazone (TRIPOD) and pioglitazone (PIPOD) markedly reduced IGT progression to T2DM.[90–92] In the ACT NOW study, pioglitazone decreased by 72% ($p < 0.00001$) the conversion rate of IGT to T2DM.[40]

4.3. Preservation of β-Cell Function

Because progressive β-cell failure is the principal factor responsible for the progression of IGT to T2DM and the development of hyperglycemia, interventions that improve β-cell function in IGT individuals should be very effective in preventing the incidence of T2DM in IGT individuals. Although TZDs markedly improve insulin sensitivity in IGT individuals, enhanced β-cell function is the strongest predictor of T2DM prevention. Studies in diabetic humans[84–90,92] and animals[93] demonstrate that troglitazone,[85,88–90] pioglitazone,[84,86,91] and rosiglitazone[84,87] augment β-cell function by (i) improving insulin sensitivity, thereby unloading the β-cells; (ii) decreasing the plasma free fatty acid concentration; (iii) mobilizing toxic lipid metabolites (fatty acyl CoAs, diacylglycerol and ceramides) out of β-cells (reversal of lipotoxicity); and (iv) direct β-cell effect mediated via the PPARγ receptor.[20,48,83,84] Because TZDs both preserve β-cell function and improve insulin sensitivity, they are very effective in preventing IGT progression to T2DM and producing a durable HbA1c reduction in T2DM.[23] However, because of fat weight gain, fluid retention, and cost,[38,39,94] the ADA Consensus Statement recommended metformin, not TZDs, for the treatment of IGT/IFG,[80] although TZDs consistently have been at least twice as effective as metformin in reducing IGT conversion to T2DM. In ACT NOW, the pioglitazone dose was titrated to 45 mg/d. However, lower doses (15–30 mg/d) have been shown to improve insulin sensitivity and insulin secretion in T2DM[95] and are associated with less weight gain and fluid retention.[96] Of note, in native Canadians with IGT,[97] low-dose rosiglitazone (2 mg/d) plus metformin (1,000 mg/d) reduced IGT conversion to T2DM by 71% without weight gain or fluid retention.

TZDs have been shown to effectively decrease and maintain a durable reduction in HbA1c in T2DM subjects in eight of eight long-term (≥1.5 years) studies (reviewed in Ref. [23]). In ADOPT, the HbA1c decrement with rosiglitazone was maintained for 5 years.[78] This sustained HbA1c reduction implies that TZDs must exert a long-term effect to preserve β-cell function. Consistent with this, in 61 T2DM subjects, pioglitazone and rosiglitazone similarly increased β-cell function, measured with the gold standard insulin secretion/insulin resistance index.[84]

In summary, in addition to their insulin-sensitizing effect, TZDs improve and preserve β-cell function, cause a durable HbA1c reduction in T2DM, and markedly reduce IGT conversion to T2DM.

4.3.1. *Glucagon-like Peptide-1 (GLP-1) Analogs*

After glucose ingestion, the increase in plasma insulin response is two- to three-fold greater than after the same level of hyperglycemia produced with intravenous glucose, i.e., the incretin effect.[98–100] Together, GLP-1, released by L cells, and glucose-dependent insulinotropic polypeptide (GIP), released by K cells, account for 90% of the incretin effect.[98–100] Both GLP-1 and GIP are potent insulin secretagogues. In addition to augmenting insulin secretion, GLP-1 also inhibits glucagon secretion, delays gastric emptying, and promotes weight loss by suppressing appetite and decreasing food intake.[98,99] Because both GLP-1 and GIP are rapidly cleaved (half-life = 1–2 m) by dipeptidyl peptidase-IV, both peptides are inappropriate for therapeutic use in T2DM and IGT subjects. Liraglutide and exenatide are GLP-1 receptor agonists that mimic the actions of GLP-1 and are resistant to dipeptidyl peptidase-IV degradation.[101,102] Similar to endogenous GLP-1, both agonists are potent insulin secretagogues,[98–100] inhibit glucagon secretion, promote weight loss and effectively reduce PG levels in T2DM.[98–102] In a long-term (3 years) extension study, exenatide produced a durable HbA1c reduction, improved β-cell function, and caused progressive weight loss.[103]

Hypoglycemia is uncommon with GLP-1 analogs because they only augment insulin secretion in the presence of hyperglycemia. Glucose is the physiologic stimulus for insulin release. It stimulates insulin secretion by increasing the production of ATP leading to closure of the ATP-dependent potassium channel. This causes depolarization of the β-cell membrane followed by calcium influx, which triggers the exocytosis of insulin-containing vesicles.[104] Both GLP-1 and GIP mediate their β-cell effects via a mechanism that is completely distinct from hyperglycemia. Following binding to their respective receptors, GLP-1 and GIP activate adenylate cyclase, which convert ATP to cAMP, which, in turn, "amplifies" an insulin secretory system that has been activated by hyperglycemia.[105] In the absence of hyperglycemia, neither GLP-1 nor GIP increases insulin secretion.

Subjects with IGT and T2DM are characterized by severely impaired β-cell function[16,18,20,22,23,37,41] and markedly reduced incretin effect in response to meal/glucose ingestion.[98–100] Studies from our group and others have demonstrated that the primary defect in IGT and T2DM is an inability of the β-cell to respond to glucose,[15] and this β-cell "blindness" to glucose, at least in part, can be restored by the incretin hormones.[106] In IGT, most studies have reported no change or slightly impaired total

GLP-1 response to a mixed meal,[49,100,107–109] but the early (0–10 m) GLP-1 response is diminished,[49,100,107–109] indicating a phasic defect in GLP-1 secretion; GIP secretion is normal or slightly increased (reviewed in Ref. [100]). In contrast, marked β-cell resistance to the stimulatory effect of GLP-1 on insulin secretion is well-documented in T2DM.[50,51,100,110] In addition, the β-cells manifest severe resistance to the stimulatory effect of GIP on insulin secretion.[50,100] β-cell sensitivity to GIP, unlike GLP-1, can be restored after normalization of glycemia with insulin.[50]

In the presence of hyperglycemia, NGT subjects manifest a robust insulin secretory response to a physiologic increase in GLP-1 concentration. In contrast, the same physiologic GLP-1 infusion in T2DM fails to augment insulin secretion in the presence of hyperglycemia.[50,51] However, if the GLP-1 infusion is increased to cause a pharmacological rise in plasma GLP-1 concentration, a normal insulin response to the hyperglycemic stimulus is achieved (Fig. 6). These results indicate that pharmacological levels of plasma GLP-1 are capable of correcting β-cell "blindness" to glucose and restoring normal β-cell function to glucose in IGT and T2DM individuals. Although the stimulatory effect of the GLP-1 analogs on β-cell function weans rapidly upon washing out the drug, a recent study reported that, if exenatide is continued for 3 years, its ability to enhance β-cell responsiveness to glucose is partially retained.[111]

Because relentless β-cell failure is responsible for progression from NGT to IGT to T2DM (Figs. 1 and 2),[15,18,23,24,41] and because exenatide

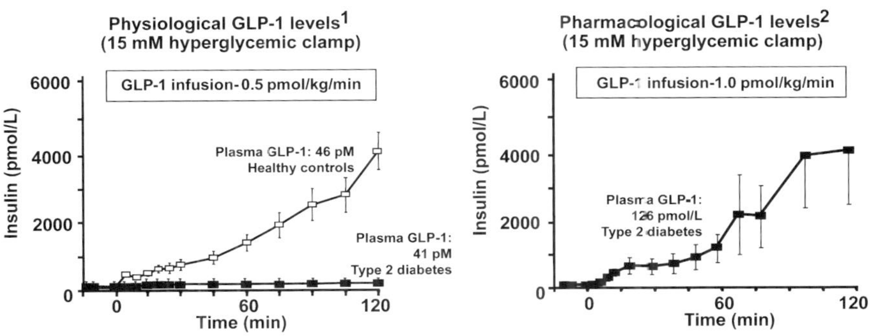

Fig. 6. Effect of physiologic (left) and pharmacologic (right) doses of GLP-1 on insulin secretion in NGT individuals and in subjects with T2DM.

(i) improves β-cell function in subjects with T2DM by restoring beta cell glucose sensitivity; (ii) promotes weight loss; (iii) does not cause hypoglycemia; (iv) can be given once weekly (exenatide extended-release), it is likely to be an ideal agent for decreasing the progression of IFG/IGT to T2DM and reverting glucose tolerance to normal. Although the effect of GLP-1 analogs on the progression of IGT to T2DM has yet to be tested on a large scale, long-term outcome study, in a 20-week study, liraglutide was administered to 564 non-diabetic obese individuals, 31% of whom had IGT.[112] In IGT subjects, liraglutide decreased the conversion to T2DM by 84–96%. Sixty-one percent of subjects lost at least 5% of body weight, and 19% lost at least 10% of body weight. The incidence of metabolic syndrome was reduced by 60%, and systolic/diastolic blood pressure declined by 5.7/3.7 mmHg.

Long-acting GLP-1 analogs, because they are administered once weekly, augment β-cell function, and promote weight loss, could prove to be ideal for preventing IGT progression to T2DM.[113]

4.3.2. *DPP-IV inhibitors*

Members of this class of drug inhibit the dipeptidyl peptidase-IV (DPP-IV), the enzyme that cleaves GLP-1 and thereby causes an increase in plasma GLP-1 levels. However, because the increase in GLP-1 level achieved with DPP-IV inhibitors highly depends upon the endogenous GLP-1 secretion, the magnitude of increase in plasma GLP-1 is modest compared to those achieved with GLP-1 analogs, and it is sufficient only to modestly increase insulin secretion and inhibits glucagon.[98] Studies in IGT individuals have demonstrated a small increase in β-cell function following vildagliptin administration. However, the effect of vildagliptin was completely reversible upon washing out the drug.[104] No outcome studies have examined the effect of DPP-IV inhibitors on the conversion rate of IGT to T2DM. Because the effect of DPP-IV inhibitors on β-cell function is modest and unlike GLP-1 analogs, this class of drugs does not promote weight loss, we favor GLP-1 analogs over DPP-IV inhibitors for the treatment of IGT.

4.4. α-Glucosidase Inhibitors

Both acarbose in STOP-NIDDM[114] and voglibose in a Japanese trial[115] were reported to modestly (~25%) decrease IGT conversion rate to T2DM. Although this preventive effect was believed to result from inhibition of carbohydrate absorption, α-glucosidase inhibitors have been shown to augment incretin secretion,[116] and this could explain in part their beneficial effects on glucose homeostasis. By altering gut microbiota flora, α-glucosidase inhibitors also could exert a beneficial effect on glucose tolerance.[117]

5. IDENTIFICATION OF HIGH-RISK IGT INDIVIDUALS FOR PHARMACOLOGICAL THERAPY

Prediabetic individuals, at high-risk to develop T2DM and atherosclerotic cardiovascular disease, are maximally/near-maximally insulin resistant, have lost up to 70–80% of β-cell function, and at least 10% have diabetic retinopathy with an HbA1c of ~6%[118,119]; a similar percentage have peripheral neuropathy.[120] β-cell dysfunction and insulin resistance are the characteristic antecedents of the diabetic state. In clinical practice, however, it is not feasible to screen individuals for defects in insulin sensitivity or insulin secretion with the gold standard methods, i.e., euglycemic insulin clamp and hyperglycemic clamp, respectively. Predictive models[121] have demonstrated that anthropometric measurements (body mass index, waist-to-hip ratio), combined with commonly measured components of the metabolic syndrome, have equivalent predictive value to the 2-hr PG during OGTT for IGT conversion to T2DM. IGT subjects whose sum of PG during OGTT is in the upper 50th percentile or who have a FPG of at least 95 mg/dL (5.3 mmol/L) are at especially high-risk to develop T2DM.[122] In the Botnia[54] and San Antonio Heart[43,123] studies, a 1-hr PG >155 mg/dL (8.61 mmol/L) was the best predictor of future T2DM in IGT subjects and it identified subjects at increased future T2DM risk independent of their glucose tolerance status. A biomarker panel (HbA1c, FPG, insulin, IL-2 receptor A, adiponectin, ferritin, high-sensitivity C-reactive protein) also has high predictive value for future diabetes.[124] Selecting individuals with IGT having additional risk factors for progression to T2DM can identify those most likely to benefit from pharmacological intervention observations confirmed in the DPP[37] and ACT NOW[40] studies.

6. APPROACH TO THE PATIENT WITH PREDIABETES

Since individuals with IGT are maximally/near maximally insulin resistant and manifest 50–80% decrease in β-cell function, and given the importance of maintaining normoglycemia as early as possible in the course of T2DM to prevent the development of vascular complications, the optimal strategy is to intervene at the stage of IGT to prevent the development of hyperglycemia and revert glucose tolerance back to NGT. Moreover, intervening at the IGT stage to prevent the progression to T2DM has been shown to be cost-effective. The DPP Research Group[133,134] concluded that: "Over 3 years, metformin was clinically effective (in preventing diabetes in IGT subjects) and cost-effective from the perspective of a health system and society, especially if implemented with generic medication pricing." A similar conclusion has been reached using model-simulated data.[135,136]

No data on the cost-effectiveness of pioglitazone or GLP-1 receptor agonists are available. Because pioglitazone[40] has been shown to be twice as effective as metformin[37] in reducing IGT conversion to T2DM, it is reasonable to extrapolate that pioglitazone, like metformin, also would be cost-effective. However, the costs of monitoring and treating the side effects of this, TZDs would also need to be considered. These include the management of edema if it occurs and the potential need to monitor and treat any bone loss in women. A small risk of fractures in long bones has been reported in postmenopausal women and this also should be considered.[78] Although some observational studies have suggested possible increased risk of bladder cancer in subjects who received 45 mg pioglitazone > 2 years, the recent interim analysis of 8 years of follow-up of the Kaiser Permanente data, the prospective study mandated by the Food and Drug Administration (FDA) to assess the long-term safety of pioglitazone, has reported a hazard risk ratio of 0.98 for diabetic subjects who received pioglitazone compared to those who never used pioglitazone.

Because of the high price of the GLP-1 analogs, which are not expected to be generically available for several years, their cost-effectiveness for the treatment of prediabetes would need to be carefully examined. From the standpoint of the individual (as opposed to the societal perspective), any intervention that prevents/delays the onset of hyperglycemia would be expected to prevent/reduce the incidence of microvascular complications (retinopathy, nephropathy, neuropathy). It is impossible to set a price on the prevention of reduction in the incidence of blindness, end-stage renal disease, and amputation for the individual.

Rather than treating individuals with prediabetes, one could opt to wait until they develop overt diabetes and initiate therapy at this stage. Although this represents a potential option, it does have several limitations. First, it requires that these prediabetic individuals be followed sequentially so that the time of onset of diabetes can be identified. Second, intensive blood glucose control at the time of diagnosis of diabetes, i.e., UKPDS, decreased but did not prevent the development of microvascular complications.[8] Moreover, the time of onset of diabetes as defined by the PG level (FPG or 2-hr PG) or the HbA1c, is somewhat arbitrary as conversion from a euglycemic status to dysglycemia is a continuous and insidious process. Approximately 10% of prediabetic individuals already have evidence of diabetic microvascular complications. Third, and most importantly, studies by Butler *et al.*[137] have demonstrated a significant reduction in β-cell mass at the prediabetic stage with a further decline with progression to overt T2DM. At present, there are no therapies that have been shown to increase β-cell mass in humans. Fourth, individuals in the upper tertile of IGT are maximally/near maximally insulin resistant, have lost 70–80% of their β-cell function, and have a significant reduction (30–40%) in β-cell volume.

Hence, as prediabetic individuals manifest all of the pathophysiological abnormalities present in overt T2DM, and a significant minority (~10%) manifest diabetic microvascular complications, it seems reasonable, therefore, to institute intervention (lifestyle plus pharmacological therapy) at the prediabetic stage in high-risk individuals rather than wait for the diagnosis of diabetes, which is somewhat arbitrary and based on the PG level and not on pathophysiology, loss of β-cell mass, or presence of microvascular complications. Since no study has compared or is likely to compare therapy instituted at the prediabetic stage vs. diabetic stage because of the large sample size and length of time required to observe the onset and demonstrate a difference in the incidence of diabetic microvascular complications, a definitive answer concerning when to institute pharmacological therapy, i.e., in high-risk prediabetic subjects or in diabetic subjects at time of diagnosis, is unlikely to be forthcoming. Therefore, we recommend the institution of pharmacologic therapy in combination with diet/exercise in high-risk IGT individuals for the reasons discussed above.

Lastly, individuals with prediabetes are at increased risk, not only to develop T2DM, but also to develop cardiovascular disease (CVD) (myocardial infarction, stroke, CV death). As discussed earlier, subjects with IGT are maximally insulin resistant and, therefore, they manifest a cluster of metabolic abnormalities (dysglycemia, dyslipidemia, hypertension, obesity, insulin resistance, procoagulant state, endothelial dysfunction, inflammation) characteristic of insulin resistance, all of which are risk factors for CVD.[20,23] Moreover, the underlying insulin resistance also is an independent risk factor for atherosclerosis above and beyond the associated risk factors.[83] These abnormalities place subjects with prediabetes at greater risk for CVD than those with NGT. Some interventions that lower diabetes risk also have been shown to decrease some of the CVD risk

Table 1. Summary of pharmacologic intervention trials in individuals with IGT.

Study	Ref.	Number	Intervention	Duration (years)	Incidence of DM in controls (%)	Relative risk reduction (%)
IDPP	79	269	Metformin	2.5	18.3	26
US DPP	37	2151	Metformin	2.8	11	31
US DPP	38	1172	Troglitazone	0.9	11	75
TRIPOD	90	236	Troglitazone	2.5	13.1	55
PIPOD	92	89	Pioglitazone	3	13.1	65
DREAM	39	5269	Rosiglitazone	3	6.5	60
ACT NOW	40	602	Pioglitazone	2.8	6	70
CANOE	97	207	Rosiglitazone	3.9	10.1	66
STOP NIDDM	114	1368	Acarbose	3.2	8.1	36
XENDOS	70	3305	orlistat	4	2.2	37

factors. For example, weight loss lowers blood pressure and improves lipid profile,[37] and pioglitazone lowers triglycerides and raises high-density lipoproteins (HDL). However, in addition to interventions that lower the risk of T2DM, special attention should also be placed on treating CVD risk factors to target, e.g., blood pressure, dyslipidemia, and to reduce CVD risk as well.

7. SUMMARY

Although behavioral modification (diet/exercise) is effective in preventing the conversion of IGT and/or IFG to T2DM, weight loss is difficult to achieve and maintain and, when achieved, often is not sufficient to prevent progression of IGT to T2DM. Pharmacological interventions (combined with diet/exercise) that improve and preserve β-cell function and enhance insulin sensitivity represent logical choices for treatment of high-risk individuals with IGT. TZDs (DREAM, DPP, ACT NOW, TRIPOD, PIPOD)[38–40,90–92,125,126] unequivocally have been shown to effectively prevent the development of T2DM in subjects with IGT and/or IFG. In the U.S. DPP[37] and Indian DPP,[79] metformin also delayed IGT conversion to T2DM, and an ADA Consensus Conference Statement[80] recommended metformin for high-risk IGT individuals. However, the efficacy of metformin in preventing IGT conversion to T2DM is half that (31 vs 72 and 62%) observed with pioglitazone[40] and rosiglitazone.[34] A recent trial demonstrated that combined therapy with low-dose rosiglitazone (2 mg/d) plus metformin (850 mg/d) was particularly effective in reducing IGT conversion to T2DM and was associated with few side effects.[97] Because of cardiovascular safety concerns with rosiglitazone,[127] we believe that low-dose pioglitazone (15–30 mg/d) plus metformin (500–1,000 mg/d) would be an ideal choice for treatment of IGT/IFG. Moreover, there is evidence to suggest that pioglitazone may decrease cardiovascular events.[94]

Because GLP-1 analogs (1) are effective in treating T2DM; (2) reduce IGT conversion to T2DM; (3) improve β-cell function; (4) promote weight loss; (5) improve cardiovascular risk factors; (6) do not cause hypoglycemia; and (7) are given once daily (liraglutide), or once weekly (exenatide extended-release), we feel that GLP-1 analogs, especially long-acting release formulations,[113] would be ideal agents for treating IGT. Combination therapy with a once weekly GLP-1 receptor agonist (to preserve β-cell function and promote weight loss) plus low-dose pioglitazone (to ameliorate insulin resistance and enhance β-cell function) is likely to be especially efficacious in preventing diabetes in people with IGT and/or IFG.

The benefit of pharmacotherapy must be weighed against the side effects of the medication. Metformin rarely causes lactic acidosis and is contraindicated if the serum creatinine is above 1.4 mg/dL in females and 1.5 mg/dL in males. Approximately 10–15% of individuals cannot tolerate metformin because of gastrointestinal side effects (nausea, vomiting, diarrhea). Pioglitazone can cause fat weight gain, fluid retention, and congestive heart failure. Paradoxically, the greater the fat weight gain, the greater is the reduction in HbA1c and the greater is the improvement in insulin sensitivity and β-cell function.[83,84,128] Peripheral edema provides a readily identifiable clinical sign of fluid retention that responds well to distally acting diuretics (amiloride, spironolactone).[129] Because the fat weight gain and fluid retention are dose-response related,[96] limiting the pioglitazone dose to 30 mg/d will provide most of the efficacy while minimizing side effects. Moreover, the combination of metformin and/or GLP-1 agonist with pioglitazone will minimize the weight gain and even promote weight loss. An increased incidence (2.6 vs 1.7% in women receiving the comparator) of trauma-related fractures has been observed in postmenopausal women treated with pioglitazone,[130] and therefore should be used with caution in this group.

The major side effects of the GLP-1 receptor agonists are nausea and vomiting, which occur in 20–30% of individuals. These gastrointestinal side effects are usually mild and transient,[131] but approximately 5% of individuals cannot tolerate exenatide/liraglutide. Pancreatitis is listed as a potential side effect of the GLP-1 receptor agonists, but an increased incidence of pancreatitis has not been substantiated in retrospective analyses of large national databases.[132]

8. CONCLUSION

In conclusion, we recommend the institution of pharmacologic therapy with low-dose pioglitazone in combination with metformin or a long-acting GLP-1 analog plus diet/exercise in high-risk IGT individuals. Each component of this approach has been shown to be efficacious in preventing the development of T2DM and reverting impaired glucose tolerance to NGT. Further, we believe, based upon pathophysiologic considerations described above, that combination therapy will be especially effective and prevents the development of diabetic microvascular complication with minimal side effects. The use of generic medications is also likely to be cost-effective.

REFERENCES

1. National Diabetes Data Group (1979) Classification and diagnosis of diabetes mellitus and other categories of glucose intolerance. *Diabetes* **28**: 1039–1057.
2. Unwin N, Shaw J, Zimmet P, Alberti KGMM. (2002) Impaired glucose tolerance and impaired fasting glycemia: The current status on definition and intervention. *Diabet Med* **19**: 708–723.
3. The Expert Committee on the Diagnosis and Classification of Diabetes Mellitus (1997) Report of the expert committee on the diagnosis and classification of diabetes mellitus. *Diabetes Care* **20**: 1183–1197.
4. Abdul-Ghani MA, DeFronzo RA. (2009) Pathophysiology of prediabetes. *Curr Diab Rep* **9**: 193–199.
5. Wild S, Roglic G, Green A, Sicree R, King H. (2004) Global prevalence of diabetes: Estimates for the year 2000 and projections for 2030. *Diabetes Care* **27**: 1047–1053.
6. The Diabetes Control and Complications Trial Research Group. (1993) The effect of intensive treatment of diabetes on the development and progression of long-term complications in insulin-dependent diabetes mellitus. *N Engl J Med* **329**: 977–986.
7. UK Prospective Diabetes Study Group. (1998) Intensive blood-glucose control with sulphonylureas or insulin compared with conventional treatment and risk of complications in patients with type 2 diabetes (UKPDS 33). *Lancet* **352**: 837–853.
8. UK Prospective Diabetes Study. (1998) Effect of intensive blood-glucose control with metformin on complications in overweight patients with type 2 diabetes (UKPDS 34). *Lancet* **352**: 854–865.
9. Ohkubo Y, Kishikawa H, Araki E, Miyata T, Isami S, Motoyoshi S, Kojima Y, Furuyoshi N, Shichiri M. (1995) Intensive insulin therapy prevents the progression of diabetic microvascular complications in Japanese patients

with non-insulin-dependent diabetes mellitus: A randomized prospective 6-year study. *Diabetes Res Clin Pract* **28**: 103–117.

10. Stratton IM, Adler AI, Neil HAW, Matthews DR, Manley SE, Cull CA, Hadden D, Turner RC, Holman RR. (2000) Association of glycaemia with macrovascular and microvascular complications of type 2 diabetes (UKPDS 35): Prospective observational study. *BMJ* **321**: 405–412.
11. Holman RR, Paul SK, Bethel MA, Matthews DR, Neil HA. (2008) 10-year follow-up of intensive glucose control in type 2 diabetes. *N Eng J Med* **359**: 1577–1589.
12. ACCORD Study Group; ACCORD Eye Study Group, Chew EY, Ambrosius WT, Davis MD, Danis RP, Gangaputra S, Greven CM, Hubbard L, Esser BA, Lovato JF, Perdue LH, Goff DC Jr, Cushman WC, Ginsberg HN, Elam MB, Genuth S, Gerstein HC, Schubart U, Fine LJ. (2010) Effects of medical therapies on retinopathy progression in type 2 diabetes. *N Engl J Med* **363**: 233–244.
13. Duckworth W, Abraira C, Moritz T, Reda D, Emanuele N, Reaven PD, Zieve FJ, Marks J, Davis SN, Hayward R, Warren SR, Goldman S, McCarren M, Vitek ME, Henderson WG, Huang GD; VADT Investigators. (2009) Glucose control and vascular complications in veterans with type 2 diabetes. *N Engl J Med* **360**: 129–139.
14. American Diabetes Association. (2011) Standards of Medical Care in Diabetes. *Diabetes Care* **34**: S11–S61.
15. Ferrannini E, Gastaldelli A, Miyazaki Y, Matsuda M, Mari A, DeFronzo RA. (2005) Beta cell function in subjects spanning the range from normal glucose tolerance to overt diabetes mellitus: A new analysis. *J Clin Endocrinol Metab* **90**: 493–500.
16. Abdul-Ghani M, Tripathy D, DeFronzo RA. (2006) Contribution of beta cell dysfunction and insulin resistance to the pathogenesis of impaired glucose tolerance and impaired fasting glucose. *Diabetes Care* **29**: 1130–1139.
17. Abdul-Ghani M, Jenkinson C, Richardson D, Tripathy D, DeFronzo RA. (2006) Insulin secretion and insulin action in subjects with impaired fasting glucose and impaired glucose tolerance: Results from the Veterans Administration Genetic Epidemiology Study (VAGES). *Diabetes* **55**: 1430–1435.
18. Weyer C, Tataranni PA, Bogardus C, Pratley RE. (2000) Insulin resistance and insulin secretory dysfunction are independent predictors of worsening of glucose tolerance during each stage of type 2 diabetes development. *Diabetes Care* **24**: 89–94.

19. Lillioja S, Mott DM, Howard BV, Bennett PH, Freymond D, Swinburn B, Bogardus C. (1988) Impaired glucose tolerance as a disorder of insulin action. Longitudinal and cross-sectional studies in Pima Indians. *N Eng J Med* **318**: 1217–1225.
20. DeFronzo RA. (1997) Pathogenesis of type 2 diabetes: Metabolic and molecular implications for identifying diabetes genes. *Diabetes Rev* **5**: 177–269.
21. Lee ET, Howard BV, Savage PJ, Cowman LD, Fabsitz RR, Copik AJ, Yeh J, Go O, Robbins DC, Welty TK. (1995) Diabetes and impaired glucose tolerance in three American Indian populations aged 45–74 years. *Diabetes Care* **18**: 599–610.
22. DeFronzo RA. (1988) Lilly Lecture. The triumvirate: Beta cell, muscle, liver. A collusion responsible for NIDDM. *Diabetes* **37**: 667–687.
23. DeFronzo RA. (2009) Banting Lecture. From the triumvirate to the ominous octet: A new paradigm for the treatment of type 2 diabetes. *Diabetes* **58**: 773–795.
24. Saad MF, Knowler WC, Pettitt DJ, Nelson RG, Charles MA, Bennett PH. (1991) A two-step model for development of non-insulin-dependent diabetes. *Am J Med* **90**: 229–235.
25. Jallut D, Golay A, Munger R, Frascarolo P, Schutz Y, Jéquier E, Felber JP. (1990) Impaired glucose tolerance and diabetes in obesity: A 6-year follow-up study of glucose metabolism. *Metabolism* **39**: 1068–1075.
26. DeFronzo RA, Ferrannini E. (1991) Insulin resistance: A multifaceted syndrome responsible for NIDDM, obesity, hypertension, dyslipidemia, and ASCVD. *Diabetes Care* **14**: 173–194.
27. Reaven G. (1988) Banting Lecture. Role of insulin resistance in human disease. *Diabetes* **37**: 1595–1607.
28. Bajaj M, DeFronzo RA. (2003) Metabolic and molecular basis of insulin resistance. *J Nuclear Cardiol* **10**: 311–323.
29. Abdul-Ghani MA, DeFronzo RA. (2010) Pathophysiology of insulin resistance in skeletal muscle. *J Biomed Biotechol* **2010**: 476279.
30. DeFronzo RA, Ferrannini E, Simonson DC. (1989) Fasting hyperglycemia in non-insulin dependent diabetes mellitus: Contributions of excessive hepatic glucose production and impaired tissue glucose uptake. *Metabolism* **38**: 387–395.
31. Abdul-Ghani MA, Matsuda M, DeFronzo RA. (2008) Strong association between insulin resistance in liver and skeletal muscle in non-diabetic subjects. *Diabetes Med* **25**: 1289–1294.

32. Groop LC, Bonadonna RC, DelPrato S, Ratheiser K, Zyck K, Ferrannini E, DeFronzo RA. (1989) Glucose and free fatty acid metabolism in non-insulin-dependent diabetes mellitus. Evidence for multiple sites of insulin resistance. *J Clin Invest* **84**: 205–213.
33. Saad MF, Knowler WC, Pettitt DJ, Nelson RG, Mott DM, Bennett PH. (1988) The natural history of impaired glucose tolerance in the Pima Indians. *N Engl J Med* **319**: 1500–1505.
34. Haffner S, Stern M, Mitchell B, Hazuda H, Patterson J. (1990) Incidence of type II diabetes in Mexican Americans: Predicted by fasting insulin and glucose, obesity and body fat distribution. *Diabetes* **39**: 283–288.
35. Pratipanawatr W, Pratipanawatr T, Cusi K, Berria R, Jenkinson CP, Maezono K, DeFronzo RA, Mandarino L. (2001) Skeletal muscle insulin resistance in normoglycemic subjects with a strong family history of type 2 diabetes is associated with decreased insulin-stimulated IRS-1 tyrosine phosphorylation. *Diabetes* **50**: 2572–2578.
36. Pimenta W, Korytkowski M, Mitrakou A, Jenssen T, Yki-Jarvinen H, Evron W, Dailey G, Gerich J. (1995) Pancreatic beta-cell dysfunction as the primary genetic lesion in NIDDM: Evidence from studies in normal glucose-tolerant individuals with a first-degree NIDDM relative. *JAMA* **273**: 1855–1861.
37. Knowler WC, Barrett-Connor E, Fowler SE, Hamman RF, Lachin JM, Walker EA, Nathan DM; Diabetes Prevention Program Research Group. (2002) Reduction in the incidence of type 2 diabetes with lifestyle intervention or metformin. *N Eng J Med* **346**: 393–403.
38. The Diabetes Prevention Program Research Group. (2005) Prevention of type 2 diabetes with troglitazone in the diabetes prevention program. *Diabetes* **54**: 1150–1156.
39. Dream Trial Investigators. (2006) Effect of rosiglitazone on the frequency of diabetes in patients with impaired glucose tolerance or impaired fasting glucose: A randomized controlled trial. *Lancet* **368**: 1096–1105.
40. DeFronzo RA, Tripathy D, Schwenke DC, Banerji MA, Bray GA, Buchanan TA, Clement SC, Henry RR, Hodis HN, Kitabchi AE, Mack WJ, Mudaliar S, Ratner RE, Williams K, Stentz FB, Musi N, Reaven PD for the ACT NOW Study. (2011) Pioglitazone for diabetes prevention in impaired glucose tolerance. *N Eng J Med* **364**: 1104–1115.
41. Polonsky KS, Sturis J, Bell GI. (1996) Non-insulin-dependent diabetes mellitus: A genetically programmed failure of the beta cell to compensate for insulin resistance. *N Engl J Med* **334**: 777–783.

42. Weyer C, Bogardus C, Mott DM, Pratley RE. (1999) The natural history of insulin secretory dysfunction and insulin resistance in the pathogenesis of type 2 diabetes mellitus. *J Clin Invest* **104**: 787–794.
43. Abdul-Ghani MA, Williams K, DeFronzo RA, Stern M. (2007) What is the best predictor of future type 2 diabetes? *Diabetes Care* **30**: 1544–1548.
44. Abdul-Ghani MA, Matsuda M, Jenkinson C, Richardson D, Kaku K, DeFronzo RA. (2008) The relationship between fasting hyperglycemia and insulin secretion in subjects with normal or impaired glucose tolerance. *Am J Physiol* **295**: E401–E406.
45. Godsland IF, Jeffs JA, Johnston DG. (2004) Loss of beta cell function as fasting glucose increases in the non-diabetic range. *Diabetologia* **47**: 1157–1166.
46. Diamond MP, Thornton K, Connolly-Diamond M, Sherwin RS, DeFronzo RA. (1995) Reciprocal variation in insulin-stimulated glucose uptake and pancreatic insulin secretion in women with normal glucose tolerance. *J Soc Gynecol Invest* **2**: 708–715.
47. Rossetti L, Giaccari A, DeFronzo RA. (1990) Glucose toxicity. *Diabetes Care Rev* **13**: 610–630.
48. Bays H, Mandarino L, DeFronzo RA. (2004) Role of the adipocytes, FFA, and ectopic fat in the pathogenesis of type 2 diabetes mellitus: PPAR agonists provide a rational therapeutic approach. *J Clin Endocrinol Metab* **89**: 463–478.
49. Toft-Nielsen MB, Damholt MB, Madsbad S, Hilsted LM, Hughes TE, Michelsen BK, Holst JJ. (2001) Determinants of the impaired secretion of glucagon-like peptide-1 in type 2 diabetic patients. *J Clin Endocrinol Metab* **86**: 3717–3712.
50. Højberg PV, Vilsbøll T, Rabøl R, Knop FK, Bache M, Krarup T, Holst JJ, Madsbad S. (2009) Four weeks of near-normalisation of blood glucose improves the insulin response to glucagon-like peptide-1 and glucose-dependent insulinotropic polypeptide in patients with type 2 diabetes. *Diabetologia* **52**: 199–207.
51. Vilsbøll T, Krarup T, Madsbad S, Holst JJ. (2002) Defective amplification of the late phase insulin response to glucose by GIP in obese Type II diabetic patients. *Diabetologia* **45**: 1111–1119.
52. Abdul-Ghani MA, Williams K, DeFronzo R, Stern M. (2006) Risk of progression to type 2 diabetes based upon relationship between post-load plasma glucose and fasting plasma glucose. *Diabetes Care* **29**: 1613–1618.

53. Grant RW, Buse JB, Meigs JB. (2005) Quality of diabetes care in U.S. academic medical centers. *Diabetes Care* **28**: 337–442.
54. Abdul-Ghani MA, Lyssenko V, Tuomi T, DeFronzo RA, Groop L. (2009) Fasting versus postload plasma glucose concentration and the risk for future type 2 diabetes: Results from the Botnia Study. *Diabetes Care* **32**: 281–286.
55. Abdul-Ghani MA, Stern MP, Lyssenko V, Tuomi T, Groop L, Defronzo RA. (2010) Minimal contribution of fasting hyperglycemia to the incidence of type 2 diabetes in subjects with normal 2-h plasma glucose. *Diabetes Care* **33**: 557–561.
56. Cowie CC, Harris MI, Silverman RE, Johnson EW, Rust KF. (1993) Effect of multiple risk factors on differences between blacks and whites in the prevalence of non-insulin-dependent diabetes mellitus in the United States. *Am J Epidemiol* **137**: 719–732.
57. Jarret RJ, Keen H, McCartney P. (1984) The Whitehall study: Ten year follow-up report on men with impaired glucose tolerance with reference to worsening to diabetes and predictors of death. *Diabetic Med* **1**: 279–283.
58. Eriksson KF, Lindgarde R. (1991) Prevention of Type 2 diabetes by diet and physical exercise: The 6-year Malmo feasibility study. *Diabteologia* **34**: 891–898.
59. Jani R, Molina M, Matsuda M, Balas B, Chavez A, DeFronzo RA, Abdul-Ghani MA. (2008) Decreased non-insulin-dependent glucose clearance contributes to the rise in fasting plasma glucose in the nondiabetic range. *Diabetes Care* **31**: 311–315.
60. Abdul-Ghani MA, Lyssenko V, Tuomi T, DeFronzo RA, Groop L. (2010) The shape of plasma glucose concentration curve during OGTT predicts the risk for future type 2 diabetes. *Diabete Metab Res Rev* **26**: 280–286.
61. Kanat M, Norton L, Winnier D, Jenkinson C, Defronzo RA, Abdul-Ghani MA. (2011) Impaired early- but not late-phase insulin secretion in subjects with impaired fasting glucose. *Acta Diabetol* **48**: 209–217.
62. Meyer C, Pimenta W, Woerle HJ, Van Haeften T, Szoke E, Mitrakou A, Gerich J. (2006) Different mechanisms for impaired fasting glucose and impaired post-prandial glucose tolerance in humans. *Diabetes Care* **29**: 1909–1914.
63. DECODE Study Group, the European Diabetes Epidemiology Group. (2001) Glucose tolerance and cardiovascular mortality: Comparison of fasting and 2-hour diagnostic criteria. *Arch Int Med* **161**: 397–405.
64. Keen H, Jarrett RJ, McCArtney P. (1982) The ten-year follow-up of the Bedford Survey (1962–1972): glucose tolerance and diabetes. *Diabetologia* **22**: 73–78.

65. Tuomilehto J, Lindstrom J, Eriksson JG, Valle TT, Hamalainen H, Ilanne-Parikka P, Keinanen-Kiukaanniemi S, Laakso M, Louheranta A, Rastas M, Salminen V, Uusitupa M; Finnish Diabetes Prevention Study Group. (2001) Prevention of type 2 diabetes mellitus by changes in lifestyle among subjects with impaired glucose tolerance. *N Engl J Med* **344**: 1343–1350.
66. The Diabetes Prevention Program Research Group (2005) Role of insulin secretion and sensitivity in the evolution of type 2 diabetes in the Diabetes Prevention Program. Effects of lifestyle intervention and metformin. *Diabetes* **54**: 2404–2414.
67. Li G, Zhang P, Wang J, Gregg EW, Yang W, Gong Q, Li H, Li H, Jiang Y, An Y, Shuai Y, Zhang B, Zhang J, Thompson TJ, Gerzoff RB, Roglic G, Hu Y, Bennett PH. (2008) The long-term effect of lifestyle interventions to prevent diabetes in the China Da Qing Diabetes Prevention Study: A 20-year follow-up study. *Lancet* **371**: 1783–1789.
68. Wing RR, Goldstein MG, Acton KJ, Birch LL, Jakicic JM, Sallis JF, Smith-West D, Jeffrey RW, Surwit RS. (2001) Behavioral science research in diabetes: Lifestyle changes related to obesity, eating behavior, and physical activity. *Diabetes Care* **24**: 117–123.
69. Venditti EM, Bray GA, Carrion-Petersen ML, Delahanty LM, Edelstein SL, Hamman RF, Hoskin MA, Knowler WC, Ma Y; Diabetes Prevention Program Research Group. (2008) First versus repeat treatment with a lifestyle intervention program: Attendance and weight loss outcomes. *Int J Obes (Lond)* **32**: 1537–1554.
70. Torgerson JS, Hauptman J, Boldrin MN. (2004) XENical in the prevention of diabetes in obese subjects (XENDOS) study: A randomized study of orlistat as an adjunct to lifestyle changes for the prevention of type 2 diabetes in obese patients. *Diabetes Care* **27**: 155–161.
71. Pi-Sunyer FX, Aronne LJ, Heshmati HM, Devin J, Rosenstock J; RIO-North America Study Group. (2006) Effect of rimonabant, a cannabinoid-1 receptor blocker, on weight and cardiometabolic risk factors in overweight or obese patients: RIO-North America: A randomized controlled trial. *JAMA* **295**: 761–775.
72. Diabetes Prevention Program Research Group, Knowler WC, Fowler SE, Hamman RF, Christophi CA, Hoffman HJ, Brenneman AT, Brown-Friday JO, Goldberg R, Venditti E, Nathan DM. (2009) 10-year follow-up of diabetes incidence and weight loss in the Diabetes Prevention Program Outcomes Study. *Lancet* **374**: 1677–1686.

73. Saaristo T, Moilanen L, Korpi-Hyövälti E, Vanhala M, Saltevo J, Niskanen L, Jokelainen J, Peltonen M, Oksa H, Tuomilehto J, Uusitupa M, Keinänen-Kiukaanniemi S. (2010) Lifestyle intervention for prevention of type 2 diabetes in primary health care: One-year follow-up of the Finnish national diabetes prevention program (FIN-D2D). *Diabetes Care* **33**: 2146–2151.
74. DeFronzo RA, Goodman AM. (1995) Efficacy of metformin in patients with non-insulin dependent diabetes mellitus. *N Eng J Med* **333**: 541–549.
75. DeFronzo RA, Barzilai N, Simonson DC (1991) Mechanisms of metformin action in NIDDM. *J Clin Endocrinol Metab* **73**: 1294–1301.
76. Cusi K, DeFronzo RA. (1998) Metformin: A review of its metabolic effects. *Diabetes Rev* **6**: 89–131.
77. Turner RC, Cull CA, Frighi V, Holman RR. (1999) Glycemic control with diet, sulfonylurea, metformin, or insulin in patients with type 2 diabetes mellitus: Progressive requirement for multiple therapies (UKPDS 49). UK Prospective Diabetes Study (UKPDS) Group. *JAMA* **281**: 2005–2012.
78. Kahn S, Haffner SM, Heise MA, Herman WH, Holman RR, Jones NP, Kravitz BG, Lachin JM, O'Neill MC, Zinman B, Viberti G; ADOPT Study Group. (2006) Glycemic durability of rosiglitazone, metformin, or glyburide monotherapy. *N Eng J Med* **355**: 2427–2443.
79. Ramachandran A, Snehalatha C, Mary S, Mukesh B, Bhaskar AD, Vijay V, Indian Diabetes Prevention Programme (IDPP). (2006) The Indian Diabetes Prevention Program shows that lifestyle modification and metformin prevent type 2 diabetes in Asian Indian subjects with impaired glucose tolerance (IDPP-1). *Diabetologia* **49**: 289–297.
80. Nathan DM, Davidson M, DeFronzo RA, Heine RJ, Henry RR, Pratley R, Zimman B. (2007) Impaired fasting plasma glucose and impaired glucose tolerance: Implications for care. Consensus Statement from American Diabetes Association. *Diabetes Care* **30**: 753–759.
81. Yki-Jarvinen H. (2004) Thiazolidinediones. *New Engl J Med* **351**: 1106–1118.
82. Spiegelman BM. (1998) PPAR-gama : Adipogenic regulator and thiazolidinedione receptor. *Diabetes* **47**: 507–514.
83. DeFronzo RA. (2010) Insulin resistance, lipotoxicity, type 2 diabetes, and atherosclerosis: The missing links. The Claude Bernard Lecture. *Diabetologia* **53**: 1270–1287.
84. Gastaldelli A, Ferrannini E, Miyazaki Y, Matsuda M, Mari A, DeFronzo RA. (2007) Thiazolidinediones improve beta-cell function in type 2 diabetic patients. *Am J Physiol* **292**: E871–E883.

85. Inzucchi SE, Maggs D, Spollet GR, Page SL, Rife FS, Walton V, Shulman GI . (1998) Efficacy and metabolic effects of metformin and troglitazone in type II diabetes mellitus. *N Engl J Med* **338**: 867–872.
86. Miyazaki Y, Mahankali A, Matsuda M, Glass L, Mahankali S, Ferrannini E, Cusi K, Mandarino L, DeFronzo RA. (2001) Improved glycemic control and enhanced insulin sensitivity in liver and muscle in type 2 diabetic subjects treated with pioglitazone. *Diabetes Care* **24**: 710–719.
87. Miyazaki Y, He H, Mandarino LJ, DeFronzo RA. (2003) Rosiglitazone improves downstream insulin-receptor signaling in type 2 diabetic patients. *Diabetes* **52**: 1943–1950.
88. Nolan JJ, Ludvik B, Beerdsen P, Joyce M, Olefsky J. (1994) Improvement in glucose tolerance and insulin resistance in obese subjects treated with troglitazone. *N Engl J Med* **331**: 1188–1193.
89. Cavaghan MK, Ehrmann DA, Byrne MM, Polonsky KS. (1997) Treatment with the oral antidiabetic agent troglitazone improves beta cell responses to glucose in subjects with impaired glucose tolerance. *J Clin Invest* **100**: 530–537.
90. Berkowitz K, Peters R, Kjos SL, Goico J, Marroquin A, Dunn ME, Xiang A, Azen S, Buchanan TA. (1996) Effect of troglitazone on insulin sensitivity and pancreatic beta-cell function in women at high risk for NIDDM. *Diabetes* **45**: 1572–1579.
91. Xiang AH, Peters RK, Kjos SL, Marroquin A, Goico J, Ochoa C, Kawakubo M, Buchanan TA. (2006) Effect of pioglitazone on pancreatic β-cell function and diabetes risk in Hispanic women with prior gestational diabetes. *Diabetes* **55**: 577–522.
92. Buchanan TA, Xiang AH, Peters RK, Kjos SL, Marroquin A, Goico J, Ochoa C, Tan S, Berkowitz K, Hodis HN, Azen SP. (2002) Preservation of pancreatic beta cell function and prevention of type 2 diabetes by pharmacologic treatment of insulin resistance in high-risk Hispanic women. *Diabetes* **51**: 2796–2803.
93. Higa M, Zhou YT, Ravazzola M, Baetens D, Orci L, Unger RH. (1999) Troglitazone prevents mitochondrial alterations, beta cell destruction, and diabetes in obese prediabetic rats. *Proc Natl Acad Sci* **96**: 11513–11518.
94. Dormandy JA, Charbonnel B, Eckland DJ, Erdmann E, Massi-Benedetti M, Moules IK, Skene AM, Tan MH, Lefebvre PJ, Murray GD, Standl E, Wilcox RG, Wilhelmsen L, Betteridge J, Birkeland K, Golay A, Heine RJ, Koranyi L, Laakso, Mokan M, Norkus A, Pirags V, Podar T, Scheen A, Scherbaum W, Schernthaner G, Schmitz O, Skrha J, Smith U, Taton J.

PROactive investigators. (2005) Secondary prevention of macrovascular events in patients with type 2 diabetes in the PROactive Study (PROspective pioglitAzone Clinical Trial In macroVascular Events): A randomized controlled trial. *Lancet* **366**: 1279–1289.

95. Miyazaki Y, Matsuda M, DeFronzo RA. (2002) Dose response effect of pioglitazone on insulin sensitivity, and insulin secretion in type 2 diabetes mellitus. *Diabetes Care* **25**: 517–523.
96. Aronoff S, Rosenblatt S, Braithwaite S, Egan JW, Mathisen AL, Schneider RL. (2000) Pioglitazone hydrochloride monotherapy improves glycemic control in the treatment of patients with type 2 diabetes: A 6-month randomized placebo-controlled dose-response study. The Pioglitazone 001 Study Group. *Diabetes Care* **23**: 1605–1611.
97. Zinman B, Harris SB, Neuman J, Gerstein HC, Retnakaran RR, Raboud J, Qi Y, Hanley AJ. (2010) Low-dose combination therapy with rosiglitazone and metformin to prevent type 2 diabetes mellitus (CANOE trial): A double-blind randomised controlled study. *Lancet* **376**: 103–111.
98. Holst JJ. (2006) Glucagon-like peptide-1: From extract to agent. The Claude Bernard Lecture, 2005. *Diabetologia* **49**: 253–260.
99. Triplitt C, DeFronzo RA. (2006) Exenatide: First-in-class incretin mimetic for the treatment of type 2 diabetes mellitus. *Expert Rev Endocrinol Metab* **1**: 329–341.
100. Nauch MA, Vardarli I, Deacon CF, Holst JJ, Meier JJ. (2011) Secretion of glucagon-like peptide-1 (GLP-1) in type 2 diabetes: What is up, what is down? *Diabetologia* **54**: 10–18.
101. DeFronzo RA, Ratner RE, Han J, Kim DD, Fineman MS, Baron AD. (2005) Effects of exenatide (synthetic exendin-4) on glycemic control and weight over 30 weeks in metformin-treated patients with type 2 diabetes mellitus. *Diabetes Care* **28**: 1092–1100.
102. Nauck M, Frid A, Hermansen K, Shah NS, Tankova T, Mitha IH, Zdravkovic M, During M, Matthews DR; LEAD-2 Study Group. (2009) Efficacy and safety comparison of liraglutide, glimepiride, and placebo, all in combination with metformin, in type 2 diabetes: The LEAD (liraglutide effect and action in diabetes)-2 study. *Diabetes Care* **32**: 84–90.
103. Klonoff DC, Buse JB, Nielsen LL, Guan X, Bowlus CL, Holcombe JH, Wintle ME, Maggs DG. (2008) Exenatide effects on diabetes, obesity, cardiovascular risk factors and hepatic biomarkers in patients with type 2 diabetes treated for at least 3 years. *Curr Med Res Opin* **24**: 275–286.

104. Henquin DC. Regulation of insulin secretion: A matter of phase control and amplitude modulation. *Diabetologia* **52**: 739–751.
105. Baggio LL, Drucker DJ. (2007) Biology of incretins: GLP-1 and GIP. *Gastroenterology* **132**: 2131–2157.
106. Chang AM, Jakobsen G, Sturis J, Smith MJ, Bloem CJ, An B, Galecki A, Halter JB. (2003) The GLP-1 derivative NN2211 restores beta-cell sensitivity to glucose in type 2 diabetic patients after a single dose. *Diabetes* **52**: 1786–1791.
107. Rask E, Olsson T, Soderberg S, Holst JJ, Tura A, Pacini G, Ahren B. (2004) Insulin secretion and incretin hormones after oral glucose in non-obese subjects with impaired glucose tolerance. *Metabolism* **53**: 624–631.
108. Byrne MM, Gliem K, Wank U, Anrold R, Katschinski M, Polonsky KS, Goke B. (1998) Glucagon-like peptide 1 improves the ability of the beta-cell to sense and respond to glucose in subjects with impaired glucose tolerance. *Diabetes* **47**: 1259–1265.
109. Ahren B, Larsson H, Holst. JJ. (1997) Reduced gastric inhibitory polypeptide but normal glucagon-like peptide 1 response to oral glucose in post-menopausal women with impaired glucose tolerance. *Eur J Endocrinol* **137**: 127–131.
110. Knop FK, Vilsboll T, Hojberg PV, Larsen S, Madsbad S, Voluna A, Holst JJ, Krarup T. (2007) Reduced incretin effect in type 2 diabetes: cause or consequence of the diabetic state? *Diabetes* **56**: 1951–1959.
111. Bunck MC, Cornér A, Eliasson B, Heine RJ, Shaginian RM, Taskinen MR, Smith U, Yki-Järvinen H, Diamant M. (2011) Effects of exenatide on measures of β-cell function after 3 years in metformin-treated patients with type 2 diabetes. *Diabetes Care* **34**: 2041–2047.
112. Astrup A, Rössner S, Van Gaal L, Rissanen A, Niskanen L, Al Hakim M, Madsen J, Rasmussen MF, Lean ME; NN8022-1807 Study Group. (2009) Effects of liraglutide in the treatment of obesity: A randomised, double-blind, placebo-controlled study. *Lancet* **374**: 1606–1616.
113. Drucker DJ, Buse JB, Taylor K, Kendall DM, Trautmann M, Zhuang D, Porter L; DURATION-1 Study Group. (2008) Exenatide once weekly versus twice daily for the treatment of type 2 diabetes: A randomised, open-label, non-inferiority study. *Lancet* **372**: 1240–1250.
114. Chiasson JL, Josse RG, Gomis R, Hanefeld M, Karasik A, Laakso M; STOP-NIDDM Trail Research Group. (2002) Acarbose for prevention of type 2 diabetes mellitus: The STOP-NIDDM randomised trial. *Lancet* **359**: 2072–2077.

115. Kawamori R, Tajima N, Iwamoto Y, Kashiwagi A, Shimamoto K, Kaku K; Voglibose Ph-3 Study Group. (2009) Voglibose for prevention of type 2 diabetes mellitus: A randomised, double-blind trial in Japanese individuals with impaired glucose tolerance. *Lancet* **373**: 1607–1614.
116. Moriya R, Shirakura T, Ito J, Mashiko S, Seo T. (2009) Activation of sodium-glucose cotransporter 1 ameliorates hyperglycemia by mediating incretin secretion in mice. *Am J Physiol Endocrinol Metab* **297**: E1358–E1365.
117. Slack E, Hapfelmeier S, Stecher B, Velykoredko Y, Stoel M, Lawson MA, Geuking MB, Beutler B, Tedder TF, Hardt WD, Bercik P, Verdu EF, McCoy KD, Macpherson AJ (2009) Innate and adaptive immunity cooperate flexibly to maintain host-microbiota mutualism. *Science* **325**: 617–620.
118. Diabetes Prevention Program Research Group. (2007) The prevalence of retinopathy in impaired glucose tolerance and recent-onset diabetes in the Diabetes Prevention Program. *Diabetic Med* **24**: 137–144.
119. Massin P, Lange C, Tichet J, Rosilio M, Vol S, Erginay A, Cailleau M, Eschwege E, Balkau B, The DESIR Study Group. (2009) HbA1c and fasting plasma glucose are predictors of retinopathy at ten years: The French desire study. *Arch Ophthalmol* **129**: 188–195.
120. Zieger D, Rathmann W, Dickhaus T, Meisinger C, Mielck A, KORA Study Grou. (2007) Prevalence of polyneuropathy in pre-diabetes and diabetes is associated with abdominal obesity and macroangiopathy: The MONICA/KORA Augsburg Surveys S2 and S3. *Diabetes Care* **31**: 464–469.
121. Abdul-Ghani MA, DeFronzo RA. (2009) Plasma glucose concentration and prediction of future risk of type 2 diabetes. *Diabetes Care* **32**: S194–S198.
122. Edelstein SL, Knowler WC, Bain RP, Andres R, Barrett-Connor EL, Dowse GK, Haffner SM, Pettitt Dj, Sorkin JD, Muller DC, Collins VR, Hamman RF. (1997) Predictors of progression from impaired glucose tolerance to NIDDM: An analysis of six prospective studies. *Diabetes* **46**: 701–710.
123. Abdul-Ghani MA, Abdul-Ghani T, Ali N, DeFronzo RA. (2009) One-hour plasma glucose concentration and the metabolic syndrome identify subjects at high risk for future type 2 diabetes. *Diabetes Care* **31**: 1650–1655.
124. Kolberg JA, Jørgensen T, Gerwien RW, Hamren S, McKenna MP, Moler E, Rowe MW, Urdea MS, Xu XM, Hansen T, Pedersen O, Borch-Johnsen K. (2009) Development of a type 2 diabetes risk model from a panel of serum biomarkers from the Inter99 cohort. *Diabetes Care* **32**: 1207–1212.
125. Buchanan TA, Xiang AH, Peters RH, Kjos SL, Marroquin A, Goico J, Ochoa C, Tan S, Berkowtiz K, Hodis HN, Azen SP. (2002) Preservation of

pancreatic beta-cell function and prevention of type 2 diabetes by pharmacological treatment of insulin resistance in high-risk Hispanic women. *Diabetes* **51**: 2796–2803.
126. Buchanan TA, Xiang AH, Peters RK, Kjos SL, Berkowitz K, Marroquin A, Goico J, Ochoa C, Azen SP. (2000) Response of pancreatic beta-cells to improved insulin sensitivity in women at high risk for type 2 diabetes. *Diabetes* **49**: 782–788.
127. Nissen SE, Wolski K. Effect of rosiglitazone on the risk of myocardial infarction and death from cardiovascular cause. *N Engl J Med* **356**: 2457–2471.
128. Miyazaki M, De Filippis E, Bajaj M, Wajcberg E, Glass L, Triplitt C, Cersosimo E, Mandarino LJ, DeFronzo RA. (2005) Predictors of improved glycaemic control with rosiglitazone therapy in type 2 diabetic patients: A practical approach for the primary care physician. *Br J Diabetes Vasc Dis* **5**: 28–35.
129. Karalliedde J, Buckingham R, Starkie M, Lorand D, Stewart M, Viberti G, Rosiglitazone Fluid Retention Study Group. (2006) Effect of various diuretic treatments on rosiglitazone-induced fluid retention. *J Am Soc Nephrol* **17**: 3482–3490.
130. Derosa G. (2010) Efficacy and tolerability of pioglitazone in patients with type 2 diabetes mellitus. Comparison with other oral antihyperglyccaemic agents. *Drugs* **70**: 1945–1961.
131. Gallwitz B. (2010) Benefit-risk assessment of exenatide in the therapy of type 2 diabetes mellitus. *Drug Safety* **33**: 87–100.
132. Garg R, Chen W, Pendergrass M. (2010) Acute pancreatitis in type 2 diabetes treated with exenatide or sitagliptin: A restospective observational pharmacy claims analysis. *Diabetes Care* **33**: 2349–2354.
133. Diabetes Prevention Program Research Group. (2003) Within-trial cost-effectiveness of lifestyle intervention or metformin for the primary prevention of type 2 diabetes. *Diabetes Care* **26**: 2518–2523.
134. Herman WH, Hoerger TJ, Brandie M, Hicks K, Sorensen S, Zhang P, Hamman RF, Ackermann RT, Engelgau MM, Ratner RE, Diabetes Prevention Program Research Group. (2005) The cost effectiveness of lifestyle modification or metformin in preventing type 2 diabetes in adults with impaired glucose tolerance. *Ann Intern Med* **142**: 323–332.
135. Gillies CL, Lambert PC, Abrams KR, Sutton AJ, Cooper NJ, Hsu RT, Davies MJ, Khunti K. (2008) Different strategies for screening and prevention of type 2 diabetes in adults: cost effectiveness analysis. *Br Med J* **336**: 1180–1185.

136. Kahn R, Alperin P, Eddy D, Borch-Johnsen K, Buse J, Feigelman J, Gregg E, Holman RR, Kirkman MS, Stern M, Tuomilehto J, Wareham NJ. (2010) Age at initiation and frequency of screening to detect type 2 diabetes: A cost-effectiveness analysis. *Lancet* **375**: 1365–1374.
137. Butler AE, Janson J, Bonner-Weir S, Ritzel R, Rizza RA, Butler PC. (2003) Beta-cell deficit and increased beta-cell apoptosis in humans with type 2 diabetes. *Diabetes* **52**: 102–110.

Chapter 6: Diabetes Prevention and Nutrition Policies from a Global Perspective

Eleanore Alexander[*,†], *Deepak Patel*[‡], *Katherine Tryon*[†], *Marieke Loubser*[‡], *and Derek Yach*[†]

1. INTRODUCTION

No country is spared the serious global health burden of diabetes mellitus, which will continue to increase in the absence of effective management and prevention strategies.[1] Diabetes is a rapidly evolving epidemic. In high-income countries, 85% to 90% of all diabetes is constituted by type 2, which until recently was considered to be a Western disease that affected wealthy adults. However, the disease has spread rapidly, particularly in the developing world, and increasingly affects the poor. It is estimated that Asia now accounts for about 60% of all individuals with diabetes.[2] The rapidly changing face of the epidemic is a consequence of increasing urbanization, aging populations, rapid social and cultural changes, changes in dietary intake, reduced physical activity, along with other unhealthy lifestyle behaviors.[1]

The association between obesity and diabetes has been confirmed in several longitudinal studies, and the relationship between physical inactivity and poor nutrition with obesity and diabetes is clear.[1] Consequently, the prevention of diabetes is dependent upon controlling these risk factors.

The importance of improving diet and increasing physical activity cannot be underestimated, as research has shown that lifestyle interventions are at least as effective as pharmacological interventions, see Table 1 for comparison.[3–5] Globally, several programs have been implemented at a

*Corresponding author. Email: ealexander@thevitalitygroup.com
†The Vitality Institute
‡Discovery Vitality

Table 1. Diabetes prevention strategies.[5]

Strategy	RR reduction (%)
Lifestyle	58
Metformin	31
Acarbose	25–33
Orlistat	37
Troglitazone	56
Rosiglitazone	60
Pioglitazone	0–72

national level, with promising results, to prevent diabetes among high-risk individuals. Furthermore, promising results have also been shown in the arena of secondary prevention, where lifestyle interventions have been shown to improve glucose control and reduce morbidity in individuals with established type 2 diabetes.

The role of behavior change in risk modification has increased on the agenda as a critical tool in addressing this global epidemic, and learnings from early successes may be able to guide further interventions. However, for sustained success at a community or even a national level policy level support is needed, and at a global level this remains woefully inadequate.

2. PRIMARY PREVENTION

There is compelling epidemiological evidence that several modifiable lifestyle factors, namely overweight and obesity, physical inactivity/sedentary behavior, and unhealthy eating are driving the diabetes epidemic. There is general agreement that to reduce the overall incidence and prevalence of diabetes, everyone should be encouraged to maintain a favorable body mass, be physically active, and eat a healthy and prudent diet.

2.1. Addressing Overweight and Obesity

Obesity is the single most important risk factor for the development of type 2 diabetes. A complex set of social, environmental, and economic factors have led to an ever-increasing global epidemic of obesity. It is widely accepted that the global increase in diabetes prevalence has occurred in the wake of the obesity epidemic.

The association between obesity and diabetes has been confirmed in several longitudinal cohort studies. In a collaborative analysis of 57 prospective studies with close to 900,000 participants mostly in western Europe and North America, mortality was lowest at a body-mass index (BMI) of 22.5–25 kg/m^2, with overall mortality risk increasing nearly 30% for each additional 5 kg/m^2.[6]

In the Nurse's Health Study, the relative risk of developing diabetes was 38.8 for women with a BMI of ≥35 kg/m^2 and 20.1 for a BMI of 30.0 to 34.9 kg/m^2, compared to women with BMI less than 23 kg/m^2.[7] In this cohort, 61% of type 2 diabetes cases could be attributed to overweight and obesity.

Similarly, in the Women's Health Study, the relative risks for developing type 2 diabetes were 3.22 for overweight women and 9.06 for obese women compared with normal weight women.[8]

Several studies indicate that abdominal obesity, assessed by waist circumference, predicts risk of diabetes independent of BMI.[9] In the Nurses' Health Study, controlling for BMI and other potentially confounding factors, the relative risk of developing diabetes was 5.1 for subjects above the 90th percentile of waist circumference (≥92 cm) compared to those in the tenth percentile (≤67 cm).

Moreover, weight gain, independent of initial body weight, is associated with increased risk of diabetes. In the Health Professional Follow-Up Study, every kilogram of weight gained increased the risk of developing diabetes by 7.3% among men.[10]

In Asians, diabetes develops at BMI levels that are lower than among Europeans. According to Hu *et al.*,[2] even a modest gain in weight increases the risk of diabetes considerably. It has also been shown that compared to Caucasians, Asians and people of Asian descent living in the West have greater visceral fat at the same waist circumference.[11,12]

Weight loss not only requires an energy-restricted diet and lifestyle modification, which bring about weight loss, but also long-term weight maintenance.[13] The USA National Weight Control Registry, established in 1994 consisting of a database of more than 10,000 individuals 18 years of age or older, offers insight into successful tools for weight loss maintenance.[14,15] Some of the key factors associated with long-term weight loss success are listed in Table 2.

Table 2. US National Weight Control Registry Key Factors Associated with Long-term Weight Loss Success.[13,14]

– Making realistic, gradual and sensible long-term lifestyle changes
– Eating breakfast regularly; 78% report eating breakfast every day and the typical breakfast consists of cereal and fruit
– Weighing oneself on a regular basis (varying from once a day to once a week). Frequent monitoring allows individuals to identify small weight gains and to take the necessary corrective action
– Engaging in high levels of physical activity (1 hr per day of moderate intensity, such as brisk walking). The most frequent type of exercise reported is walking
– Developing a consistent eating pattern, across weekdays and weekends
– Reducing television viewing time (62% watch less than 10 hr of television a week).

Initial body composition affects body mass changes resulting from weight loss; individuals with higher levels of body fat initially lose more body fat versus lean muscle tissue than those with low levels of body fat.[16] Modeling has been done by Hall and colleagues, showing that the timing of weight change is dynamic rather than linear and depends on initial body composition. The modeling also suggests that energy equivalent changes in physical activity versus calorie intake can lead to varying degrees of weight change, as diet leads to greater weight loss when the scale of each intervention increases.

2.2. Increasing Physical Activity and Reducing Sedentary Behavior

Numerous epidemiologic studies have shown that physical inactivity and sedentary behavior increase the risk of developing diabetes. For instance, in the Nurse's Health Study, prolonged television watching was associated with the highest risk of developing diabetes. Each 2-hr/day increment of time spent watching television was associated with a 14% increase in diabetes risk.[17]

In the Health Professionals' Follow-Up Study, men who watched television more than 40 hr per week had a nearly three-fold increase in the risk of type 2 diabetes compared with those who spent less than 1 hr per week watching TV.[18]

Conversely, convincing epidemiologic data also supports the role of physical activity in preventing diabetes. In the Nurse's Health Study, each 2-hr/day increment of standing or walking was associated with a 12% reduction in the risk of diabetes while brisk walking for 1 hr/day was associated with a 34% reduction in risk. It was estimated that 30% (95% CI, 24–36%) of new cases of obesity and 43% (95% CI, 32–52%) of new cases of diabetes could be prevented by adopting a relatively active lifestyle (<10 hr/wk of TV watching and ≥30 min/day of brisk walking).

Thus, in order to reduce the risk of obesity and type 2 diabetes, public health campaigns should not only promote increasing exercise levels but should also discourage sedentary behaviors, especially prolonged TV watching.

2.2.1. *Improving nutrition*

Eating a healthy diet with moderate portions and maintaining a healthy weight can help prevent type 2 diabetes in the general population.[19]

In addition to weight, diet quality is associated with diabetes risk. A meta-analysis found that healthy diet patterns including whole grains, fruit, and vegetables may decrease the risk of diabetes, while unhealthy diet patterns including red meats, high fat dairy, refined grains, and sweets may increase the risk of diabetes; this is consistent with previous meta–analyses.[20,21] Debate exists around the role of increasing sugar intake in modern diets contributing to obesity, diabetes, and other chronic diseases.[22]

The Institute of Medicine (IOM) at the National Academy of Sciences in the United States has highlighted recommendations to create healthy food and beverage environments to ensure the healthy option is the easy option as part of a report on Accelerating Progress in Obesity Prevention.[23] The IOM recommends that government and the private sector work to reduce unhealthy food options while increasing affordable healthier options. Specific recommendations are outlined in Table 3 and include actions for government, private sector, schools, nongovernmental organizations, and health care providers.

Table 3. IOM strategies and actions to prevent obesity in the United States.[22]

1.	Reduce overconsumption of sugar-sweetened beverages
2.	Increase lower-calorie options for children in restaurants
3.	Utilize strong nutritional standards for foods and beverages provided by the government
4.	Create and implement health-promoting food and beverage retail and distribution policies
5.	Understand the implications of US agriculture policy for the population diet.

2.3. Addressing Overweight and Obesity in Children and Adolescents

Numerous studies have highlighted the detrimental effects of obesity and overweight in early years of life on metabolic diseases in adults.

Tirosh *et al.* prospectively followed 37,674 apparently healthy young men, aged 17 years, for incident angiography-proven coronary heart disease and diabetes.[24] In a mean follow-up period of 17.4 years, they documented 1,173 incident cases of type 2 diabetes and 327 cases of coronary heart disease. Elevated adolescent BMI was a significant predictor of both diabetes (hazard ratio 2.76 for the highest vs. the lowest decile) and angiography-proven coronary heart disease (hazard ratio, 5.43). However, further adjustment for BMI at adulthood completely nullified the association of adolescent BMI with diabetes but not the association with coronary heart disease. This finding suggests that BMI in adolescence has a more reversible or shorter term effect on the risk of diabetes compared with its effect on risk of coronary heart disease.

Juonala *et al.* reported similar findings from a combined analysis of four prospective cohort studies (total 6,328 subjects) that measured body-mass index from childhood for a mean follow-up of 23 years.[25] They found that subjects with consistently high adiposity status from childhood to adulthood, compared with those having a normal BMI as children and were nonobese as adults, had an increased risk of type 2 diabetes [relative risk, 5.4; 95% confidence interval (CI), 3.4–8.5]. Individuals who were overweight or obese during childhood but were nonobese as adults had similar risks to those who had a consistently normal BMI from childhood to adulthood ($p>0.20$ for all comparisons). This suggests that the risk of developing diabetes diminishes in overweight and obese adolescents if they lose weight going into adulthood. Strategies to reduce overweight and obesity in children and adolescents are likely to have the greatest payoff in terms of containing the diabetes epidemic.

2.3.1. *Primary prevention in high-risk individuals*

There is strong and consistent evidence from several randomized controlled trials that type 2 diabetes can be prevented or delayed through lifestyle interventions that improve diet, increase physical activity, and reduce weight in people at high risk of developing the disease. People at highest risk of developing diabetes (prediabetes) have a long quiescent period of abnormal glucose metabolism with blood glucose levels lower than those diagnostic of diabetes.[26] Individuals with prediabetes have impaired fasting glucose (IFG) with fasting glucose levels between 6.1 and 6.9 mmol/L (109.8 to 124.2 mg/dL) and/or impaired glucose tolerance (IGT) with 2-hr glucose values during the oral glucose tolerance test between 7.8 and 11.0 mmol/L (140.4 to 198 mg/dL).[27] Obese individuals, especially with abdominal or visceral obesity, are at particular risk of developing prediabetes and have a relatively high-risk for the future development of diabetes and other manifestations of the metabolic syndrome, namely, dyslipidemia with high triglycerides and/or low HDL cholesterol, and hypertension.

The Dutch Hoorn study found that individuals who have prediabetes constituted about 16% of the population but at the end of a 6-year follow-up, they contributed to more than 60% of the new cases of diabetes.[28] Several randomized prospective studies, conducted in both developed and developing countries, found that the onset of diabetes can be delayed or prevented in those at greatest risk.

The major programs that have been implemented to directly address diabetes in high-risk individuals include the United States Diabetes Prevention Program (DPP), Finnish Diabetes Prevention Study (DPS), the Chinese Da Qing Study, the Indian Diabetes Prevention Program, and the DE-PLAN prevention and management program in Europe. These programs are highlighted in Table 4.[29]

The most effective diabetes prevention program to date focusing on lifestyle intervention is the Diabetes Prevention Program (DPP). The DPP

Table 4. Major community-based interventions for type 2 diabetes prevention.

Study, Location	Intervention	Size of study	Age	Sex	Length	Impact % DM Risk Reduction
DPP, USA[30]	Lifestyle intervention on diet, physical activity and behavior modification training Metformin (850 mg 2x/day) Placebo	3,234 participants	Mean age 51 years	68% women	Average 2.8 years	Lifestyle: 58%; significantly more effective than metformin
DPS, Finland[43]	Intensive lifestyle intervention with nutritionist counseling and training sessions Control	522 participants	Mean age 51 years	67% female	3.2 years (most intensive in year 1)	58%
Da Qing, China[42]	Diet intervention Exercise intervention Diet + exercise intervention	577 participants	Mean age 45		6 years	Diet only: 31% PA only" 46% Diet + PA: 42%
DPP, India[47]	Lifestyle modification advice Metformin Lifestyle + metformin	531 participants	Mean age 45.9	21% female	3 years	Lifestyle: 28.5% reduction Metformin: 26.4% Lifestyle + metformin: 28.2%
Malmo Sweden	Lifestyle intervention	222 participants	Ages 47–49	Men only	5 years	Men who participated in the lifestyle intervention had a lower incidence of type 2 diabetes, and had a greater reversal of glucose intolerance compared to men who received usual care.
DE-PLAN Europe						No systematic results published

demonstrated a significant benefit in the incidence of diabetes in a population with prediabetes, reducing the risk by 58%.[30] After a 10-year follow-up period, diabetes incidence was reduced by 34%. The program combines intensive lifestyle coaching (weekly for 4 months, followed by monthly for 6 months) with physical activity. The specific goal was a 5–7% weight reduction and normalization of insulin sensitivity.

2.3.2. *The Diabetes Prevention Program*

The landmark Diabetes Prevention Program (DPP) was a major multi-center clinical research study aimed at investigating whether weight loss through dietary changes and increased physical activity or treatment with the oral diabetes drug metformin (Glucophage) could prevent or delay the onset of type 2 diabetes in study participants who were overweight and had prediabetes.[31] The DPP included 3,234 adults with IGT randomized to four groups: placebo control, lifestyle management, metformin, and troglitazone. The troglitazone group was withdrawn within a year because of adverse effects.

The DPP found that participants who lost 7% of initial body weight and expended 700 kcal of energy per week through moderate physical activity (equivalent to approximately 2 ½ hr per week of brisk walking) reduced their chances of developing diabetes by 58% in 3 years compared to controls in all ethnic groups including men and women. Lifestyle changes worked particularly well for participants aged 60 and older reducing their risk by 71%. About 5% of the lifestyle intervention group developed diabetes each year during the study period compared with 11% of those in the placebo group.

A recent follow-up study of the DPP has shown that the benefits of lifestyle intervention persisted over 10 years with a reduction in the incidence of diabetes of 34% in the lifestyle intervention group compared to control.[32]

Below is a summary of the key features of the lifestyle intervention in the DPP[33]:

- *Goal-based behavioral intervention*: To provide an intervention that would be appropriate for the diverse population, participants at all study centres were given the same weight loss and physical activity goal, but individualization was allowed to achieve these goals.

- *Individual case managers or "coaches"*: For the most part, the DPP used an individual model of treatment, rather than a group-based approach. Each lifestyle subject was assigned an individual case manager or "coach" who delivered the curriculum and ensured that participants were motivated to achieve lifestyle goals. An average of one-and-a-half to two lifestyle coaches were assigned to each clinical center responsible for approximately 40 participants. The majority of lifestyle coaches were registered dietitians or had a qualification in exercise physiology, behavioral psychology, or health education.
- *Frequent contact and ongoing intervention*: The lifestyle intervention offered 16 core sessions to be completed within the first 24 weeks after randomization (Table 5).
- *Adherence/maintenance intervention*: After completing the 16-session core curriculum, participants were seen face-to-face at least once every 2 months for the remainder of the trial and were contacted by phone at least once between visits.
- *Supervised activity sessions*: Each clinical centre offered voluntary supervised physical activity sessions at least two times per week throughout the trial. The types of supervised activity sessions varied across centres and included group walks, aerobic classes, and one-on-one personal training.
- *Individualization through "toolbox"*: To help participants achieve and maintain lifestyle goals, a "toolbox" of strategies was developed that could be used with individual participants.

On the whole, a deliberately intensive approach to lifestyle was used in the DPP trial. The DPP was not designed to compare different behavioral approaches for long-term behavior change or to test the effectiveness of a lifestyle intervention that could be "translated" for use in community settings.

Altogether, the cost of delivering the intervention in its first year was estimated at $1,399 per participant. This cost poses a major challenge for scaling such a program to a broader population.[34]

Table 5. DPP 16-session core curriculum.[32]

Session	Title	Description
1	Welcome to the Lifestyle Balance Program	Build commitment to the DPP lifestyle change program by recording personal reasons for joining the DPP and perceived benefits to self, family, and others. Highlight the two study goals: 7% weight loss and 150 min of weekly physical activity and review key aspects of the relationship between the lifestyle coach and participant in working toward these goals. Introduce self-monitoring of food intake.
2	Be a Fat Detective	Introduce regular self-monitoring of weight at home. Help participants find the main sources of fat in their diet through self-monitoring fat grams using the "DPP Fat Counter" and by reading food labels. Assign a fat gram goal based on starting weight.
3	Three Ways to Eat Less Fat	Practice self-monitoring skills, including weighing and measuring foods and estimating portion size of foods. Teach three ways to eat less fat: eat high-fat foods less often, eat smaller portions, and substitute lower fat foods and cooking methods.
4	Healthy Eating	Emphasize the importance of a regular meal pattern and eating slowly. Use the Food Guide Pyramid (USDA) as a model for healthy eating and compare personal eating patterns to these recommendations. Recommend specific low-fat, low-calorie substitutes at each level of the Food Pyramid.
5	Move Those Muscles	Introduce physical activity and begin to build to 150 min of physical activity over the next 4 weeks, using activities such as brisk walking. Begin self-monitoring of physical activity as well as food intake. Review personal activity history and likes and dislikes about physical activity. Encourage attendance at group supervised activity sessions.
6	Being Active: A Way of Life	Help participants learn to find the time to be physically active each day by including short bouts (10–15 min) and healthy lifestyle activities, e.g., climbing stairs and walking extra blocks from the bus stop. Teach the basic principles for exercising safely, what to do in the event of injury, and knowing when to stop.

(*Continued*)

Table 5. (*Continued*)

Session	Title	Description
7	Tip the Calorie Balance	Teach the fundamental principle of energy balance and what it takes to lose 1–2 lbs per week. For those individuals who have made little progress with weight loss, assign self-monitoring of calories as well as fat grams or provide a structured meal plan at reduced calorie levels.
8	Take Charge of What's Around You	Introduce the principle of stimulus control. Identify cues in the participant's home environment that lead to unhealthy food and activity choices and discuss ways to change them.
9	Problem Solving	Present the five-step model of problem solving: describe the problem as links in a behavior chain, brainstorm possible solutions, pick one solution to try, make a positive action plan, evaluate the success of the solution. Apply the problem-solving model to eating and exercise problems.
10	The Four Keys to Healthy Eating Out	Introduce four basic skills for managing eating away from home: anticipating and planning ahead, positive assertion, stimulus control, and making healthy food choices.
11	Talk Back to Negative Thoughts	Practice identifying common patterns of self-defeating, negative thoughts and learn to counter these thoughts with positive statements.
12	The Slippery Slope of Lifestyle Change	Stress that slips are normal and learning to recover quickly is the key to success. Teach participants to recognize personal triggers for slips, their reactions to those slips, and what it takes to get back on track.
13	Jump Start Your Activity Plan	Introduce the basic principles of aerobic fitness: frequency, intensity, time, type of activity (FITT). Teach participants to measure their heart rate and perceived level of exertion as a way of determining the appropriate levels of activity. Discuss ways to cope with boredom by adding variety to the physical activity plan.
14	Make Social Cues Work for You	Present strategies for managing problem social cues, e.g., being pressured to overeat, and help participants learn to use social cues to promote healthy behaviors, e.g., making regular dates with a walking partner or group. Review specific strategies for coping with social events such as parties, vacations, and holidays.

(*Continued*)

Table 5. *(Continued)*

Session	Title	Description
15	You Can Manage Stress	Highlight the importance of coping with stress, including stress caused by the DPP, by using all of the skills previously taught, e.g., positive assertion, engaging social support, problem solving, planning, talking back to negative thoughts, and being physically active.
16	Ways to Stay Motivated	Enhance motivation to maintain behavior change by reviewing participants' personal reasons for joining DPP and by recognizing personal successes thus far. Introduce other strategies for staying motivated including posting signs of progress, setting new goals, creating friendly competition, and seeking social support from DPP staff and others.

Various researchers have modified the findings of the DPP with the aim of making it less intensive and more applicable in the community setting. Ali *et al.* conducted a systematic review and meta-analysis of 28 US-based studies applying the findings of the DPP.[35] They reported that across diverse settings, lifestyle intervention programs that adapted the DPP achieved significant weight loss of 4–5%. There was no convincing evidence that fewer or more than the 16 sessions of the DPP were more cost effective in achieving weight loss. In general, the greater the number of core sessions offered, the greater were attendance and weight loss. The use of lay educators appeared to achieve similar weight loss as medical and allied health personnel.

Efforts are currently underway in the United States to offer the basic components of the Diabetes Prevention Program in a community setting. The CDC has partnered with the United Health Group to offer the program through the YMCA (The Y). Vojta *et al.* reported that the YMCA's DPP was effectively scaled to 46 communities in 23 states in less than 2 years.[36] In this initiative, 1,723 participants completed the core program at an average service-delivery cost of about $400 each. For those completing the program, the average weight loss was about 5%.

In a recent review of the YMCA program, Ackermann stated that "offering the DPP in the community holds much promise to improve health for a reasonable cost, but this will not provide a solution for everyone."[37] Much is yet to be learned about those "left out," why some individuals do not succeed, and how successes might be maintained over an extended period of time.

The DPP has been duplicated in other forms, including an online version by the private company, Omada Health. However, this medium, while performing well in pilot trials and producing an initial success rate for weight reduction similar to the DPP, lacks long-term follow-up data. The Healthy Living Partnerships to Prevent Diabetes (HELP PD) has also replicated the successful methodology from the DPP but done so within a cheaper and existing community health structure. HELP PD has two-year follow-up data demonstrating 46.5% of participants maintaining a 5% or more weight reduction.[38] These programs represent great opportunities to execute a proven lifestyle change curriculum across different subpopulations. Diet, lifestyle, and behavior therapy are considered the three primary key components for weight loss and comprehensive lifestyle modification will typically provide weekly individual or group sessions to assist with changing eating and activity habits. This approach has been supported by published outcomes from the DPP and adaptations of the DPP.[31,32,35]

Commercially available interventions, such as Weight Watchers, have been shown to be effective in producing an approximate 15–25% reduction in baseline weight. However, follow-up data indicates that commercially available programs are less impactful with 1 year or longer follow-up. In addition, these programs can be costly for participants and carry a high probability of regaining 50% or more of initial weight lost within 1 to 2 years.[39] Recent data shows Weight Watchers to be cost-effective when compared to standard care offered by general practitioners.[40]

In addition to national level programs, community programs have seen promising results in several countries. Community Interventions in Health (CIH) is a multicomponent study on chronic disease prevention in India, China, and Mexico. CIH focused on community mobilization and also included health education and social marketing in locations including schools, worksites, health care areas, and the broader community.[41] Results of the 16–24 month intervention to improve diet, physical activity, and reduce smoking found that while the control group showed poorer health behaviors over time, the intervention group maintained their health behaviors.[42] The intervention group also reduced salt added in cooking. Separately from CIH, there are ongoing community level projects underway in Sri Lanka, China, South Africa, Malaysia, and the United Kingdom.

In the Chinese Da Qing study, conducted among 577 adults with impaired glucose tolerance, subjects were randomized to a control group or to one of three active treatment groups: diet, exercise, or diet plus exercise. Follow-up evaluation examinations were conducted at 2-year intervals over a 6-year period to identify subjects who developed diabetes. After adjustment for differences in baseline BMI and fasting glucose, the diet, exercise, and diet-plus-exercise interventions were associated with 31% ($p < 0.03$), 46% ($p < 0.0005$), and 42% ($p < 0.005$) reductions in risk of developing diabetes, respectively.[43]

The US and Finnish studies achieved a 58% reduction in diabetes incidence through lifestyle modification among those with prediabetes compared to controls.[31,44] Follow-up studies have demonstrated long-term maintenance of reduced diabetes risk.[45,46]

Several studies performed in other countries have shown similar benefits.[47,48] The Indian Diabetes Prevention program was a community-based randomized controlled study in 531 participants with persistent impaired glucose tolerance.[48] The four arms of the study included control, moderate intensity lifestyle management, metformin, and a combination of lifestyle management and metformin. In a median follow-up period of 30 months, the rate of conversion to diabetes was 18.3% in the control group compared to relative risk reduction of about 29% in all interventions arms.

In summary, lifestyle interventions in primary care settings and recently in community settings have shown encouraging results in preventing or delaying the onset of diabetes in people at greatest risk. However, much still needs to be learned about wide-scale prevention methods that are affordable and sustainable at community and individual levels.[49,50] Challenges remain in scaling up smaller interventions that have shown efficacy as well as producing a cost-effective model at a national level. There are only a few studies that have addressed the cost-effectiveness of diabetes prevention. In the Diabetes Prevention Program study, it was found that lifestyle intervention was more cost-effective than treatment with metformin. It was estimated that to prevent one case of diabetes, the intensive lifestyle intervention cost was $15,700 while the metformin treatment cost was $31,000. Although the cost of prevention was high, the intervention was deemed to be cost-effective.

Using a simulation model, Zhuo *et al.* projected that a nationwide roll-out of a community-based version of the DPP using group-sessions and trained lay health educators would prevent or delay about 885,000 cases of type 2 diabetes and produce savings of $5.7 billion in the United States over 25 years.[51] The authors claim that implementing such a nationwide program would be an efficient use of health care resources. Although a prevention program would lead to cost savings in both younger and older people, it would achieve greater health and economic gains if it were directed at people under the age of 65.

2.3.3. *Drugs in primary prevention*

Metformin is the drug that has been studied most extensively for diabetes prevention. In the DPP trial, 1,073 participants with IGT were allocated to 850 mg of metformin twice daily and 1,082 to placebo.[31] At the mean follow-up period of 2.8 years, metformin reduced the incidence of diabetes by 31% compared with placebo (see Table 1). Metformin was most effective in individuals who had a baseline BMI of 35 kg/m^2 or more. In this group, the incidence was reduced by approximately 50%. The beneficial effects of metformin were most evident in younger participants and induced a moderate loss of weight, which may have contributed to the positive outcome. Other trials of metformin have also yielded positive results in terms of preventing diabetes in those at high risk.[48,49]

Several other drugs — acarbose, thiazolidinediones, and rosiglitazone — have shown to be effective in preventing diabetes in high-risk individuals but many of these drugs exhibit significant side effects such as gastrointestinal symptoms and hepatotoxicity, thereby limiting their wide use.[52–54]

It should be noted that lifestyle intervention reduced the incidence of diabetes by 58% and in contrast to lifestyle intervention, where the beneficial effects were evident long after cessation of the active intervention, the positive effects of drug treatment waned soon after withdrawal.[55]

3. SECONDARY PREVENTION

Nutrition, particularly calorie intake, plays an important role in weight balance; if more calories are consumed than are burned, weight gain occurs. In individuals with type 2 diabetes, maintaining a healthy diet is even more important because excess calorie intake can lead to hyperglycemia, a condition associated with long-term complications. Individuals with diabetes are encouraged by the Mayo Clinic to include complex carbohydrates, high fiber foods, mono- and polyunsaturated fats such as olive oil and heart healthy fish in the diet while avoiding foods high in saturated or trans-fats, cholesterol, and sodium.[56]

Lifestyle interventions have also been shown to improve control and reduce morbidity in those with type 2 diabetes.

The most comprehensive secondary prevention program with a principal emphasis on lifestyle interventions is the Look AHEAD (Action for Health in Diabetes) study launched in June 2001 by the National Institutes of Health.[57] The study sought to provide a definitive assessment of the long-term health consequences of intentional weight loss through caloric restriction and increased physical activity. The study was conducted across 16 centers in the United States and enrolled 5,145 overweight individuals with type 2 diabetes. Participants were randomly allocated to a Diabetes Support and Education (DSE) group and a Lifestyle Intervention Group. Individuals in the DSE group received usual medical care which was provided by their own primary care physicians. In addition, they were offered three group educational sessions per year for the first 4 years. Participants in the Lifestyle Intervention group received usual medical care combined with an intensive 4-year program designed to increase physical activity and reduce initial weight by 7% or more.[58]

The primary end point was the first occurrence of a composite cardiovascular outcome, which included death from cardiovascular causes, nonfatal myocardial infarction, and nonfatal stroke. Death from any cause, myocardial infarction, stroke, hospitalization for angina, coronary-artery bypass grafting, percutaneous coronary intervention, hospitalization for heart failure, or peripheral vascular disease were secondary outcomes. The planned follow-up period was initially set at 11.5 years but was extended to 13 years.

The lifestyle intervention in the Look AHEAD Study was based on the DPP protocol but was adapted for use in individuals with type 2 diabetes. The Look AHEAD protocol diverged from the DPP lifestyle interventions in the following ways[58]:

- The interventions in Look AHEAD were offered in group-based rather than individual treatment during the first year.
- The program offered liquid meal replacements to achieve weight loss.
- The program offered the option of weight loss medication after the first 6 months in selected individuals.

At 1 year, participants in the intervention (intensive lifestyle intervention, ILI) arm showed significant weight loss (8.6% vs 0.7%), significantly improved diabetes control, and reduced CVD risk factors and medication use compared to the Diabetes Support and Education (DSE) arm. Mean HbA1c dropped from 7.3% to 6.6% in the ILI arm versus from 7.3% to 7.2% in DSE.

Gregg and colleagues further reported that ILI was superior to conventional diabetes education and treatment for inducing a transient, partial remission of type 2 diabetes.[58] At 2, 3, and 4 years, 9.2%, 6.4%, and 3.5%, respectively, of ILI participants ($n = 2262$) had partial diabetes remission compared with 1.7%, 1.3%, and 0.5% of participants, respectively, in the DSE group ($n = 2241$). Participants with early-stage diabetes were most likely to benefit from the intensive lifestyle intervention.

At 4 years, ILI participants maintained greater improvements than DSE participants in weight, fitness, HbA1c levels, systolic blood pressure, and high-density lipoprotein cholesterol levels.[59] However, these improved risk factor profiles did not translate into lower rates of nonfatal myocardial infarction, nonfatal stroke, hospitalization for angina, or death compared with conventional diabetes treatment. This has recently led the National Institutes of Health to halt the Look AHEAD intervention group at a median follow-up of 9.6 years because it did not decrease the occurrence of cardiovascular events, which was the primary goal of the study.[60]

Despite this finding, there is evidence that lifestyle interventions are important for improving risk factors and outcomes at all stages of the metabolic spectrum from prediabetes to type 2 diabetes. The challenge is to translate this evidence into cost-effective, large-scale programs with increased recognition that the best way to do so is through studies that are performed in a clearly defined context and have an explicit focus on feasibility, scalability, and cost.

The TODAY study compared the efficacy of three treatment regimens to achieve durable glycemic control in 699 children and adolescents aged 10 to 17 years with recent-onset type 2 diabetes.[61] Eligible patients were treated with metformin to attain a HbA1c level of less than 8% and were randomly assigned to continued treatment with metformin alone or to metformin combined with rosiglitazone or a metformin plus lifestyle-intervention program focusing on weight loss through eating and activity. The primary outcome was loss of glycemic control defined by HbA_{1c} of at least 8% for 6 months or sustained metabolic decompensation requiring insulin. In the metformin group, 51.7% failed to maintain glycemic control compared to 38.6% in the metformin plus rosiglitazone group and 46.6% for the metformin plus lifestyle intervention group.

In an accompanying editorial, Allen wrote:

> For a substantial proportion of those millions of children at risk for largely preventable type 2 diabetes, the findings of the TODAY study reinforce the idea that medications and even procedures will not stave off a lifetime of illness. The stark message from the TODAY study is that, tomorrow and beyond, public-policy approaches — sufficient economic incentives to produce and purchase healthy foods and to build safe environments that require physical movement — and not simply the prescription of more and better pills will be necessary to stem the epidemic of type 2 diabetes and its associated morbidity.[62]

4. BEHAVIOR CHANGE

Reversing the escalating rates of obesity and diabetes around the globe will require significant changes on the personal, community, and overarching policy levels for success. On a personal level, education is needed to promote healthier choices but education alone is not enough for successful, lasting behavior change.[63] Effectively tailored education for specific audiences can help inform individuals about health issues (such as diabetes) and risk factors (such as nutrition and physical activity). The development of social marketing, adapting learning from marketing and applying them to social issues, has made health messaging even more sophisticated. However, education alone is not enough to elicit behavior change. The social environment where we make our decisions needs to encourage appropriate actions. For example, a public education campaign on sugary drinks and large portion size informed New Yorkers of the amount of sugar and calories in many beverages; this has the potential for increased effectiveness if combined with changing the food environment such as changing the default sizes or offering incentives to purchase lower calorie beverages.

The US federal government is working to create environments that support improving nutrition and increasing physical activity. For example, the Let's Move Campaign launched by First Lady Michelle Obama includes incorporating nutrition and physical activity education into the academic curriculum. Opportunities include teaching children their colors using fruits and vegetables and teaching older students about nutrition through calorie counts and daily nutritional value charts.[64]

4.1. Behavioral Economics

Behavioral economics, a field focused on the social, cognitive, and emotional effects of personal economic decisions, is rapidly gaining attention as an innovative opportunity to help improve consumer choices and behaviors. Leaders in the field include Daniel Kahneman, the Nobel Prize winner for his work on behavioral economics and more recently, Richard Thaler, and Cass Sunstein, publishing about opportunities for building choice architecture to promote certain decisions, termed "nudges."[65] Sunstein has also suggested simplification of US policy and regulation to promote ease of understanding and better decision making using nudges.[66]

Nudges are approaches that influence decisions while preserving freedom of choice examples including[65,66]:

1. The provision of clear and simple information to guide certain choices — e.g., the shift from the Food Pyramid to MyPlate in 2010 (Figs. 1 and 2).

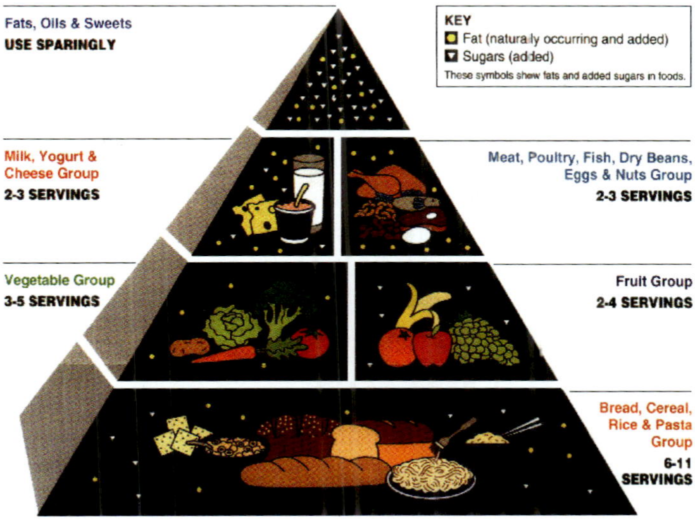

Fig. 1. Food pyramid.[65]

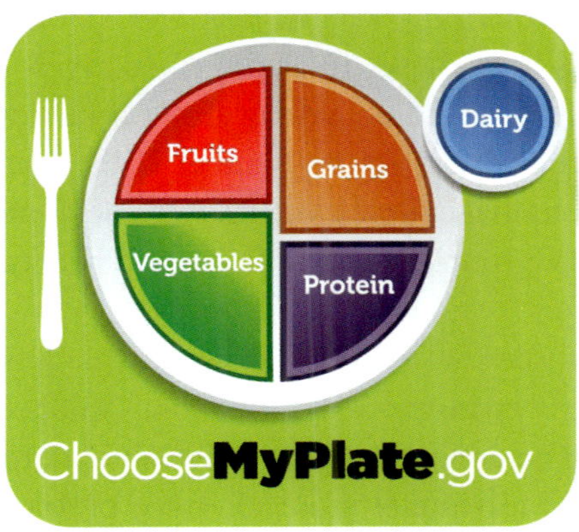

Fig. 2. MyPlate.[65]

MyPlate provides a clear graphic representation of food groups to enable individuals to follow a balanced diet.

2. The framing of information to influence the decision — e.g., If told that 90% of those that have undertaken an operation are alive in 5 years,

individuals are more likely to consent to procedures than if they are told that after 5 years, 10% are dead.

3. The use of default settings so that other choices need to be actively selected — e.g., organ donation is >99% in Austria and only 12% in Germany mainly due to Austria using opt-out techniques and Germany using opt-in techniques to promote organ donation.
4. The changing of environmental design to make certain choices easier — e.g., supermarkets placing fruit and vegetables in prominent positions in the front.
5. The provision of comparable information — e.g., individuals are more likely to pay taxes on time if aware that others do.

In addition to creating optimal choice architecture to encourage certain decisions, highlighted by Thaler and Sunstein, incentives have great potential to increase participation and achievement of outcomes that are currently very challenging to achieve normally. For example, weight loss and smoking cessation are extremely challenging outcomes to achieve and require sustained behavior change. Kevin Volpp and colleagues have seen success in studies promoting weight loss and smoking cessation using financial incentives.[67–69] These financial incentives include monetary rewards for participation and achieving desired outcomes, lottery-based systems that only reward the lottery winner if they achieved the desired outcome and a system that couples lottery with social participation, further rewarding the lottery group if most of the group had achieved the desired outcome.

Success has been seen with financial incentives to encourage behavior change and, more controversially, financial disincentives are being increasingly used. The concept of loss aversion underpins the use of disincentives whereby individuals more strongly prefer avoiding losses to obtaining gain. Therefore, positioning incentives in terms of a penalty is likely to have a stronger effect on modifying behavior than positioning positively. While disincentives are much more controversial than positive incentives, they are increasingly being used. CVS Caremark's decision to penalize ($600 annually) employees that do not take part in a "wellness review" that includes height, weight, body fat, blood pressure, and other health indicators brought this issue into popular discussion.[70] However, many companies have or plan to impose penalties. Aon Hewitt's survey found that 58% of employers plan to "impose consequences on participants who do not take appropriate actions for improving their health."[71]

4.2. Environmental Aspects

The surrounding environment, including urban design, public transportation, and food availability, has the potential to enhance or discourage behaviors related to obesity and diabetes such as healthy and unhealthy food consumption and physical activity.[72] The powerful effects of environments on behaviors and physiology have been highlighted as opportunities for environments to promote health rather than disease. Swinburn and colleagues have published a framework categorizing obesity determinants and solutions from environmental, behavioral, and physiological levels (Fig. 3).

A review by the American Heart Association of population approaches for improving diet and increasing physical activity identified interventions in media and education, labeling and information, economic incentives, schools, workplaces, the local environment, and restrictions and mandates.[73] The approaches were classified according to evidence for agreement and evidence levels based on study strengths. Dietary interventions

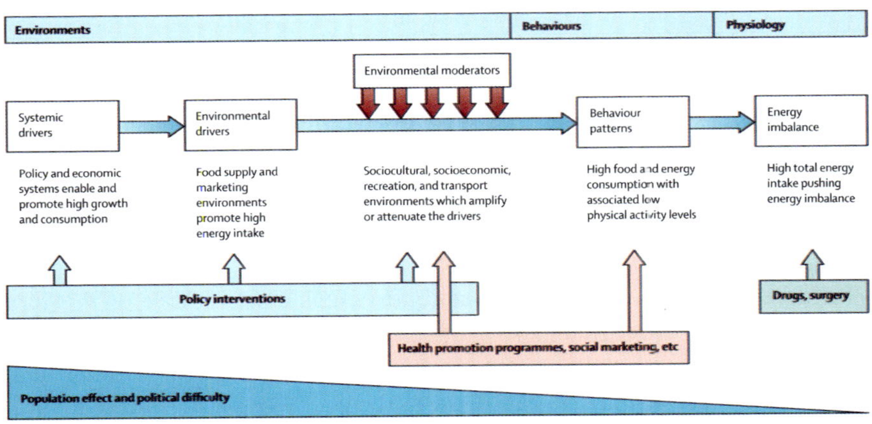

Fig. 3. Framework of obesity determinants and solutions.[71]

with effective and beneficial evidence for agreement supported by well-designed research studies include subsidy strategies to lower the price of healthier foods and beverages and multicomponent interventions to improve nutrition and physical activity. Interventions with less evidence strength (evidence from a single randomized trial or nonrandomized studies) include sustained media and educational campaigns with multiple modes for increasing specific healthy food consumption and decreasing specific unhealthy food consumption, restrictions on television advertisements for unhealthy foods and beverages advertised to children, and regulatory policies to reduce specific nutrients in foods, e.g., trans-fats.

Physical activity interventions with evidence from a single randomized trial or nonrandomized studies include increased availability and types of school playground spaces and equipment.

5. GOVERNMENT POLICY

To promote health by increasing the nutritional quality of diets, many policy options have been discussed and proposed, and several implemented. Policies range from government restrictions or taxes on foods high in sugar, salt, or fat, to government and industry subsidies to promote healthy food purchasing and consumption, to requiring nutrition labeling of foods and limiting portion sizes. Internationally, most countries have policies to address obesity and diet-related noncommunicable diseases (NCDs), including diabetes, although the policies are often not comprehensive and focused on education. The World Health Organization (WHO) reports that popular policies include dietary guidelines, nutrition counseling at primary care centers, and food labeling.[74] Healthy eating media communications are popular in Eastern Mediterranean and South East Asia regions, and national programs to promote fruit and vegetable consumption are common in the Americas region.

Marketing regulations on food and beverages exist in 58% of Western Pacific Region countries and 50% of Eastern Mediterranean Region countries. Other policies include increasing prices on unhealthy foods and workplace interventions. Tax policies have been frequently discussed and have been implemented in several countries, for example in Denmark for products with saturated fat, France for sugary drinks, and Hungary in products containing salt, sugar, and caffeine. Denmark recently ended the tax on products with saturated fat, due to unforeseen challenges such as consumers crossing country lines to buy products and higher prices on lean meats as well as fattier cuts.[75] The United States has debated taxing sugary drinks for several years, and New York city mayor Michael Bloomberg tried to limit soda containers to a maximum of 16 ounces.

On an international level, led by the WHO, diabetes and obesity targets have been established to reduce the burden of disease. Resulting from the United Nations High Level Meeting on Non-Communicable Disease, a 0% increase in diabetes and obesity is included as one of the nine voluntary global targets for reducing NCDs by 2025.[76]

The UK has taken a slightly different track to tackle unhealthy lifestyle behaviors and, in March 2011, launched the Responsibility Deal. This had four main working groups: nutrition, physical activity, alcohol, and health at work. In each working group, companies were asked to voluntarily sign up to pledges, such as calorie labeling, salt reduction, trans-fat removal from products, promotion of active travel to and from work, promotion of Department of Health physical activity guidelines, and offering healthy employee restaurants. While some have praised this as industry and government working together for social good, others have said that it is ineffective and has prevented stronger, potentially more effective, interventions from being implemented.

Behavioral economic interventions offer an opportunity for unique sites (such as worksites or schools) to encourage fruit consumption by placing fruit in a pleasing, eye-catching bowl or in a well-lit part of the cafeteria, and promote weight loss and smoking cessation through incentive programs. However, sustained success nationally or in communities requires support at the policy level to facilitate making healthy behaviors and choices. For example, agricultural policies in the United States currently favor mass production of corn for animal feed and ethanol production, and analyzing the subsidy structure of food groups supported by agricultural policy versus food groups supported by the dietary guidelines highlights the discrepancy between agriculture and health policies at the federal level.[77] The opportunities for synergistic benefits on behavior change resulting from combined industry and government efforts are immense. For example, consider a healthy eating campaign promoting specific nutrition changes to reduce calorie intake that is implemented a few months in advance of industry rolling out smaller portion size products. The campaign would educate and prime the population for behavior change by encouraging adoption of smaller portion sizes, especially if the new products were advertised by respected role models and incentivized with a price discount.

On the federal level, nutrition and agriculture policies should align with policies and goals to improve population nutrition and health. Rather than subsidies supporting mass production of corn, wheat, soybeans, rice, and cotton, which currently receive more than 90% of agricultural subsidies, support should go to fruit and vegetable crops that are encouraged by nutrition policies, yet are currently designated as "specialty crops" in agricultural policy.[78]

5.1. Further Policy Considerations

Regulations that target environmental drivers of the obesity pandemic are critical in strategies directed at obesity control.[72] Examples include reducing the cost of healthy foods, increasing the cost of unhealthy foods, enforcing bans on unhealthy food marketing to children and involving the food industry in altering product formulations to ensure healthier food composition. Obesity needs to be addressed at all levels of the socioecological model with broad and meaningful sector-wide changes. Environments need to be created where opportunities for physical activity and healthy dietary choices are easily accessible. Scientific recommendations need to be linked with applied strategies and action steps (e.g., in schools, workplaces, etc.). Policymakers, health care practitioners, legislators, and academics should all be involved in supporting individuals, particularly at the societal level, in their endeavor to manage body weight, through the collaboration of private and public stakeholders. The food industry has a key role to play by practicing responsible marketing, decreasing the sugar and fat content of processed foods and ensuring that nutritious foods are available and affordable to consumers.

Five core principles, implemented across multiple sectors, are critical in developing a comprehensive and coherent obesity management strategy.[79] These include:

- A system-wide approach where the nation's health is defined as a societal and an economic issue
- Higher priority for the prevention of health problems, with clearer leadership, accountability, strategy and management structures
- Engagement of stakeholders within and outside government
- Long-term, sustained interventions
- Ongoing evaluation and a focus on continuous improvement.

It has become evident that there is a need for multisectoral solutions to address the global problem of overweight and obesity. Bold actions by many players acting together could slow and eventually reverse the epidemic. Agreement should be reached on the most effective measures to be taken separately and collectively, on adequate resourcing of proposed solutions and on ensuring coherent action by all stakeholders. Obesity-targeted solutions should be synergistic, coherent, comprehensive, and cost-effective. If a significant and sustained impact is to be made on the current state of overweight and obesity, complementary actions need to be taken by all players including individuals, governments, industry, and food companies in developing innovative and comprehensive solutions.

6. CONCLUSIONS

The rapidly evolving epidemic of diabetes is a global concern not only for high-income countries but also the developing world. While the analysis of primary prevention of diabetes has made the clear link between diabetes and obesity, physical inactivity and poor nutrition, targeted measures at community and national levels remain limited. Furthermore, government policies to support such measures are in their infancy. Policies must work to support healthy environments, including nutrition policies and urban design, as well as health care policies for those that need assistance from medical providers. As these processes are in their infancy, continuous evaluation is critical so that modifications can be made as necessary to ensure the most effective interventions.

Individuals with prediabetes are most likely to develop diabetes over subsequent years with several prevention programs having demonstrated promising results in high-risk individuals. These have highlighted the importance of improving diet and increasing physical activity, interventions at least and often considerably more effective than pharmacological interventions. This knowledge must be incorporated in the global agenda to ensure that focus does not remain on medication alone.

The role of behavior change in both risk modification and treatment adherence is critical to making the healthy choice the easy choice. However, while much progress can be made both at local and national levels without policy support, to fully capitalize on the impact that behavior change can have, policy support is needed for initiatives, particularly around environmental aspects.

For global policies in diabetes prevention to be effective, it is critical that a system-wide approach is taken, that there is an effective balance in focusing on prevention as well as on cure, that a wide range of stakeholders are engaged both within and outside government, and that ongoing evaluation is implemented from the start with a focus on continuous improvement. With the body of evidence growing on what could be done, now is the time for action.

REFERENCES

1. International Diabetes Federation (IDF), http://www.idf.org/diabetesatlas/5e/diabetes, accessed April 30, 2013.
2. Hu FB. (2011) Globalization of diabetes: The role of diet, lifestyle, and genes. *Diabetes Care* **34**: 1249–1257.
3. Ahmad LA, Crandall JP (2010) Type 2 diabetes prevention: A review. *Clin Diabetes* **28**: 53–59.
4. Gillies CL, Abrams KR, Lambert PC, *et al.* (2007) Pharmacological and lifestyle interventions to prevent or delay type 2 diabetes in people with impaired glucose tolerance: Systematic review and meta-analysis. *BMJ* **334**: 299.
5. Excellence in diabetes conference. Istanbul, Turkey. February 6–9, 2013.

6. Prospective Studies Collaboration. (2009) Body-mass index and cause specific mortality in 900,000 adults: Collaborative analysis of 57 prospective studies. *Lancet* **373**: 1083–1096.
7. Zhang P, Zhang X, Brown J, *et al.* (2010) Global healthcare expenditure on diabetes for 2010 and 2030. *Diabetes Res Clin Pract* **87**: 293–301.
8. Weinstein AR, Sesso HD, Lee IM, *et al.* (2004) Relationship of physical activity vs body mass index with type 2 diabetes in women. *JAMA* **292**: 1188–1194.
9. Carey VJ, Walters EE, Colditz GA, *et al.* (1997) Body fat distribution and risk of non-insulin-dependent diabetes mellitus in women. The Nurses' Health Study. *Am J Epidemiol* **145**: 614–619.
10. Koh-Banerjee P, Wang Y, Hu FB, Spiegelman D, Willett WC, Rimm EB. (2004) Changes in body weight and body fat distribution as risk factor for clinical diabetes in US men. *Am J Epidemiol* **159**: 1150–1159.
11. Lear SA, Humphries KH, Kohli S, Chockalingam A, Frohlich JJ, Birmingham CL. (2007) Visceral adipose tissue accumulation differs according to ethnic background: Results of the Multicultural Community Health Assessment Trial (M-CHAT). *Am J Clin Nutr* **86**: 353–359.
12. Boyko EJ, Fujimoto WY, Leonetti DL, Newell-Morris L. (2000) Visceral adiposity and risk of type 2 diabetes: A prospective study among Japanese Americans. *Diabetes Care* **23**: 465–471.
13. Lysen LK, Israel DA. (2012) Nutrition in weight management. In: Mahan LK, Escott-Stump S, Raymond JL. (eds), *Krause's Food and the Nutrition Care Process*, pp. 462–488 Ed. by 13th ed. Saunders Elsevier, St. Louis, MI.
14. National Weight Control Registry. (2013) Brown Medical School. The Mirian Hospital Weight Control & Diabetes Research Centre. http://www.nwcr.ws/ Accessed April 13, 2013.
15. Wing RR, Phelan S. (2005) Long-term weight loss maintenance. *Am J Clin Nutr* **82**: 222S–225S.
16. Hall KD, *et al.* (2011) Quantification of the effect of energy imbalance on bodyweight. *Lancet* **378**: 826–837.
17. Hu FB, Li TY, Colditz GA, Willett WC, Manson JE. (2003) Television watching and other sedentary behaviors in relation to risk of obesity and type 2 diabetes mellitus in women. *JAMA* **289**: 1785–1791.
18. Hu FB, Leitzmann MF, Stampfer MJ, Colditz GA, Willett WC, Rimm EB. (2001) Physical activity and television watching in relation to risk for type 2 diabetes mellitus in men. *Arch Intern Med* **161**: 1542–1548.
19. Harvard School of Public Health. Preventing diabetes: The bottom line. http://www.hsph.harvard.edu/nutritionsource/diabetes-prevention/

20. Alhazmi A, Stojanovski E, McEvoy M, Garg ML. (2013) The association between dietary patterns and type 2 diabetes: A systematic review and meta-analysis of cohort studies. *J Hum Nutr Diet* **27**: 251–260.
21. Esposito K, Kastorini CM, Panagiotakos DB, Giugliano D. (2010) Prevention of type 2 diabetes by dietary patterns: A systematic review of prospective studies and meta-analysis. *Metab Syndr Relat Disord* **8**: 471–476.
22. Taubes G. (2011) Is sugar toxic? *New York Times* http://www.nytimes.com/2011/04/17/magazine/mag-17Sugar-t.html?pagewanted=all&_r=0
23. IOM. (2012) *Accelerating Progress in Obesity Prevention: Solving the Weight of the Nation*. The National Academies Press, Washington DC.
24. Tirosh A, Shai I, Afek A, *et al.* (2011) Adolescent BMI trajectory and risk of diabetes versus coronary disease. *N Engl J Med* **364**: 1315–1325.
25. Juonala M, Magnussen CG, Berenson GS, *et al.* (2011) Childhood adiposity, adult adiposity, and cardiovascular risk factors. *N Engl J Med* **365**: 1876–1885.
26. Standards of medical care in diabetes — 2013. *Diabetes Care* **36**: S11–S66.
27. World Health Organization (2006) Definitions and Diagnosis of Diabetes Mellitus and Intermediate Hyperglycemeia: Report of the WHO/IDF Consultation. Author, Geneva.
28. de VF, Dekker JM, Jager A, *et al.* (2001) Relation of impaired fasting and postload glucose with incident type 2 diabetes in a Dutch population: The Hoorn Study. *JAMA* **285**: 2109–2113.
29. International Diabetes Federation. Prevention studies. http://www.idf.org/diabetes-prevention/prevention-studies/studies
30. Wadden TA, Webb VL, Moran CH, Bailer BA. (2012) Lifestyle modifications for obesity: New developments in diet, physical activity, and behavior therapy. *Circulation* **135**: 1157–1170.
31. Knowler WC, Barrett-Connor E, Fowler SE, *et al.* (2002) Reduction in the incidence of type 2 diabetes with lifestyle intervention or metformin. *N Engl J Med* **346**: 393–403.
32. Knowler WC, Fowler SE, Hamman RF, *et al.* (2009) 10-year follow-up of diabetes incidence and weight loss in the Diabetes Prevention Program Outcomes Study. *Lancet* **374**: 1677–1686.
33. The Diabetes Prevention Program (DPP) Research Group. (2002) The Diabetes Prevention Program (DPP): Description of lifestyle intervention. *Diabetes Care* **25**: 2165–2171.
34. Hernan WH, Brandle M, Zhang P, *et al.* (2003) Costs associated with the primary prevention of type 2 diabetes mellitus in the diabetes prevention program. *Diabetes Care* **26**: 36–47.

35. Ali MK, Echouffo-Tcheugui J, Williamson DF. (2012) How effective were lifestyle interventions in real-world settings that were modeled on the Diabetes Prevention Program? *Health Aff* (Millwood) **31**: 67–75.
36. Vojta D, Koehler TB, Longjohn M, Lever JA, Caputo NF. (2013) A coordinated national model for diabetes prevention: Linking health systems to an evidence-based community program. *Am J Prev Med* **44**: S301–S306. doi: 10.1016/j.amepre.2012.12.018.
37. Ackermann R. (2013) Working with the YMCA to Implement the Diabetes Prevention Program. *Am J Prev Med* **44**: S352–S356.
38. Tucker ME. (2013) Lifestyle interventions for prediabetes is successful. *Am J Prev Med* Published online, March 18.
39. Tsai AG, Wadden TA. (2005) Systematic review: An evaluation of major commercial weight loss programs in the United States. *Ann Intern Med* **142**: 56–66.
40. Fuller NR, Colagiuri S, Schofield D, *et al.* (2013) A within-trial cost-effectiveness analysis of primary care referral to a commercial provider for weight loss treatment, relative to standard care — An international randomised controlled trial. *Int J Obes* (*Lond*) **37**: 828–834.
41. O'Connor Duffany K, Finegood DT, Matthews D, *et al.* (2011) Community interventions for health (CIH): A novel approach to tackling the worldwide epidemic of chronic disease. *CVD Prevent Control* **6**: 47–56.
42. Dyson P, Matthews D. (2013) Overview of results of CIH. Istanbul Convention and Exhibition Center, Istanbul, Turkey, February 8.
43. Pan XR, Li GW, Hu YH, *et al.* (1997) Effects of diet and exercise in preventing NIDDM in people with impaired glucose tolerance. The Da Qing IGT and Diabetes Study. *Diabetes Care* **20**: 537–544.
44. Tuomilehto J, Lindstrom J, Eriksson JG, *et al.* (2001) Prevention of type 2 diabetes mellitus by changes in lifestyle among subjects with impaired glucose tolerance. *N Engl J Med* **344**: 1343–1350.
45. Li G, Zhang P, Wang J, *et al.* (2008) The long-term effect of lifestyle interventions to prevent diabetes in the China Da Qing Diabetes Prevention Study: A 20-year follow-up study. *Lancet* **371**: 1783–1789.
46. Lindstrom J, Ilanne-Parikka P, Peltonen M, *et al.* (2006) Sustained reduction in the incidence of type 2 diabetes by lifestyle intervention: Follow-up of the Finnish Diabetes Prevention Study. *Lancet* **368**: 1673–1679.
47. Kosaka K, Noda M, Kuzuya T. (2005) Prevention of type 2 diabetes by lifestyle intervention: A Japanese trial in IGT males. *Diabetes Res Clin Pract* **67**: 152–162.

48. Ramachandran A, Snehalatha C, Mary S, Mukesh B, Bhaskar AD, Vijay V. (2006) The Indian Diabetes Prevention Programme shows that lifestyle modification and metformin prevent type 2 diabetes in Asian Indian subjects with impaired glucose tolerance (IDPP-1). *Diabetologia* **49**: 289–297.
49. Ramachandran A, Snehalatha C. (2011) Diabetes prevention programs. *Med Clin North Am* **95**: 353–372, viii.
50. Kahn R. (2012) Reducing the impact of diabetes: Is prevention feasible today, or should we aim for better treatment? *Health Affairs* **31**: 76–83.
51. Zhuo X, Zhang P, Gregg EW, *et al.* (2012) A nationwide community-based lifestyle program could delay or prevent type 2 diabetes cases and save $5.7 billion in 25 years. *Health Aff (Millwood)* **31**: 50–60.
52. Chiasson JL, Josse RG, Gomis R, Hanefeld M, Karasik A, Laakso M. (2002) Acarbose for prevention of type 2 diabetes mellitus: The STOP-NIDDM randomised trial. *Lancet* **359**: 2072–2077.
53. Knowler WC, Hamman RF, Edelstein SL, Barrett-Connor E, *et al.* (2005) Prevention of type 2 diabetes with troglitazone in the Diabetes Prevention Program. *Diabetes* **54**: 1150–1156.
54. Gerstein HC, Yusuf S, Bosch J, *et al.* (2006) Effect of rosiglitazone on the frequency of diabetes in patients with impaired glucose tolerance or impaired fasting glucose: A randomised controlled trial. *Lancet* **368**: 1096–1105.
55. Li CL, Pan CY, Lu JM, *et al.* (1999) Effect of metformin on patients with impaired glucose tolerance. *Diabet Med* **16**: 477–481.
56. Mayo Clinic. Diabetes diet: Create your health-eating plan. http://www.mayoclinic.com/health/diabetes-diet/DA00027
57. Wing RR. (2010) Long-term effects of a lifestyle intervention on weight and cardiovascular risk factors in individuals with type 2 diabetes mellitus: Four-year results of the Look AHEAD trial. *Arch Intern Med* **170**: 1566–1575.
58. Look AHEAD Research Group, Wadden TA, West DS, *et al.* (2006) The Look AHEAD study: A description of the lifestyle intervention and the evidence supporting it. *Obesity* **14**: 737–752.
59. Gregg EW, Chen H, Wagenknecht LE, *et al.* (2012) Association of an intensive lifestyle intervention with remission of type 2 diabetes. *JAMA* **308**: 2489–2496.
60. Wing RR, Bolin P, Brancati FL, *et al.* (2013) Cardiovascular effects of intensive lifestyle intervention in type 2 diabetes. *N Engl J Med* **369**: 145–154.
61. TODAY study group. (2012) A clinical trial to maintain glycemic control in youth with type 2 diabetes. *N Engl J Med* **366**: 2247–2256.
62. Allen DB. (2012) TODAY — a stark glimpse of tomorrow. *N Engl J Med* **366**: 2315–2316.

63. WHO. The Ottawa Charter for Health Promotion (1986) http://www.who.int/healthpromotion/conferences/previous/ottawa/en/index1.html#
64. Let's Move. Incorporate Nutrition and Physical Education into the curriculum. http://www.letsmove.gov/incorporate-nutrition-education-physical-education-curriculum
65. Thaler RH, Sunstein CR. (2009) *Nudge*. Penguin Books, London.
66. Sunstein CR. (2013) *Simpler*. Simon & Schuster, New York.
67. Volpp KG, John LK, Troxel AB, *et al.* (2008) Financial incentive-based approaches for weight loss: a randomized trail. *JAMA* **300**: 2631–2637.
68. Volpp KG, Troxel AB, Pauly MV, *et al.* (2009) A randomized, controlled trial of financial incentives for smoking cessation. *N Eng J Med* **360**: 699–709.
69. Loewenstein G, Asch DA, Volpp KG. (2013) Behavioral economics holds potential to deliver better results for patients, insurers and employers. *Health Aff* **32**: 1244–1250.
70. Berman J. (2013) CVS to penalize workers who don't disclose weight, body fat. *Huffington Post*. http://www.huffingtonpost.com/2013/03/20/cvs-workers-insurance_n_2915006.html
71. Aon Hewitt. (2013) Aun Hewitt survey highlights important role of incentives in US employers' efforts to improve workforce health and performance. http://aon.mediaroom.com/2013-03-25-Aon-Hewitt-Survey-Highlights-Important-Role-of-Incentives-in-U-S-Employers-Efforts-to-Improve-Workforce-Health-and-Performance
72. Swinburn BA, Sacks G, Hall KD, *et al.* (2011) The global obesity pandemic: Shaped by global drivers and local environments. *Lancet* **378**: 804–814.
73. Mozaffarian Dm Afshin A, Benowitz NL, *et al.* (2012) Population approaches to improve diet, physical activity, and smoking habits: A scientific statement from the American Heart Association. *Circulation* **126**: 1514–1563.
74. WHO. (2010) Global Nutrition Policy Review: What does it take to scale up nutrition action? http://apps.who.int/iris/bitstream/10665/84408/1/9789241505529_eng.pdf
75. *The Economist* (2012) Denmark's food taxes: A fat chance. http://www.economist.com/news/europe/21566664-danish-government-rescinds-its-unwieldy-fat-tax-fat-chance
76. WHO. Set of 9 voluntary global NCD targets for 2025. http://www.who.int/nmh/global_monitoring_framework/gmf1_large.jpg
77. Produce for Better Health Foundation. 2010 gap analysis: How federal spending falls short of addressing public health needs. http://www.pbhfoundation.org/pdfs/about/res/pbh_res/2010gapanalysis.pdf

78. USDA. (2013) Specialty Crop Block Grant Program — Farm Bill. http://www.ams.usda.gov/AMSv1.0/ams.fetchTemplateData.do?template=TemplateN&rightNav1=SpecialtyCropBlockGrant0Program&topNav=&leftNav=CommodityAreas&page=SCBGP&resultType
79. FORESIGHT Report. (2002) *Tackling Obesities: Future Choices — Project Report*, 2nd ed. Government Office for Science, http://www.bournemouth.gov.uk/PlanningBuildings/Planning/Policy/Local-Plan/CoreStrategy/CoreStrategyFiles/SubmissionFiles/BackgroundDocs/Websiteversions/3-17-TacklingObesitiesFutureChoices.pdf, accessed April 30, 2013.

Chapter 7: Global Health and Governmental Policies in Diabetes Prevention

Jean Claude Mbanya and Renee Bowers†*

1. INTRODUCTION

Diabetes and other noncommunicable diseases (NCDs) have been silent global killers for many decades. Recently, the silence was broken when global advocacy efforts brought noncommunicable diseases to the fore, demanding international attention and action. Besides diabetes, NCDs consist of cancer, cardiovascular disease, and chronic respiratory disease. They are united not only by their contribution to mortality but also by common behavioral risk factors, including unhealthy eating, physical inactivity, smoking, and harmful use of alcohol.[1] This chapter will describe global advocacy efforts to bring diabetes and noncommunicable diseases to the global stage, the success achieved to date, and demonstrate why this important work must continue. Additionally, the importance of prevention and the pivotal role of governments and policy will be highlighted as their actions impact the way forward for the diabetes and NCD epidemics the world is facing.

2. GLOBAL BURDEN OF DIABETES AND NONCOMMUNICABLE DISEASES

Noncommunicable diseases (NCDs) caused an estimated 36 million deaths in 2008 and are the leading cause of death globally. Of the deaths, 80%

*Corresponding author. Biotechnology Center, Faculty of Medicine and Biomedical Sciences, University of Yaounde I, Yaounde, Cameroon. Email: jcmbanya@yahoo.co.uk
†Chronic Disease Consultant, Ottawa, Ontario, Canada

occur in low- to middle-income countries (LMICs). Moreover, they affect the young, with 29% of deaths occurring in those under the age of 60. This is more than double the rate of 13% found in high-income countries. NCD rates are expected to rise by an average of 15% globally between 2010 and 2020, with the greatest increase expected in the World Health Organization (WHO) regions of Africa, South East Asia, and the Mediterranean where an increase of 20% is predicted. In fact, by 2030, NCDs are expected to surpass communicable, maternal, perinatal disease, and nutrition-related disease as a cause of death.[2]

The International Diabetes Federation (IDF) Atlas figures showed that diabetes has the most staggering effect when separated from other NCDs. In 2012, more than 371 million people had diabetes; by 2030 this is expected to rise to 552 million people. Of the people with diabetes, 80% will be living in LMICs. What is more alarming is that we are only realizing part of the picture as half of those with diabetes, approximately 183 million people, are undiagnosed. The effect of this epidemic is being realized mostly in LMICs as they harbor three out of four cases of diabetes. The presence of diabetes means more people are not just living with diabetes, but are also dying from the devastating complications. In 2011, 4.7 million people died due to diabetes.[3]

The human toll is not the only impact of NCDs. The combined economic losses in LMICs from the four major NCDs are estimated to exceed $7 trillion from the period 2011–2025 (an average of $50 billion per year). For diabetes alone, more than $471 billion per year is spent, representing approximately 11% of total health care expenditures in adults.[3]

On a per person basis, the annual losses amount to an average of $25 in a low-income country, $50 million in a middle-income country and $139 in an upper middle-income country. In fact, of all the NCDs, diabetes can thrust, and will certainly keep individuals, in poverty due to the cost of medications and supplies required to manage their disease.[3–5]

Both the human and economic cost demand an urgent need for action and demonstrate the integral link between development and diabetes and NCDs. The combined human and economic toll of diabetes and NCDs created the impetus for international attention and a sense of urgency for international action.

3. GLOBAL HEALTH, DIABETES, AND NONCOMMUNICABLE DISEASES

One of the main venues for bringing attention to global health issues is through United Nations (UN) processes, namely the Millennium Development Goals (MDGs). The Millennium Project was commissioned by the United Nations Secretary-General in 2002 to develop a concrete action plan for the world to achieve the MDGs and to reverse the grinding poverty, hunger, and disease affecting billions of people.[5] MDGs aim was to encourage development by improving social and economic conditions in the world's poorest countries. The first set of MDGs focused on the eradication of poverty, improving maternal health, strengthening health systems, and reducing infectious diseases such as HIV/AIDS, tuberculosis, and malaria.[5] While substantive efforts have been made in achieving these goals, the success has been hampered by factors affecting development including the very presence of diabetes and NCDs.

The specific effects of diabetes and the current MDGs has been brought to international attention in the International Diabetes Federation Atlas. This report provided the evidence that diabetes is also an issue of poverty, is related to gender inequality, and can be a threat to maternal and child health due to uncontrolled diabetes and pregnancy, possibly compromising the health of the mother and child and even result in death. Finally, diabetes and infectious diseases such as HIV/AIDS and tuberculosis are inextricably linked as the presence of these infectious diseases increases the risk of developing diabetes.[3]

Diabetes and NCDs were not considered as part of the health goals for the first set of MDGs. This was in part due to the myriad of myths surrounding diabetes and NCDs and their associated risk factors. The myths consisted of diabetes and NCDs being diseases of wealth and not poverty, that they were primarily diseases of older age, and were caused by individual lifestyle choices. In LMICs, it was erroneously believed that actions were (i) unnecessary as the burden was not high, (ii) not affordable, (iii) unattainable due to lack of health and physical resources, and (iv) inappropriate as resources needed to address diabetes and NCDs would have to be diverted from other areas. The lack of leadership and the sense of competing priorities were also issues. Policymakers and governments perceived they had to choose between the double burden of communicable and NCDs. These choices seemed impossible in an already overburdened health system. These myths resulted in a lack of action in LMICs that were needed to address diabetes and NCDs.[6]

The global community started to mobilize around diabetes in 2006, through the United Nations Resolution 61/225 on Diabetes.[7] This resolution was the beginning of governments acknowledging that diabetes was an epidemic and a serious global health threat. This UN resolution brought together over 195 IDF member associations who joined forces to unite for diabetes. Their efforts resulted in the World Diabetes Day, which continues to unite the global diabetes community on November 14 every year. The World Diabetes Day campaign is led by IDF. The first years of the campaign focussed on diabetes in the disadvantaged and the vulnerable in 2006, and diabetes in children and adolescents in 2007 and 2008. The current campaign has focused on the need for diabetes prevention and education since 2009.[8,9]

However, the actions leading up to this UN resolution made the global diabetes community realize that in order to fully realize the vision of the prevention of diabetes additional partners were required since diabetes shares common risk factors with other NCDs. Therefore, the actions required to achieve this vision involves multiple sectors. For global advocacy efforts to continue, the IDF joined with partners namely the Union for International Cancer Control, World Heart Federation, International Union against Tuberculosis and Lung Disease to form the NCD Alliance. Together these international nongovernmental organizations (NGOs) mobilized over 880 member associations and formed an international civil movement to advocate for NCDs, the NCD Alliance, which focused their efforts to create a global advocacy.[10]

In May 2010, a UN high-level meeting was announced and global advocacy efforts were increased. IDF led a series of discussion papers to bring attention on diabetes and the *Lancet* featured a series focusing on NCDs — not just on the size and importance of the issue — but also suggestions for solutions. Several IDF publications highlighted the need for action such as the Global Diabetes Plan and other advocacy materials. This was quite an important step as the meeting was a success but there had to be actions following the meeting.

In September 2011, the historical United Nations High Level Meeting on Non-communicable Diseases was held, which represented a turning point for addressing diabetes and NCDs and their corresponding risk factors. Not only did this meeting dispel many of the myths noted above, but it presented a forum for the global community to meet and discuss the issues and actions. International advocacy efforts culminated at this point when the General Assembly adopted the United Nations Resolution 66/10 titled the "Political Declaration of the High-level Meeting of the General Assembly on the Prevention and Control of Non-communicable Diseases."[10] UN declarations are important as they provide a framework for action and discussion related to necessary resources. They also provide the platform for governments to become accountable for actions. However, they are declarations of intent and not a guarantee of action. Therefore, while this meeting was historic in nature, it was one important step in a continuing journey toward actions to stem the current diabetes and NCD epidemic. The global advocacy efforts had to continue to make the outcomes of this meeting a reality.

3.1. The Global Response to the Diabetes and Noncommunicable Disease Epidemic

The global community has responded positively to the call for action on diabetes and NCDs. The pivotal meeting in September 2011 demonstrated there was consensus that diabetes and NCDs constitute a major challenge for development and threaten the achievement of the current MDGs. The political declaration issued a clear call for integrating diabetes and NCD policies and programs into health planning processes of the member states. The political declaration included 22 political commitments to global action on diabetes and NCDs and shifted the responsibility to governments. Most importantly, this document was the beginning of committing governments to setting targets and indicators towards diabetes and NCDs.

In May 2012, the World Health Organization's 65th World Health Assembly (WHA) agreed to the first voluntary global targets for a 25% reduction in premature mortality from NCDs by 2025.[11] Subsequently, in November 2012, nine global targets (see Table 1) and 25 indicators (see

Table 1. Voluntary global targets for noncommunicable diseases.

1. A 25% relative reduction in the overall mortality from cardiovascular diseases, cancers, diabetes or chronic respiratory diseases
2. At least 10% relative reduction in the harmful use of alcohol, as appropriate, within the national context
3. A 10% relative reduction in prevalence of insufficient physical activity
4. A 30% relative reduction in mean population intake of salt/sodium
5. A 30% relative reduction in current tobacco use in person aged 15+ years
6. A 25% relative reduction in the prevalence of raised blood pressure or contain the prevalence of raised blood pressure, according to national circumstances
7. Halt the rise in diabetes and obesity
8. At least 50% of eligible people receive drug therapy and counseling (including glycemic control) to prevent heart attack and strokes
9. An 80% availability of the affordable basic technologies and essential medicines, including generics, required to treat major noncommunicable diseases in both public and private facilities

Table 2) were agreed upon and subsequently adopted in May 2013 by the World Health Assembly.

Preventing diabetes and NCDs became a focal point and this was reflected in the outcomes and indicators for the WHO Global Action Plan for the Prevention and Control of Non-communicable Diseases 2013–2020.[12] Historically, governments agreed to halt the rise in obesity and diabetes by 25% and agreed to targets on primary prevention such as alcohol, tobacco, salt, and physical inactivity and secondary prevention through drug therapy and counseling. The most lifesaving of all targets is the 80% availability of essential medicines. This will not only save lives but improve the quality of life through decreasing further complications of diabetes.[1] The agreed upon indicators will track mortality and morbidity, assess progress in addressing risk factors, and evaluate the implementation of national strategies and plans.[12]

The indicators are based on the World Health Organization's set of best buys. Best buys are interventions that are cost-effective and have the possibility of being implemented in LMICs.[4] The best buys range from population health measures such as taxation on tobacco, advertising bans on alcohol, nutrition policies to reduce sodium and fats, and promoting physical activity. Other suggestions include improving access to medication and improved screening of lesions for cancer among others. The total

Table 2. Global indicators for noncommunicable diseases.

Target	Indicator
1	1. Unconditional probability of dying between ages 30 and 70 years from cardiovascular diseases, cancer, diabetes or chronic respiratory diseases 2. Cancer incidence, by type of cancer per 100,000 population
2	3. Age standardized prevalence of current tobacco use among person aged 15+ years 4. Prevalence of current tobacco use among adolescents
3	5. Age-standardized prevalence of insufficiently active persons aged 18+ years (defines as less than 150 min of moderate-intensity activity per week, or equivalent) 6. Prevalence of insufficiently physically active adolescents defined as less than 60 min of moderate to vigorous intensity activity daily
4	7. Total (recorded and unrecorded) alcohol per capita (15+ years old) consumption within a calendar year in litres of pure alcohol as appropriate within the national context 8. Age-standardized prevalence of heavy episodic drinking among (adolescents and adults) as appropriate, within the national context 9. Alcohol-related morbidity and mortality among adolescents and adults, as appropriate within the national context
5	10. Age-standardized mean population intake of salt (sodium chloride) per day in grams persons aged 18+
6	11. Age-standardized prevalence of raised blood pressure among persons aged 18+ years (defined as systolic blood pressure >140 mmHg and/or diastolic blood pressure >90 mmHg)
7	12. Age-standardized prevalence of raised blood glucose/diabetes among adults aged 18+ years (defined as fasting plasma glucose value ≥7.0 mmol/L (126 mg/dL) or on medication for raised blood glucose) 13. Age-standardized prevalence of overweight and obesity in adults aged 18+ years (defined as body mass index greater than 25 kg/m^2 for overweigh or 30 kg/m^2 for obesity) 14. Prevalence of overweight and obesity in adolescents (defined according to the WHO Growth Reference, overweight- one standard deviation BMI for age and sex and obese-two standard deviations body mass index for age and sex)

(Continued)

Table 2. *(Continued)*

Target	Indicator
Additional indicators under risk factors	15. Age-standardized prevalence of adult (aged 18+ years) population consuming less than five total servings (400 g) of fruit and vegetables per day 16. Age-standardized prevalence of raised total cholesterol among persons aged 18+ years (defined as total cholesterol ≥ 5.0 mmol/L or 190 mg/dL) and mean total cholesterol 17. Age-standardized mean proportion of total energy intake from saturated fatty acids in persons aged 18+ years.
8	18. Availability and affordability of quality, safe and efficacious essential NCD medicines, including generics, and basic technologies in both public and private facilities Drug therapy to prevent heart attack and stroke
9	19. Proportion of eligible persons (defined as aged 40 years and over with a 10-year cardiovascular risk greater than or equal to 30% including those with existing cardiovascular disease) receiving drug therapy and counseling (including glycemic control) to prevent heart attacks and strokes
Additional indicators under National Systems Response	20. Access to palliative care assessed by morphine-equivalent consumption of strong opioid analgesics (excluding methadone) per death from cancer 21. Proportion of women between the ages of 30–49 screened for cervical cancer at least once, or more often, and for lower or higher age groups according to national programs or policies 22. Adoption of national policies that limit saturated fatty acids and virtually eliminate partially hydrogenated vegetable oils in the food supply as appropriate within the national context and national programs 23. Policies to reduce the impact on children of marketing on foods and nonalcoholic beverages high in saturated fats, trans fatty acids, free sugars, or salt 24. Vaccination coverage against hepatitis B virus monitored by number of third doses of Hep-B vaccine (HepB3) administered to infants 25. Availability, as appropriate, of cost-effective, affordable, of HPV vaccines, according to national programs and policies

Source: WHO Global Action Plan for the Prevention and Control of Non-communicable Diseases, 2013–2020.

cost of implementing the full suggested set of best buy interventions across all LMICs is estimated to be $170 billion, at an average of $11.4 billion per year. Per person this comes to under $1 in low-income countries, $1.50 in lower middle-income, and $3 in upper middle-income countries.[4] While they are demonstrated to be cost-effective and feasible to implement, the actions require political will to develop a strong policy and support implementation. This is often where there are conflicting interests and reduced capacity to develop the policies required to guide action on a national level. However, actions cannot be achieved without strong policies to set the course.

3.2. The Need for Governmental Policies in Diabetes Prevention

The Political Declaration of the High Level Meeting of the General Assembly on the Prevention and Control of Non-communicable Diseases stated that "prevention is the cornerstone of the global response to non-communicable disease"(paragraph 34) and to achieve this, a "whole of government" and "whole of society effort" are required.[10] This is particularly relevant when focusing on prevention of NCDs, namely diabetes.

Strong policies are required at the country level to guide action from the national to local level to address both the risk factors and management of diabetes. Policies need to focus on all levels of prevention — primordial, primary, secondary, and tertiary as these types of activities mutually support chronic disease prevention and management efforts. Primordial prevention aims to establish healthy environments where people live and decrease the risk of disease. This is usually the purview of policy and health promotion. Primary prevention aims to protect health through personal and community-based efforts and is usually the focus of public health interventions. Secondary prevention aims to provide early detection and interventions and tertiary prevention strives to minimize the impact of the established disease on the person's quality of life. Essentially when viewed as a mutually supportive effort, people have the conditions to be healthy, understand and act upon their risk, and manage their condition.[13] The importance of primary prevention cannot be minimized as the WHO estimates that approximately 80% of NCDs could be avoided if people changed risky behaviors. In the developing world alone that could lead to 6 million avoided deaths.[1] Secondary and tertiary prevention interventions are equally important as they strive to reduce the burden of the disease, through promoting management and treatment to minimize progression and maintain quality of life.[14,15]

The call for this broad approach is related to the key drivers, namely economic growth, globalization, and unplanned urbanization, responsible for the increase in both risk factors and prevalence of diabetes and NCDs. Globally, NCDs, especially diabetes, have a more severe impact on the poor and as a result require a policy context to alleviate this effect.[16,17] The drivers of diabetes and NCDs necessitate that policies to prevent diabetes and NCDs must also be present outside of health and are a key consideration in other public policy domains such as transportation, agriculture, education and finance, social services, and trade.[10] They must be structured to support both population level intervention and strengthen health systems to promote equity.

It is imperative to understand that primary prevention cannot be the focus while neglecting management; nor can the reverse be considered an option. This is particularly relevant for diabetes and NCDs where it is known that exposure to risk throughout the life course has a cumulative effect.[18] To minimize risk through addressing risk factors, the appropriate positive environment must be present to ensure promoting and facilitating living a healthy lifestyle. Otherwise, providing health education in a context where it cannot be actualized is nothing more than an exercise in futility and sets up the person to fail when the failure is a reflection of the system and not the person.

To direct policies, the Global Strategy for the Prevention and Control of Non-communicable Disease 2013–2020 can serve as the basis for action. Further to this, specific actions for risk factor reduction can be guided by frameworks such as the World Health Organization Framework Convention on Tobacco Control,[19] the World Health Organization Global Strategy on Diet, Physical Activity and Health,[20] and World Health Organization Global Strategy to reduce the Harmful use of Alcohol.[21] Complementary policies to address risk factors can ensure that they provide the opportunity for early detection and treatment of risk factors and disease.

3.3. What Does This Mean for Developing Countries?

The double burden of communicable and noncommunicable disease means action toward diabetes and NCDs is even more critical as it impedes outcomes of communicable disease. However, instead of being positioned as opposing entities and competing interests, they must be viewed in as complementary and integrated. This is essential as many of the countries have scarce resources directed toward health and require enhanced financing toward diabetes and NCDs.[6]

Strong policies must be present to direct financing. Many LMICs have not started to focus on policies to promote health. The WHO Country Cooperation's strategy demonstrated that few countries identified as LMIC have dedicated policies toward risk factors for diabetes and NCDs as well as established diabetes and NCDs.[22]

Within LMICs, 54% of countries have policy areas dedicated to tobacco, 62% related to harmful use of alcohol, 26% related to healthy eating, and 44% related to physical activity.[22] Specifically, in Sub-Saharan Africa, a review of published policies related to the World Health Organization Global Strategy on Diet, Physical Activity and Health in the African Region showed only about two-thirds of countries had incorporated actions to promote healthy diets and/or physical activity in their national policies.[23]

Policies and actions related to the risk factors for diabetes and NCDs can present a challenge to LMICs. Implementing some of the best buys as indicated by the World Health Organization, such as taxation on tobacco and alcohol, can result in increased lobbying efforts by these industries that are focused on these countries. Also, in some countries where tobacco is produced, policies poised to reduce their consumption can be viewed as an economic threat.

With respect to healthy foods, globalization of food contributes to a more homogenous and cheaper diet that can be available. However, it may not always provide the healthiest food choices. This contributes to malnutrition, which is the insufficient, excessive, or imbalanced consumption of nutrients and can result in obesity as well as underweight, still present in many developing countries. This contributes to the rising over and under nutrition paradox in developing countries. Physical activity can also pose a challenge due to pollution created by urbanization and competition for space to participate in physical activity. Political will and strong leadership are paramount to the introduction and implementation of policies to improve risk factors for diabetes and NCDs.[23,24]

Diabetes- and NCD-focused policies are also lacking. The World Health Organization Country Cooperation's strategy also identified that within LMICs, only 54% of countries had policies for diabetes and cardiovascular disease, 54% of countries had policies for cancer best buys, 39% of countries had a national NCD policy, and 32% had a NCD research policy.[22]

There is a great deal of work still required to develop and implement health system policies to support secondary and tertiary prevention and to ensure equity. Traditionally, health systems in LMICs have been structured to respond to acute instead of chronic conditions.[24] Chronic conditions require a continuum of interventions spanning from primary prevention to palliative care and responding to acute responses in between. However, achieving this can be a challenge in LMICs due to lack of universal health coverage, human resources, and equipment to conduct testing and diagnostic services.[25] This prevents the scalability of many of the major well-known interventions. To overcome these barriers, innovative ways of providing services have to be investigated including alternate delivery models, task shifting among health providers, and increasing lobbying to ensure universal coverage.[26]

3.4. Future Perspectives: What does this Mean for Diabetes and Noncommunicable Diseases?

Thus far we know that diabetes and NCDs are mostly preventable, prevention measures are affordable and there is hope to decrease the unbearable burden that is taking a toll on the human, economic, and social development of LMICs.

There are still unknowns as well. Some of these are related to practice such as how to address gaps in policies and competing health priorities influencing what can be implemented.[27] This necessitates a strong research agenda related to diabetes and NCDs that include: (i) research for placing diabetes and NCDs in the global development agenda and for monitoring diabetes and NCDs and their risk factors, (ii) intersectoral and multidisciplinary research to understand influences on the macroeconomic and social determinants of diabetes and NCDs and exposure to risk factors, (iii) translation and health system research for the global application of proven cost-effective strategies, and (iv) research to enable expensive but effective interventions to become accessible and used appropriately in resource-constrained settings.[27]

The major challenge remains outside of the health sector and rests with political will to further what is known about diabetes and NCDs and transform the polices that exist into achievable actions. This requires investment of resources — economic human and social — to promote equity and scalability of interventions, to prevent and manage NCDs, and to evaluate progress.

This political will can be increased through including diabetes and NCDs in the MDGs. We have seen the gains from other areas of health such as HIV/AIDS, Maternal Child Health and Tuberculosis through their inclusion in the MDGs. Currently, the international community is not able to respond to requests to support and implement diabetes and NCD policies and programs as the resources are not available.

4. CONCLUSION

Global awareness of diabetes has achieved great gains. Diabetes and NCDs are now acknowledged as one of the major challenges for development in the 21st century and there has been agreement on voluntary targets and indicators. What remains is to include diabetes and NCDs in the future MDGs, where actions are not voluntary, and to the discretion of national and political agendas.

We must remember that it is not voluntary for any person to develop diabetes or any noncommunicable disease. Susceptible individuals are often in a situation where the environments are either disease- or health-promoting and the resources are not always there to respond.

The vision in the World Health Organization Action Plan for the Prevention and Control of Non-communicable Disease 2013–2020 states, "there should be a world free of avoidable burden of non-communicable disease."[12] The international vision of IDF for diabetes "is a world free of diabetes." Until these visions are collectively achieved, global united advocacy efforts must continue.

REFERENCES

1. World Health Organization (2011) Global Status Report on Non-communicable Diseases. WHO, Geneva.
2. World Health Organization (2008) The Global Burden of Disease: 2004 update. WHO, Geneva.
3. http://www.idf.org/diabetesatlas/5e/the-global-burden accessed on August 29, 2012.
4. World Health Organization and World Economic Forum. (2011) From Burden to 'Best Buys': Reducing the economic impact of Non-Communicable Diseases in Low- and-Middle Income Countries. World Health Organization and World Economic Forum, Geneva. www.who.int/nmh/publications/best-buys- summary, last accessed August 29, 2012.
5. http://www.un.org/millenniumgoals/bkgd.shtml accessed August 29, 2012.
6. Knaul, F.M., Frenk, J, Shulman, L. for the Global Task Force on Expanded Access to Cancer Care and Control in Developing Countries. (2011) Closing the Cancer Divide: A Blueprint to Expand Access in Low and Middle Income Countries. Harvard Global Equity Initiative, Boston, MA, November.
7. United Nations Resolution adopted by the General assembly A/Res/61/25 http://www.un.org/en/ga/search/view_doc.asp?symbol=A/RES/61/225&Lang=E (accessed August 29, 2013).
8. http://www.idf.org/sites/default/files/UN%20Resolution%20on%20World%20Diabetes%20Day%20of%20Dec%202006.pdf (accessed August 29, 2013).
9. http://www.idf.org/worlddiabetesday/about (accessed August 29, 2013).
10. United Nations General Assembly, Political Declaration of the High-Level Meeting of the General Assembly on the Prevention and Control of Noncommunicable Diseases. (2011) http://www.un.org/ga/search/view_doc.asp?symbol+A/66/L.1 (accessed August 19, 2013).
11. Anne, G. (2012) World leaders agree to cut deaths from non-communicable disease by a quarter by 2025. *Br Med J* **344**: e3768.
12. World Health Assembly. (2013) Follow-up to the Political Declaration of the High-level Meeting of the General Assembly on the Prevention and Control of Non-communicable Diseases. Geneva. World Health Organization, WHA A66/10.
13. Last, J. (2001). *A Dictionary of Epidemiology*. Oxford University Press, New York.
14. World Health Report (2008) Primary Health Care-More now than ever. World Health Organization, Geneva.

15. McCoy D, Schand S, Sridhad D. (2009) Global health funding: How much, where it come from and where it goes. *Health Policy Plan* **24**: 407–417.
16. World Health Assembly. (2000) Global Strategy for the Prevention and Control of Non-communicable diseases (NDCDS). World Health Organization, Geneva. WHA A53/14.
17. Mendis S, Chestnov O. (2013) Policy reform to realize the commitments of the Political Declaration on non-communicable disease. *Br Med Bull* **105**: 7–27.
18. Hill I, Nishida C, James W. (2004) A life course approach to diet, nutrition and the prevention of chronic diseases. *Public Health Nutrit* **7**: 101–121.
19. World Health Organization (2003) WHO Framework Convention on Tobacco Control. World Health Organization, Geneva.
20. World Health Organization (2008) 2008–2013 action plan for the global strategy for the prevention and control of non-communicable diseases: Prevent and control cardiovascular diseases, cancers, chronic respiratory diseases and diabetes. World Health Organization, Geneva.
21. World Health Organization (2010) Global strategy to reduce the harmful use of alcohol. World Health Organization, Geneva.
22. World Health Organization. WHO Country Cooperation Strategy (CCS). www.who.int/country focus/cooperation_ strategy
23. Patterns and Determinants of Fruit and vegetable Consumption in sub-Saharan Africa A multicountry Comparison http://www.who.int/entity/dietphysicalactivity publications/F&v_africa_econimcs.pdf (19 August 2013, date last accessed.
24. World Health Organization. (2009) Package of Essential Non-communicable (WHO-PEN) Disease Interventions for Primary Health Care in Low resource Settings. World Health Organization, Geneva.
25. World Health Organization. (2011) Global Status report on Non-communicable disease 2010. World Health Organization, Geneva.
26. World Health Organization. (2011) Scaling up against non-communicable diseases: How much will it cost? World Health Organization and World Economic Forum, Geneva. www.who/int/nmh/publications/best_buys_summary (accessed August 19, 2013).
27. Mendis, S, Alwan A. eds. (2011) A prioritized research agenda for non-communicable disease. World Health Organization, Geneva.

Chapter 8: Infrastructure and Capacity for Diabetes Prevention in The United States

Mohammed K. Ali and Ann L. Albright*

1. INTRODUCTION

An estimated 26 million people in the United States have diabetes[1] and 90–95% of these have type 2 diabetes.[2] Nationally, diabetes is the number one cause of adult-onset blindness, kidney failure, and nontraumatic limb amputations, a significant contributor to cardiovascular disease, as well as the seventh leading cause of death.[3] Diabetes also has sizeable economic impacts. In 2012, diabetes was associated with $245 billion in health care expenditures and productivity losses in the United States[4] and over 60% of the direct medical costs were paid by government insurance programs (Medicare, Medicaid, and the Military). In fact, diabetes is the leading driver of growing Medicare[a] expenditures in the United States.[5] Growing medical costs are largely driven by the escalating incidence of diabetes, the long-standing need for medications to control glucose and co-morbidities like high cholesterol and high blood pressure for those affected, and hospital inpatient care for major clinical events (e.g., heart attacks).[4,5]

The absolute number of people in the United States who have diabetes grew 75% between national surveys in 1988–1994 (14.9 million) and 2005–2010 (26.1 million), largely on account of population aging and growing obesity prevalence (1). Diabetes is also expected to continue to

*Corresponding author. Email: mkali@emory.edu

[a]The US federal government insurance program that covers health and preventive services for people aged 65 and older and disabled individuals.

grow as an estimated 79 million Americans have prediabetes,[6] a precursor phase where blood glucose is higher than normal but not yet in the diagnostic range for diabetes. People with prediabetes have 5 to 12 times the risk of developing type 2 diabetes than people with normal blood glucose levels.[7]

There is robust evidence from large randomized controlled trials[8–10] that structured behavioral interventions that help individuals with prediabetes sustainably modify their lifestyles can prevent or at least delay the onset of diabetes. The processes involved in translating these important findings from controlled research studies to tangible programs for US adults with prediabetes have required inputs and efforts from a variety of stakeholders. The process of institutionalizing diabetes prevention into the complex US context and reaching the scale necessary to achieve population health benefits continues to require meaningful engagement from multiple sectors. In this chapter, we share experiences of building the US National Diabetes Prevention Program. We discuss the challenges and successes, in applying research findings regarding diabetes prevention into real-life practice for the diverse US population. We utilize a framework by Brownson and colleagues[11] to contextualize and situate the individual components of implementing diabetes prevention within this vast, complex, and fast-changing society.

2. DIABETES PREVENTION AS AN EXAMPLE OF EVIDENCE-BASED PUBLIC HEALTH

The pursuit of improving population health involves several important components. Brownson and colleagues propose that evidence-based policies and programs in medicine and public health[11] are built on the confluence of:

1. Understanding population needs and disease burdens
2. Existence of evidence-based interventions
3. Contextual adaptation and interdisciplinary perspectives
4. Appropriate human, financial, and infrastructural resources
5. Supportive environmental and policy contexts.

The case for wide-scale implementation of lifestyle change programs to prevent diabetes has been supported by evidence of large burdens inflicted by diabetes and prediabetes and existence of interventions, which have begun to motivate the mobilization of resources and policy support. Each of these aspects is discussed in greater detail, along with residual challenges that hinder progress in population-level diabetes prevention efforts.

2.1. Disease Burden

US national surveillance data unambiguously demonstrate a very high burden of prediabetes in the country, which fortells of even greater health and economic burdens due to diabetes in the near future. These data have helped accentuate the urgency to act by highlighting the impacts for a variety of stakeholders. For example, employers and insurance companies may view growing numbers of employees with diabetes as a sign of reduced productivity and high health care payments.[12] This is both a stimulus to reduce health care costs from these stakeholder perspectives, but may also have implications for discrimination in the work force.[13]

2.2. Evidence-Based Intervention

There is also strong evidence supporting intervention. The US Diabetes Prevention Program (DPP) study[8] was the largest of the efficacy studies[9,10] worldwide that evaluated lifestyle interventions to reduce diabetes incidence. The DPP randomized 3,234 overweight study participants who had prediabetes to an intensive structured lifestyle intervention, metformin, or placebo. The lifestyle intervention was aimed at stimulating and supporting high participant motivation to sustainably change their behavior patterns and maintain the changes. The intervention was also resource intensive. Participants received 16 one-on-one personalized lifestyle coaching sessions by individuals with extensive training in nutrition, exercise physiology, or behavioral psychology as well as in-person maintenance sessions once every two months and unlimited telephone contact between sessions. The intervention included meal replacements and provided access to exercise facilities. This structured intensive intervention resulted in a 58% cumulative reduction in diabetes incidence compared to placebo when the trial was stopped after 3.5 years. Effects were consistent across different age and ethnic groups. Importantly, without the intervention, people with prediabetes would continue to convert to having diabetes at high rates annually, incurring higher risk of end-organ complications and increasing health care costs with time.

The collateral and long-term benefits of the intervention are also noteworthy. Structured lifestyle change programs are associated with cardiovascular risk factor benefits, improving control of blood pressure and cholesterol.[14] Furthermore, the cumulative diabetes incidence in the original lifestyle intervention group remains 34% lower even 10 years after randomization even though the intervention was provided to the placebo and metformin study groups upon discontinuation of the randomized trial.[15]

Important insights have emerged from the study that laid a foundation for wide-scale implementation of lifestyle interventions to prevent diabetes. First, the DPP's package of lifestyle principles — 150 minutes of moderate physical activity per week, lower total calorie intake, and reducing fat intake in one's daily diet — offers an easy-to-convey set of lifestyle messages.[16,17] Second, the study showed that moderate weight loss — 5 to 7% of one's baseline weight — was an important factor in reducing diabetes incidence.[16] This offers another powerful messaging opportunity, that drastic weight reduction is not necessary to prevent diabetes in this high-risk population.[18,19] This also aligned with the literature[70] showing that drastic weight reduction is often unsustainable. Third, the study and many that followed demonstrate that populations at high-risk for diabetes (such as those with prediabetes) are the most likely to experience benefit from intervention.[35] In this group, detection and intervention are highly cost-effective.[20,21] Fourth, since the one-year cost to deliver this intervention was $1,399 per person,[22] it is unlikely to be adopted more widely in its original resource-intensive form. However, this has stimulated further research into seeking alternative lower-cost approaches or adopting delivery of lifestyle change interventions that nonetheless maintain the original program's effectiveness.

2.3. Contextual Adaptation

Since the 3.5-year findings of the DPP were presented in 2002, US government agencies have supported a variety of translation studies testing different adaptations of the DPP lifestyle intervention for real-life community and clinical settings.[23] Very few of these studies were designed with adequate sample size and duration of follow-up to demonstrate reductions in diabetes incidence, which is reasonable given that the DPP trial had already provided strong proof of principle. The adaptations, therefore, were focused on lowering costs, increasing appeal to diverse population subgroups (e.g., people of different ethnicities or living in different circumstances), and achieving weight reduction. The studies utilized group lifestyle sessions, which lowered the volume and total cost of health coaches needed. The type of health coaches varied from higher-cost medically trained personnel (formally trained physicians, nurses, nurse practitioners or case managers, educators, dietitian/nutritionists, exercise physiologists, or behavioral psychologists), to lower-cost lay volunteers, as well as the use of virtual media (online, telephonic, automated calls, or digital video) to deliver lifestyle intervention training and keep participants engaged. The choice of coach or session moderator was also aligned to the population preference and setting, which included clinical, community, religious, workplace, or home settings. To counter potential participant fatigue and attrition, some studies modified and delivered the lifestyle intervention training curriculum via a reduced number of sessions.

Aggregating 28 of these studies that were published by 2011, an average of 4 to 5% weight reduction from baseline was observed, and there was no significant difference in weight loss achieved by the type of intervention delivery approach (medically trained, lay worker, or virtual medium) used.[23] This finding remained similar when limited to studies with longer than 9 months of follow-up. Greater weight reduction was seen with higher number of sessions attended and there was no evidence of participant fatigue as the number of sessions offered correlated well with the number of sessions attended. More studies investigating different virtual methods of engagement are ongoing and include cable television delivery and online media where group dynamics of lifestyle change programs can be technologically simulated.

2.4. Human, Financial, and Infrastructure Resources

The United States has a market-based, multipayer health system. Revenue generation, coverage agreements, and reimbursement mechanisms are complex. In this context, there are many stakeholders who sometimes have competing interests. It is especially tough to integrate preventive services amid an abundance of curative services and complex coverage and reimbursement stipulations and systems.[24,25] As such, any significant change in this system requires collective resolve and action from numerous influential stakeholder groups.

In 2009, a meeting of federal government, nonprofit, state government officials, public and private payers, and academic representatives was convened to discuss wide-scale implementation of diabetes prevention lifestyle change programs to curtail growth of the diabetes epidemic. The combination of national surveillance data showing sizeable impending diabetes burdens and the body of work showing an effective and adaptable lifestyle intervention to forestall diabetes has been instrumental in motivating action to implement diabetes prevention more widely in the United States. At this 2009 meeting, some private payers (employers and insurance companies) had estimated that preemptive prevention may offer a significant opportunity to lower long-term health costs.[12] Also, translation studies were showing that the program could be effectively delivered by community-based organizations.[23,26,27] This heightened awareness and readiness from different stakeholder groups had reached a critical juncture, signaling a rare opportunity for decisive action. In particular, private payers like United Health Group and community organizations like the YMCA of the United States were among the first private payer and nonprofit community delivery organizations, respectively, to form a partnership.[28–30]

This signaled the start of a clinical-community-payer public–private partnership model (Fig. 1) to support the delivery of lifestyle change programs in geographically and financially accessible community infrastructure. This model involves government- and private sector–funded efforts to (1) build human resource capacity, specifically, training lay lifestyle coaches in motivational techniques and delivery of the lifestyle change curriculum; (2) deliver lifestyle change programs, which are both efficient and potentially sustainable[26,31]; and (3) increase program referrals and participation. This was supported in 2010 by the US Congress authorizing the Centers for Disease Control and Prevention (CDC) to establish a National Diabetes Prevention Program (PHSA, SEC 399 V-3 National Diabetes Prevention Program) (Fig. 2). Since quality of health and

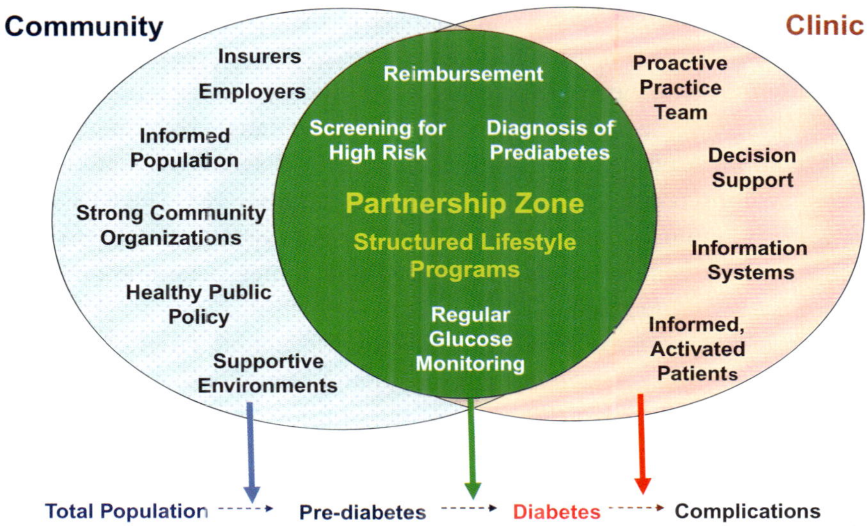

Fig. 1. The US community–clinic–payer–agency partnership model.

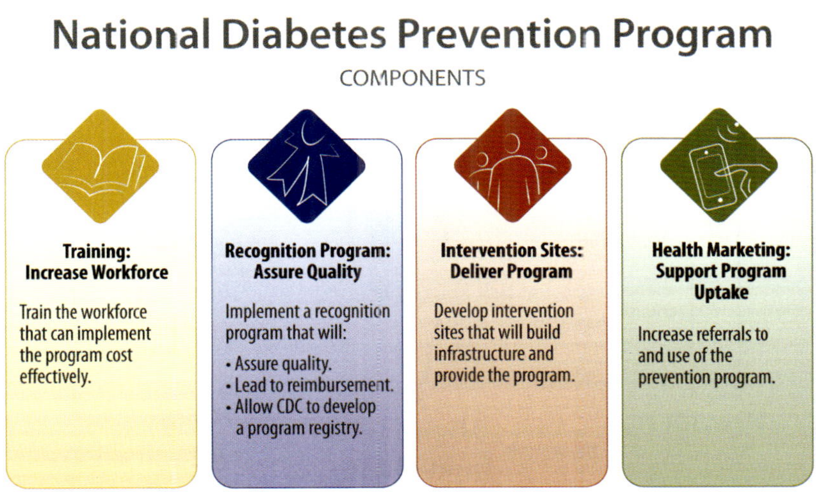

Fig. 2. Four pillars of Center for Disease Control and Prevention's Role in the US National Diabetes Prevention Program.

preventive services can vary considerably in the open market, standards were needed to protect users from asymmetries of information and maintain emphasis on cohesive expansion of the program. Using a process that included a public comment period, the CDC set standards to be met by organizations aspiring to be certified to deliver diabetes prevention services, assuring consistency and effectiveness of programs. The CDC recognition program provides technical assistance to organizations and also will become a centralized data repository and source regarding program performance and location.

In implementing the National Diabetes Prevention Program, a new infrastructure was created to link community-based program delivery organizations to insurance payers. In addition, there has been an emergence of intermediary organizations that provide services to both program delivery organizations and insurers/employers including technology, business processes, and participant identification, engagement, and enrollment (Fig. 3). To motivate goal achievement, some private payer groups have established processes for payment based on performance.

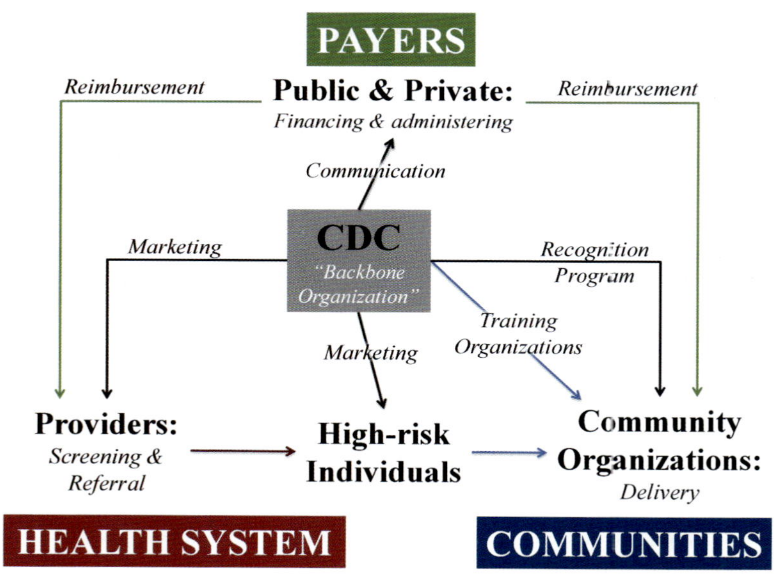

Fig. 3. Interactions among and between stakeholders in the US National Diabetes Prevention Program.

This new infrastructure allows organizations that were previously unable to participate in health care delivery and reimbursement to provide critical diabetes prevention services and interact with the traditional payers of health care services.

As has been demonstrated, although the name National Diabetes Prevention Program connotes an all-encompassing single institutional endeavor, it is actually an example of a collective impact initiative.[32] Collective impact is more than a partnership, or a network. It refers to the committed efforts of actors from different sectors that (1) share a common agenda, (2) are supported by shared measurement systems, (3) mutually reinforce each other's activities, (4) regularly communicate, and (5) have a backbone support organization.[32]

National diabetes prevention efforts in the United States have involved the collective efforts of many stakeholders that each contribute in their distinct areas of competency. No single organization or sector could develop and advance the diabetes prevention agenda alone; however, each of the organizations and sectors involved has the same understanding and has resolved to pursue a collaborative approach. Each actor's activities reinforce or are coordinated with those of other actors — for example, institutions offering diabetes prevention services can attract enrollees if these services are covered by payers while payer groups hope to benefit in the long-term by offsetting health care costs for high-risk individuals that would have converted to diabetes. Shared measurement also reinforces this collaboration as payers reimburse preventive service providers based on agreed-upon performance metrics like enrollee attendance and weight loss achieved. These metrics are the indicators that certified organizations providing diabetes prevention services are expected to report to the CDC, which serves as the coordinating backbone. Reporting these metrics is required to maintain an organization's federal certification. Various meetings and open communication among insurers, providers, third-party service providers, and the CDC have facilitated strengthening of relationships and adherence to the mission.

To date, the National Diabetes Prevention Program[33] has made significant strides but more work remains. Interest and involvement of private payers has energized growth in coverage for lifestyle change programs. Public payer groups are also evaluating the costs and feasibility of achieving health gains through lifestyle change programs. In addition, while there are community-based organizations delivering lifestyle change programs for diabetes prevention in almost all states and the District of Columbia, further expansion and reach of these programs is required to achieve higher accessibility.

2.5. Supportive Environments

Although the clearest evidence for how to prevent type 2 diabetes comes from studies conducted in high-risk adults, type 2 diabetes is often thought of as a common-source epidemic that is rooted in culture and society as much as in individual behaviors.[34] Several aspects of the etiology and evidence base of type 2 diabetes prevention suggest that approaches directed at both those at high-risk (prediabetes) and the whole population are necessary to make a major impact on the trends in the diabetes epidemic. Approaches directed to those at high-risk usually include screening and identification of people with a high probability of developing a condition.[35–37] This identification allows preventive services to be reserved for and directed to people most likely to benefit. A whole population approach aims to shift the entire distribution of a risk factor in a healthy direction, even if just by a small degree, to have a large effect on the proportion who develop disease. Opportunities to influence population risk target the food environment, the planning of communities, as well as social and economic factors.[38–42] While these broader whole population approaches are complementary to the more targeted high-risk approaches, additional evidence to better understand the impact of effective large-scale environmental changes is needed.

3. RESIDUAL CHALLENGES

Evidence from multiple trials around the world has shown that structured lifestyle programs are most effective and cost-effective in people at high-risk for diabetes. There are several challenges that continue to impede efforts to curtail the growth of diabetes and to achieve better health outcomes for people at-risk for diabetes. Addressing these obstacles will likely improve translation of the evidence-base into policy and practice implementation such that high-risk individuals will benefit and population health might improve.

3.1. Challenge 1: Identification of High-Risk Individuals

Among people with impaired glucose tolerance in the DPP study, those achieving improved beta-cell function and even transient regression to normal glucose levels experienced lower conversion to diabetes.[43] However, since early phases of dysglycemia (prediabetes and early diabetes) are asymptomatic and can only be confirmed objectively via blood glucose measurements,[44,45] 90% of those with prediabetes[46] and a quarter of those with blood glucose levels in the diabetes range in the United States are unaware of their status.[1,2] Despite these awareness gaps and despite continued growth of diabetes and prediabetes burdens in the United States,[1,6] screening for both of these conditions continues to be debated.

Current screening guidelines from expert groups [e.g., US Preventive Services Task Force (USPSTF) and American Diabetes Association (ADA)] provide divergent recommendations. Based on USPSTF recommendations, almost half of those with dysglycemia would get overlooked for glucose testing. This is an important missed opportunity as prediabetes is progressive and earlier intervention may be beneficial.[29,47] Offering earlier lifestyle modification to the intervention group compared to the metformin and control groups in the DPP Outcomes Study continues to have incremental benefits (34% lower cumulative incidence of diabetes, less need for medications, as well as better hypertension and lipid control).[15] In contrast, the ADA guidelines have a lower threshold for recommending glucose testing and potentially lead to overtesting and a low yield among those tested, which is inefficient. Fortunately, other potential harms of overtesting (e.g., pain, some anxiety) tend to be minimal and diminish with time.[36,48–51]

There is some hope that multistage screening — using risk score questionnaires or calculators — can be used fairly successfully to narrow in on those that are eligible for blood tests and reduce testing costs and inefficiencies.[52,53] Increasingly, nonlaboratory risk scores and algorithms (based on the combination of age, BMI, family history, other CVD risk factors) are being used to query health information technology databases, insurance claims data, and employee databases to identify those that should be offered blood testing or health promotion interventions.[54,55] In addition, this aspect of risk identification also highlights the importance of increasing awareness about diabetes risk across the population and among care providers that advise patients about testing.

3.2. Challenge 2: Successful Outcomes Depend on End-User Engagement and Support

Sustained lifestyle modification, at its core, requires behavior change.[56] This is not an easy proposition and involves continued engagement and varied strategies to adopt and maintain positive lifestyle behaviors.[57,58]

First, awareness, perceived risk, motivation, and financial accessibility all influence the likelihood of an individual enrolling into a lifestyle modification program. Identifying and communicating risk is important as 71–82% of those advised actually attempt to adopt lifestyle modifying behaviors.[46] A number of population-wide and focused (e.g., to health care provider groups) awareness efforts as well as health system advances (e.g., refinement of screening guidelines and consensus among public and private payers on coverage) are important aspects of increasing enrollment among high-risk individuals. In addition, understanding what informational and esthetic aspects appeal to consumers, through focus groups and other marketing research avenues, may yield more meaningful approaches.

Second, successfully delaying diabetes onset requires sustained adherence to lifestyle principles and weight management. As with most preventive interventions, health benefits for the individual accrue gradually and are often not immediately evident.[25] Lifestyle session counselors have an important role to play here in instilling a long-term perspective and supporting eligible candidates through the peaks and troughs of behavior change. Equipping lifestyle coaches with motivational interviewing skills and incentivizing performance based on the outcomes of their class enrollees may yield positive outcomes. Attention must also be given to tailoring behavior change for different sociodemographic (e.g., race/ethnicity, cultures) and personality subgroups in the population (e.g., those who prefer technology versus in-person engagement).

Further research is needed to improve our awareness and implementation efforts. Implementation research involves identifying, understanding, and addressing the barriers to adoption and maintenance of evidence-based care and prevention interventions (tools, treatments, policies, and guidelines).[59,60] Practice- and policy-oriented research of this nature can provide greater understanding of behaviors and motivations of end-users, and help us understand the resources and stakeholders needed to sustainably implement these interventions in diverse settings.[61] Importantly, we need to understand the *process* of scaling up. Successfully achieving wide-scale implementation involves learning the processes through which "early adopter" stakeholders become increasingly skillful and committed to using an intervention and assimilating it into their routine structures and functioning.[62–64] Assimilating data on costs, acceptability, and effectiveness[65,66] can also be helpful in achieving sustainable resources and policies for diabetes prevention.[67] The National Diabetes Prevention Program's data repository will have an important role to play here, providing key data about processes and outcomes.

3.3. Challenge 3: Return on Investment (ROI)

Prevention requires long-term vision for those enrolled in programs, but also for those financing the program as the health and economic gains (or rather, cost offsets) are realized over several years. In the competitive health care sector in the US, insurance companies are accountable to their shareholders and have to demonstrate rapid returns for investing in prevention. The literature suggests that, from a payer's perspective, structured lifestyle modification is and remains cost-effective at 10 years following randomization.[21] Nearly all studies found lifestyle intervention to prevent diabetes to be cost-effective or cost-saving[68]; however, the reported cost-effectiveness ratio or the ROI varies.[69] It is challenging to justify the investment when an institution or corporation may have to incur all the fixed costs up front and then the time horizon to breaking even or even accruing gains may be long. The break-even time horizon varies based on the volume and characteristics of enrollees (e.g., engagement, risk level, etc.)

as well as the intensity of the intervention and durability of the intervention effect and cost model used (e.g. pay-for-performance). As data from the national program become available, estimated ROI will be an important gauge of the sustainability of diabetes prevention initiatives that are financed by corporations and the public sector.

4. CONCLUDING REMARKS AND FUTURE DIRECTIONS

The existing and projected burden of diabetes requires that efforts to prevent diabetes be implemented on a large scale. The strongest evidence for the prevention of type 2 diabetes is among those at high-risk and involves using a structured lifestyle intervention that addresses nutrition, physical activity, and behavior change strategies to achieve moderate weight loss. Translation studies have demonstrated that lifestyle intervention can be delivered more cost-effectively and achieve similar weight loss.[23]

In response to the growing incidence of type 2 diabetes and the body of evidence supporting prevention, Congress authorized the CDC to establish the National Diabetes Prevention Program. The National Diabetes Prevention Program includes workforce training, quality assurance through program recognition, effective program delivery and payment models, and health marketing to increase program uptake necessary for reducing the incidence of type 2 diabetes.[48]

In many respects, the inherent challenges and barriers of the US context helped shape the current national program. The complicated context of interacting payers, policymakers, providers, and user stakeholders in US health and preventive services necessitated bringing together multiple stakeholders to invest their human, infrastructural, and financial resources toward a collective goal. To confront a complex multifactorial disease like diabetes within the US context, a single organization would have had limited impact; there are nearly 1.4 million nonprofit organizations in the United States that often work on their own to find solutions to major health and social problems.[32] It was the need for lower cost lifestyle program delivery mechanisms that led to government research investments and translation studies piloting innovative adaptation options.[23] Also, to implement these findings more widely to achieve real public health impact and reduce diabetes incidence, leading stakeholders and institutions had to convene and agree that the existing evidence was sufficient to act upon. Expansion of the program is now focused on achieving pervasive and sustainable intervention delivery.

Disclosure: The findings and conclusions in this chapter are those of the authors and do not necessarily represent the official position of the Centers for Disease Control and Prevention.

REFERENCES

1. Cheng YJ, Imperatore G, Geiss LS, Wang J, Saydah SH, Cowie CC, *et al.* (2013) Secular changes in the age-specific prevalence of diabetes among U.S. adults: 1988–2010. *Diabetes Care* Epub 2013/05/03.
2. Centers for Disease Control and Prevention. (2012) Diabetes Report Card 2012. CDC, Atlanta, GA.
3. Centers for Disease Control and Prevention. (2011) National diabetes fact sheet: national estimates and general information on diabetes and prediabetes in the United States, 2011. CDC, Atlanta, GA.
4. Anon (2013) Economic costs of diabetes in the U.S. in 2012. *Diabetes Care* **36**: 1033–1046. Epub 2013/03/08.
5. Thorpe KE, Ogden LL, Galactionova K. (2010) Chronic conditions account for rise in Medicare spending from 1987 to 2006. *Health Aff (Millwood)* **29**: 718–724. Epub 2010/02/20.
6. Bullard KM, Saydah SH, Imperatore G, Cowie CC, Gregg EW, Geiss LS, *et al.* (2013) Secular changes in U.S. prediabetes prevalence defined by hemoglobin A1c and fasting plasma glucose: National health and nutrition examination surveys, 1999–2010. *Diabetes Care* **36**: 2286–2293. Epub 2013/04/23.
7. Gerstein HC, Santaguida P, Raina P, Morrison KM, Balion C, Hunt D, *et al.* (2007) Annual incidence and relative risk of diabetes in people with various categories of dysglycemia: A systematic overview and meta-analysis of prospective studies. *Diabetes Res Clin Pract* **78**: 305–312. Epub 2007/07/03.
8. Knowler WC, Barrett-Connor E, Fowler SE, Hamman RF, Lachin JM, Walker EA, *et al.* (2002) Reduction in the incidence of type 2 diabetes with lifestyle intervention or metformin. *N Engl J Med* **346**: 393–403. Epub 2002/02/08.

9. Tuomilehto J, Lindstrom J, Eriksson JG, Valle TT, Hamalainen H, Ilanne-Parikka P, *et al.* (2001) Prevention of type 2 diabetes mellitus by changes in lifestyle among subjects with impaired glucose tolerance. *N Engl J Med* **344**: 1343–1350. Epub 2001/05/03.
10. Li G, Zhang P, Wang J, Gregg EW, Yang W, Gong Q, *et al.* The long-term effect of lifestyle interventions to prevent diabetes in the China Da Qing Diabetes Prevention Study: A 20-year follow-up study. *Lancet* **371**: 1783–1789. Epub 2008/05/27.
11. Brownson RC, Fielding JE, Maylahn CM. (2009) Evidence-based public health: A fundamental concept for public health practice. *Annu Rev Public Health* **30**: 175–201. Epub 2009/03/20.
12. United Health Center for Health Reform and Modernization. (2010) The United States of Diabetes: Challenges and opportunities in the decade ahead. November [cited 2013 August]; Available from: http://www.unitedhealth-group.com/hrm/unh_workingpaper5.pdf.
13. Anderson JW, Konz EC, Frederich RC, Wood CL. (2001) Long-term weight-loss maintenance: A meta-analysis of US studies. *Am J Clin Nutr* **74**: 579–584. Epub 2001/10/31.
14. Uusitupa M, Peltonen M, Lindström J, Aunola S, Ilanne-Parikka P, Keinänen-Kiukaanniemi S, *et al.* (2009) Ten-year mortality and cardiovascular morbidity in the Finnish Diabetes Prevention Study — Secondary analysis of the randomized trial. *PLoS One* **4**: e5656.
15. Diabetes Prevention Program Research G. (xxxx) 10-year follow-up of diabetes incidence and weight loss in the Diabetes Prevention Program Outcomes Study. *Lancet* **374**: 1677–1686.
16. Hamman RF, Wing RR, Edelstein SL, Lachin JM, Bray GA, Delahanty L, *et al.* (2006) Effect of weight loss with lifestyle intervention on risk of diabetes. *Diabetes Care* **29**: 2102–2107. Epub 2006/08/29.
17. Peters E, Dieckmann N, Dixon A, Hibbard JH, Mertz CK. (2007) Less is more in presenting quality information to consumers. *Med Care Res Rev MCRR* **64**: 169–190.
18. Wing RR, Hill JO. (2001) Successful weight loss maintenance. *Annu Rev Nutrition* **21**: 323–341. Epub 2001/05/26.
19. Clinical Guidelines on the Identification, Evaluation, and Treatment of Overweight and Obesity in Adults — The Evidence Report. (1998) National Institutes of Health. *Obes Res* **6**: 51S–209S. Epub 1998/11/14.
20. Herman WH, Hoerger TJ, Brandle M, Hicks K, Sorensen S, Zhang P, *et al.* (2005) The cost-effectiveness of lifestyle modification or metformin in

preventing type 2 diabetes in adults with impaired glucose tolerance. *Ann Intern Med* **142**: 323–332. Epub 2005/03/02.

21. Group TDPPR. (2012) The 10-Year Cost-effectiveness of lifestyle intervention or metformin for diabetes prevention: An intent-to-treat analysis of the DPP/DPPOS. *Diabetes Care* **35**: 723–730.
22. Hernan WH, Brandle M, Zhang P, Williamson DF, Matulik MJ, Ratner RE, *et al.* (2003) Costs associated with the primary prevention of type 2 diabetes mellitus in the diabetes prevention program. *Diabetes Care* **26**: 36–47. Epub 2002/12/28.
23. Ali MK, Echouffo-Tcheugui J, Williamson DF. (2012) How effective were lifestyle interventions in real-world settings that were modeled on the Diabetes Prevention Program? *Health Aff (Millwood)* **31**: 67–75. Epub 2012/01/11.
24. Williamson DF, Marrero DG. (2010) Scaling up type 2 diabetes prevention programs for high risk persons: Progress and challenges in the United States. In: Schwarz P, Reddy P, Greaves C, Dunbar J, Schwarz J (eds), *Diabetes Prevention in Practice*, pp. 69–82 TUMAINI Institute for Prevention Management, Dresden.
25. Fineberg HV. (2013) The paradox of disease prevention: Celebrated in principle, resisted in practice. *JAMA* **310**: 85–90. Epub 2013/07/04.
26. Ackermann RT, Finch EA, Brizendine E, Zhou H, Marrero DG. (2008) Translating the Diabetes Prevention Program into the community. The DEPLOY Pilot Study. *Am J Prev Med* **35**: 357–363. Epub 2008/09/10.
27. Katula JA, Vitolins MZ, Rosenberger EL, Blackwell CS, Morgan TM, Lawlor MS, *et al.* (2011) One-year results of a community-based translation of the diabetes prevention program: Healthy-living partnerships to prevent diabetes (HELP PD) project. *Diabetes Care* **34**: 1451–1457. Epub 2011/05/20.
28. Finch EA, Kelly MS, Marrero DG, Ackermann RT. (2009) Training YMCA wellness instructors to deliver an adapted version of the diabetes prevention program lifestyle intervention. *Diabetes Educ* **35**: 224–228, 32. Epub 2009/03/27.
29. Vojta D, Koehler TB, Longjohn M, Lever JA, Caputo NF. (2013) A coordinated national model for diabetes prevention: Linking health systems to an evidence-based community program. *Am J Prev Med* **44**: S301–S306. Epub 2013/03/27.
30. Longjohn M, Vojta D. (2012) Translating research into evidence-based practice with potential for population-wide impact. *Am J Public Health* **102**: e5; author reply e5. Epub 2012/06/16.

31. Abelson R. (2010) An insurer's new approach to diabetes. *New York Times* [Online Newspaper updated April 13; cited June 10]; Available from: http://www.nytimes.com/2010/04/14/health/14diabetes.html.
32. Kania J, Kramer M. Collective Impact. (2011) [cited Winter]; 35–41]. Available from: http://www.ssireview.org/images/articles/2011_WI_Feature_Kania.pdf.
33. Centers for Disease Control and Prevention. National Diabetes Prevention Program. (2013) [cited August 2013]; Available from: http://www.cdc.gov/diabetes/prevention/.
34. Colagiuri R, Colagiuri S, Yach D, Pramming S. (2006) The answer to diabetes prevention: Science, surgery, service delivery, or social policy? *Am J Public Health* **96**: 1562–1569. Epub 2006/07/29.
35. Williamson DF, Narayan KM. (2009) Identification of persons with dysglycemia: Terminology and practical significance. *Primary Care Diabetes* **3**: 211–217. Epub 2009/09/19.
36. Echouffo-Tcheugui JB, Ali MK, Griffin SJ, Narayan KM. (2011) Screening for type 2 diabetes and dysglycemia. *Epidemiol Rev* **33**: 63–87. Epub 2011/06/01.
37. Glumer C, Yuyun M, Griffin S, Farewell D, Spiegelhalter D, Kinmonth AL, *et al.* (2006) What determines the cost-effectiveness of diabetes screening? *Diabetologia* **49**: 1536–1544. Epub 2006/06/06.
38. Nielsen SJ, Popkin BM. (2003) Patterns and trends in food portion sizes, 1977–1998. *JAMA* **289**: 450–453. Epub 2003/01/22.
39. Brownell KD, Farley T, Willett WC, Popkin BM, Chaloupka FJ, Thompson JW, *et al.* (2009) The public health and economic benefits of taxing sugar-sweetened beverages. *N Engl J Med* **361**: 1599–1605. Epub 2009/09/18.
40. Novak NL, Brownell KD. (2011) Taxation as prevention and as a treatment for obesity: The case of sugar-sweetened beverages. *Curr Pharmaceut Design* **17**: 1218–1222. Epub 2011/04/16.
41. Christakis NA, Fowler JH. (2007) The spread of obesity in a large social network over 32 years. *N Engl J Med* **357**: 370–379. Epub 2007/07/27.
42. Elbel B, Kersh R, Brescoll VL, Dixon LB. (2009) Calorie labeling and food choices: A first look at the effects on low-income people in New York City. *Health Aff (Millwood)* **28**: w1110–w1121. Epub 2009/10/08.
43. Perreault L, Pan Q, Mather KJ, Watson KE, Hamman RF, Kahn SE. (xxxx) Effect of regression from prediabetes to normal glucose regulation on long-term reduction in diabetes risk: Results from the diabetes prevention program outcomes study. *Lancet* **379**: 2243–2251.

44. Saad MF, Knowler WC, Pettitt DJ, Nelson RG, Mott DM, Bennett PH. (1988) The natural history of impaired glucose tolerance in the Pima Indians. *N Engl J Med* **319**: 1500–1506.
45. Abdul-Ghani MA, DeFronzo RA. (2009) Pathophysiology of prediabetes. *Curr Diabetes Rep* **9**: 193–199.
46. Geiss LS, James C, Gregg EW, Albright A, Williamson DF, Cowie CC. (2010) Diabetes risk reduction behaviors among U.S. adults with prediabetes. *Am J Prev Med* **38**: 403–409. Epub 2010/03/24.
47. Albright AL, Gregg EW. (2013) Preventing type 2 diabetes in communities across the U.S.: The national diabetes prevention program. *Am J Prev Med* **44**: S346–S351.
48. Eborall H, Davies R, Kinmonth AL, Griffin S, Lawton J. (2007) Patients' experiences of screening for type 2 diabetes: Prospective qualitative study embedded in the ADDITION (Cambridge) randomised controlled trial. *BMJ* **335**: 490. Epub 2007/09/01.
49. Eborall HC, Griffin SJ, Prevost AT, Kinmonth AL, French DP, Sutton S. (2007) Psychological impact of screening for type 2 diabetes: Controlled trial and comparative study embedded in the ADDITION (Cambridge) randomised controlled trial. *BMJ* **335**: 486. Epub 2007/09/01.
50. Paddison CA, Eborall HC, Sutton S, French DP, Vasconcelos J, Prevost AT, *et al.* (2009) Are people with negative diabetes screening tests falsely reassured? Parallel group cohort study embedded in the ADDITION (Cambridge) randomised controlled trial. *BMJ* **339**: b4535. Epub 2009/12/02.
51. Rahman M, Simmons RK, Hennings SH, Wareham NJ, Griffin SJ. (2012) Effect of screening for Type 2 diabetes on population-level self-rated health outcomes and measures of cardiovascular risk: 13-year follow-up of the Ely cohort. *Diab Med* **29**: 886–892. Epub 2012/01/31.
52. Ginde AA, Cagliero E, Nathan DM, Camargo CA, Jr. (2008) Value of risk stratification to increase the predictive validity of HbA1c in screening for undiagnosed diabetes in the US population. *J Gen Intern Med* **23**: 1346–1353. Epub 2008/06/11.
53. Khunti K, Gillies CL, Taub NA, Mostafa SA, Hiles SL, Abrams KR, *et al.* (2012) A comparison of cost per case detected of screening strategies for Type 2 diabetes and impaired glucose regulation: Modelling study. *Diabetes Res Clin Prac* **97**: 505–513. Epub 2012/05/05.
54. Kelly E, Carls GS, Lenhart G, Mauceri E, Columbus D, Cavuoti A, *et al.* (2010) The Novartis health index: A method for valuing the economic impact of risk reduction in a workforce. *J Occup Environ Med* **52**: 528–535. Epub 2010/05/01.

55. Rolando L, Byrne DW, McGown PW, Goetzel RZ, Elasy TA, Yarbrough MI. (2013) Health risk factor modification predicts incidence of diabetes in an employee population: Results of an 8-year longitudinal cohort study. *J Occup Environ Med* **55**: 410–415. Epub 2013/03/28.
56. Wing RR, Gorin AA. (2003) Behavioral techniques for treating the obese patient. *Primary Care* **30**: 375–391.
57. Hill J, Wing R. (2003) The National Weight Control Registry [cited 2013 September]; Available from: http://xnet.kp.org/permanentejournal/sum03/registry.html.
58. Wing RR, Hill JO. (2001) Successful weight loss maintenance. *Ann Rev Nutrit* **21**: 323–341.
59. Narayan KM, Benjamin E, Gregg EW, Norris SL, Engelgau MM. (2004) Diabetes translation research: Where are we and where do we want to be? *Ann Intern Med* **140**: 958–963. Epub 2004/06/03.
60. Narayan KM, Gregg EW, Engelgau MM, Moore B, Thompson TJ, Williamson DF, *et al.* (2000) Translation research for chronic disease: The case of diabetes. *Diabetes Care* **23**: 1794–1798. Epub 2000/12/29.
61. Glasgow RE. (2004) Practical, practice, and policy relevant trials. *Curr Diab Rep* **4**: 111–112. Epub 2004/03/24.
62. Damschroder L, Aron D, Keith R, Kirsh S, Alexander J, Lowery J. (2009) Fostering implementation of health services research findings into practice: A consolidated framework for advancing implementation science. *Implement Sci* **4**: 50.
63. Klein K, Sorra J. (1996) The challenge of innovation implementation. *Acad Manage Rev* **21**: 1055–1080.
64. Rabin BA, Brownson RC, Haire-Joshu D, Kreuter MW, Weaver NL. (2008) A glossary for dissemination and implementation research in health. *J Public Health Manage Pract* **14**: 117–123 10.1097/01.PHH.0000311888.06252.bb.
65. Glasgow RE, McKay HG, Piette JD, Reynolds KD. (2001) The RE-AIM framework for evaluating interventions: What can it tell us about approaches to chronic illness management? *Patient Educ Counsel* **44**: 119–127. Epub 2001/08/02.
66. Jilcott S, Ammerman A, Sommers J, Glasgow RE. (2007) Applying the RE-AIM framework to assess the public health impact of policy change. *Ann Behav Med* **34**: 105–114. Epub 2007/10/12.
67. Garfield SA, Malozowski S, Chin MH, Narayan KM, Glasgow RE, Green LW, *et al.* (2003) Considerations for diabetes translational research in real-world settings. *Diabetes Care* **26**: 2670–2674. Epub 2003/08/28.

68. Li R, Zhang P, Barker LE, Chowdhury FM, Zhang X. (2010) Cost-effectiveness of interventions to prevent and control diabetes mellitus: A systematic review. *Diabetes Care* **33**: 1872–1894. Epub 2010/07/30.
69. Zhuo X, Zhang P, Gregg EW, Barker L, Hoerger TJ, Pearson-Clarke T, *et al.* (2012) A nationwide community-based lifestyle program could delay or prevent type 2 diabetes cases and save $5.7 billion in 25 years. *Health Affairs* **31**: 50–60.
70. Seagle HM, Strain GW, Makris A, Reeves RS; American Dietetic Association (2009) Position of the American Dietetic Association: Weight Management. *J Am Dietetic Assoc* **109**: 330–346.

Chapter 9: Epidemiological Trends, Risk Factors and Prevention of Diabetes: Special Focus on South Asians and Migrants

*Akhtar Hussain**,†, *Bishwajit Bhowmik**, *Fareeha Shaikh**, *Nayla Cristina do Vale Moreira** *and AKA Khan*‡

1. INTRODUCTION

Once considered a disease of affluence, type 2 diabetes (T2DM) is now a global epidemic. It is, in fact, one of the major contemporary causes of premature disability and death. In virtually every developed nation, diabetes ranks as one of the top two causes of blindness, renal failure, and lower limb amputation.[1] The life expectancy of individuals with T2DM may be shortened by as many as 15 years, with up to 80% dying of cardiovascular diseases.[1]

The onset of most cases of T2DM is preceded by a latent phase of glucose intolerance or impaired glucose regulation. Impaired glucose regulation, also termed pre-diabetes, consists of impaired fasting glucose (IFG) and/or impaired glucose tolerance (IGT). In addition to diabetes IGT and or IFG also constitute a cause of major public health concern because of its association with diabetes incidence and an increased risk for developing cardiovascular diseases (CVD). Approximately 70% of these individuals, however, are expected to develop T2DM in 10 to 15 years if there is no implementation of lifestyle or therapeutic intervention.[1]

* Corresponding author. Email: akhtar.hussain@medisin.uio.no

†Department of International Health, Institute of Health and Society, University of Oslo, Oslo, Norway.

‡Department of Endocrinology, Bangladesh Institute of Research and Rehabilitation in Diabetes, Endocrine and Metabolic Disorders (BIRDEM), Dhaka, Bangladesh.

According to the International Diabetes Federation, 77.6 million people had diabetes in South Asian (SA) countries in 2011.[1] India, Pakistan, Bangladesh, Sri Lanka, Nepal, Bhutan and Maldives are in SA and the region represents one-fifth of the world's population with diabetes.[2] More than 2 million SAs live in the United States of America (USA) and almost 1 million in Canada.[2] In the United Kingdom (UK), this ethnic group increased rapidly during the last 30 years and currently comprise the largest ethnic minority group representing 4% of the total population.[3,4] The majority belong to the lower socio-economic classes, economically and/or socially, at least in the initial phases of settling in the UK. Studies involving migrant SAs in developed countries reported a high prevalence of T2DM.[5–9] A number of factors including genetics, ethnicity, dyslipidemia, migration, stress, diet and lifestyle have been associated with prevalence of T2DM in migrant SAs.[7] The age at presentation is also significantly younger and the condition remains undiagnosed in up to 40% of SA individuals.[10–12]

2. PREVALENCE, TRENDS OF PREVALENCE AND INCIDENCE OF DIABETES AND PRE-DIABETES IN SOUTH ASIA

Although the SA Region comprises only seven countries, it is one of the most populous in the world. Close to 20% of all adults with DM in the world live in this region.[1] According to the IDF, 7.8% of the adult population, or 77.6 million people, had DM in SA in 2011, 61.3 million of whom were in India.[1] As expected, the number of people with DM in the region will increase to 127 million by 2030. An additional 30.94 million people had IGT in 2011. Bangladesh had the highest prevalence of DM among adults in the region at 10.7%, with Maldives next at 9.4%. The number of people with DM in India, Bangladesh, Pakistan and Sri Lanka make up 99% of the total for the region. Table 1 shows the number of people aged 20–79 years with DM and IGT in SA countries in 2011.[1]

It is expected that those residing in urban areas in SA will increase from 33% to 46% between 2011 and 2030.[1] Studies conducted at different times in SA countries have shown that SAs living in cities in the subcontinent

Table 1. Number of people (20–79 years) with Diabetes Mellitus (DM) & Impaired Glucose Tolerance (IGT) in South Asian (SA) countries in 2011.[1]

Country	DM people (million)	M/F (million)	Prevalence (%)	Undiagnosed DM (million)	Urban/ rural (million)	IGT people (million)	Prevalence (%)	DM related death	DM related expenditure (USD/person)
India	61.3	32.5/28.8	9.2	31.3	27.5/ 33.7	20.5	3.0	983,203	68
Bangladesh	8.4	4.1/4:3	10.7	4.0	5.5 /2.9	2.14	2.8	144,443	27
Pakistan	6.3	3.2/ 3.1	8.0	3.9	2.73/ 3.62	7.19	7.6	65,735	36
Sri Lanka	1.1	0.56/0.55	7.6	0.55	0.30/ 0.78	0.77	5.5	15,203	117
Nepal	0.49	0.26/ 0.23	3.7	0.23	0.30/ 0.19	0.32	2.2	11,297	44
Bhutan	0.02	0.019/0.002	5.8	0.01	0.01/0.01	0.01	3.0	120	174
Maldives	0.02	0.008/0.007	9.4	0.01	0.01/ 0.01	0.01	4.8	141	803

Notes: DM — diabetes mellitus; M/F — male/ female; IGT — impaired glucose tolerance; USD — US dollar.

have much higher rates of T2DM compared with rural populations but rates are increasing in both rural and urban areas as lifestyles become more westernized. In 2004, the prevalence of diabetes in rural and urban areas of Bangladesh was 2.3% and 8.8%, respectively, in various age groups.[13] In India, it was 1.9% and 7.3% in rural and urban areas, respectively, in 1999 and 2004[14,15] and in Pakistan it was 6.5% and 10.8% in rural and urban areas in 1995,[16] respectively. Studies conducted in Sri Lanka[17] and Nepal[18] also showed higher diabetes prevalence in urban areas (Table 2).

Studies evaluating temporal changes in the prevalence of diabetes and pre-diabetes were available only for Bangladesh,[19,20] India [21–25] and Sri Lanka.[26–29] The prevalence of diabetes in an urban Indian population had significantly increased from 8.3% in 1989 to 18.6% in 2005, and during the same period a similar increase from 2.2% to 9.2% was observed in a rural Indian population.[25] The age standardized prevalence of diabetes in a rural Bangladeshi population had significantly increased from 2.3% in 1999 to 7.9% in 2009.[19] Similarly, a study in Sri Lanka demonstrated that the age-standardized prevalence of diabetes had significantly increased from 2.5% in 1990 to 8.5% in 2000 in a rural community,[46] with only a slight increase in urban Sri Lanka from 5.3% to 6.5% during the same period.[26,29]

The trends for the prevalence of pre-diabetes are not as definitive. The increased prevalence observed in urban India in the period 1989 (8.3%) to 2000 (16.7%) had declined to 7.4% by 2006. A similar pattern was observed in rural Bangladesh. The prevalence of IFG increased significantly ($p = 0.011$) from 4.6% (1999) to 5.6% (2004) but declined to 5.3 by 2009.[19] Prevalence data in rural populations of India[21–25] and Sri Lanka[26–29] also showed a decline in prevalence during a similar period.

Studies evaluating incidence of diabetes and pre-diabetes were available only for India[30] and Bangladesh.[31] Mohan *et al.* conducted an 8-year follow-up study in urban South India from 1996 to 2004. The incidence rate of diabetes was 20.2 per 1,000 person-years and that of pre-diabetes was 13.1 per 1,000 person-years among subjects with NGT.[30] The overall 5-year (1999–2004) cumulative incidence of diabetes in rural Bangladesh was 16.4 per 1,000 person-years and 65.1 per 1,000 person-years in those with IFG adjusted for age and sex.[31]

Table 2. Prevalence of T2DM among Asian Indians and migrant South Asians.

Study design	Year	Setting	Sampling methods	Sample size	M/F	Age (yr)	Population	Diagnostic methods	Prevalence	Reference
Cross sectional survey[34]	2006–2007	UK	Medical practices with deprived population	34,359	26637/17772	>20	SA's, Caucasian & Blacks	Diagnostic read code for T2DM	11 (SAs), 3.5 (Caucasians) 8 (Blacks)	Dreyer *et al*, 2009
Cross sectional survey[35]	2001–2003	UK	Random	435	271/164	20–75	Migrant SAs	OGTT	20	Hanif *et al*., 2008
Population based study[36]	2001	UK	Random	1,063	517/546	35–79	Urban migrant Pakistanis, Europeans & Afro-Caribbean's	OGTT	33 (Pakistanis)* 20 (Europeans) 22 (Caribbean's)	Rise *et al*., 2001
Cross sectional survey[37]	2000	Norway	Random	2,513	1101/1412	30–67	SAs & western volunteers	Self-reported	14.3/27.5 (SAs)*α 5.9/2.9 (West)*α	Jenum *et al*., 2005
Community based study[38]	2004	USA	Random	1,046	537/509	17–87	Asian Indian migrants	Self-reported	18.3	Venkataraman *et al*., 2004

(*Continued*)

Table 2. *(Continued)*

Study design	Year	Setting	Sampling methods	Sample size	M/F	Age (yr)	Population	Diagnostic methods	Prevalence	Reference
Population cohort. 10-yr follow-up[39]	1994	South Africa	Systemic cluster	563	232/331	>15	South African Indians	OGTT	16.2*	Motala *et al.*, 2003
Cross sectional survey[40]	1984–1995	Singapore	Registry from previous surveys	5,707	2796/2911	24–64	Asian Indian, Malay, Chinese	FBG	12.8 (Indians)* 4 (Malay) 3 (Chinese)	Yeo *et al.*, 2006
Population based study[41]	1992	Singapore	Random	3,568	1712/1856	18–69	Asian Indian, Malay, Chinese	OGTT	12.2 (Indians)* 10.1 (Malay) 7.8 (Chinese)	Tan *et al.*, 1999
Population based study[42]	1996–1998	Canada	Stratified from previous survey	985	506/479	35–79	Urban ethnic SAs, Europeans & Chinese	FBG	10 (SAs)* 5 (Europeans) 2 (Chinese)	Anand *et al.*, 2000
Cross sectional survey[14]	2004	Bangladesh	Random	6,312	2768/3544	≥20	Rural & Urban	FBG & OGTT (selected number)	2.3/8.1	Hussain *et al.*, 2004
Population based study[15]	2003–2005	India	Stratified	4,4523	21816/22707	15–64	Rural & Urban	Self-reported	4.5 (3.1 & 7.3)	Mohan *et al.*, 2008

(Continued)

Table 2. *(Continued)*

Study design	Year	Setting	Sampling methods	Sample size	M/F	Age (yr)	Population	Diagnostic methods	Prevalence	Reference
Cross sectional survey[16]	1999–2002	India	Random	41,270	20534/20736	≥25	Rural & Urban	FBG	4.3 (1.9 & 4.6)	Sadikot *et al.*, 2004
Population based survey[17]	1995	Pakistan	Cluster	1,404	435/969	≥25	Rural & Urban	OGTT	6.5/10.8	Samad *et al.*, 1999
Cross sectional survey[18]	2005–2006	Srilanka	Cluster	5,000	1720/2668	≥18	Rural & Urban	FBG & OGTT	11.5 (11 & 13.6)	Katulanda *et al.*, 2008
Population based survey[19]		Nepal	—	2,006	—	≥30	Rural & Urban	FBG & OGTT	9.0/9.5	Mehta *et al.*, 2011

Notes: SAs — South Asians; OGTT — Oral glucose tolerance test; FBG — Fasting blood glucose; α — values reported as Males/Females;* adjusted for age and gender.

Not only did prevalence and incidence rates increase, the region had the second highest number of deaths (1.48 million) attributable to DM of any of the seven IDF regions in 2011. This represented 32% of total diabetic deaths in the IDF regions and approximately 15% of all deaths for the region among adults.[1] More than half of these deaths occurred in those under the age of 60. In spite of the large number of people with DM in the SA Region, healthcare expenditures due to DM was the lowest in the IDF regions, accounting for less than 1% of the global total.[1] Health care expenditure due to diabetes was lowest in Bangladesh (27 USD/person) and highest was in Maldives (803 USD/person) in 2011.[1]

3. PREVALENCE OF DIABETES IN SOUTH ASIAN IMMIGRANTS

Worldwide international migration is a large and growing phenomenon. According to the International Organization for Migration World Migration Report 2010, the number of international migrants was estimated at 214 million in 2010. If this number continues to grow at the same pace as during the last 20 years, it could reach 405 million by 2050.[32] Like most parts of the developing world, a large number of SAs have also migrated to different countries of the developed world. Migrant Asian groups have a greater susceptibility to adverse environmental influences than co-habitants of different races.[33] The reported prevalence of T2D was found to be higher in migrant SAs compared to those in their homeland. When compared to host populations in the UK, Europe, Norway, Canada, USA, South Africa, New Zealand and Singapore, prevalence rates were higher for migrant SAs.[34–43] The prevalence rate of T2DM in migrant SAs was highest in the UK (11–33%)[34–36] followed by Norway (14–28%),[37] USA (18%),[38] South Africa (16.2%),[39] Singapore (12.8%),[40,41] Canada (10%)[42] and New Zealand (8.3%)[43] (Table 2). Compared with Western populations, SAs develop DM at younger ages, at lower degrees of obesity, and at much higher rates given the same degree of weight gain.[44] For example, in Canada, a higher proportion of SAs (62.5%) were diagnosed prior to age 50 compared with approximately one-third (34.7%) of Caucasions.[45] The mean age at which diabetes was initially diagnosed was 44.6 years in

SAs and 51.4 years in Caucasions.[45] In studies performed in the USA, the mean age of diabetes diagnosis for SAs was between 50 and 57 years.[38,46] In both the UK and USA, prevalence rates of T2DM have been several times higher in SAs compared with the general and other ethnic populations.[47,48] The increased prevalence may be a consequence of strong gene-environmental interaction which is propelled by lifestyle changes caused by so-called modernization.[1]

Studies have shown that SAs have a higher rate of pre-diabetes and a three times greater risk of progression to T2DM compared to Caucasion Europeans in the UK.[49,50] In the ADDITION-Leicester study, pre-diabetes was shown to be associated with significant vascular diseases in the relatively young (mean age 59 years).[51] Data from the 2001 Census of England and Wales showed that people born in Bangladesh, followed by those born in Pakistan, had the highest rates of death due to CVD.[52] However, a review reported that among SAs, blood pressure (BP) is slightly higher in Indians, slightly lower in Pakistanis and much lower in Bangladeshis.[53]

4. RISK FACTORS FOR T2DM IN SOUTH ASIANS AND MIGRANT

IDF reported that the exponential rise in T2DM can be attributed to environmental exposure on the background of genetic susceptibility.[1] Over the last half century, there has been rapid socioeconomic development in SA countries resulting in a move from a traditional to a modern (urbanization/westernization) way of life. Virtually in all populations, a higher fat and low fiber containing diet and decreased physical activity have accompanied modernization. These changes in diet and physical inactivity, combined with increasing longevity and obesity, have formed the basis for dramatic increases in the prevalence of diabetes mellitus both in developed and developing countries.[1] Jayawardena *et al.*[54] conducted a systematic review and meta-analysis of the prevalence and trends of the diabetes epidemic in SA reported that family history, age, male gender, body mass index (BMI), wasit-to-hip ratio (WHR), systolic and diastolic blood pressures are significant risk factors for diabetes among SAs. In addition, few other studies have also demonstrated an association between diabetes and wealth/income,[22,55–57] hypercholesterolemia,[57] physical inactivity,[23,55,56,58] the presence of acanthosis nigricans,[59] graduate education[25] and office-based occupations.[56]

Various ethnic groups within the Western population have distinct differences in susceptibility to diabetes given the same environmental influences. This may refer to gene and environmental interaction for DM. There are both ethnic and economic reasons for the increasing burden of T2DM prevalence among immigrants. Ethnicity-related differences for the risk of T2DM may have been attributable to genetics, epigenetics, foetal and environmental factors (Forsdahl–Barker hypothesis), and also to the Western lifestyle with reduced physical activity and calorie dense diet.

Potential risk factors for SA and SA Immigrants are discussed below.

4.1. Generalized and Abdominal Obesity

According to International Association for the Study of Obesity, more than 1.5 billion adults worldwide are overweight, and 525 million are obese. In addition, at least 155 million children worldwide are overweight or obese.[60] Most alarming, not only in urban areas, obesity is also increasing rapidly in rural areas in SAs countries. However, Asians have lower rates of overweight and obesity than their Western counterparts using the conventional definition of WHO [body mass index (BMI) $\geq 25\,kg/m^2$ for overweight and $\geq 30\,kg/m^2$ for obese]. In rural Bangladesh,[19] general obesity (BMI $\geq 25\,kg/m^2$) increased 6 fold (4.4–26.6%) and central obesity [waist circumference (WC): male $\geq 90\,cm$ and female $\geq 80\,cm$] increased approximately 13-fold (3.9–39.7%) in the decade from (1999–2009). In rural India, the prevalence of obesity increased nearly 8.6-fold in a period of 14 years (24). Figure 1 shows the temporal changes in prevalence of obesity ($\geq 25\,kg/m^2$) in rural Bangladesh[19] and rural India.[24] Despite lower BMI, some Asian countries have similar or even higher prevalences of diabetes than Western countries.[61] Almost 80% of SA patients with T2DM are non-obese compared with 60% to 80% in the West who are obese.[62] The risk of diabetes (odds ratio) was significant for Asian Indian populations with a BMI of $>23\,kg/m^2$.[63,64] This has been confirmed by studies in migrant Indians and in other Asian populations.[65] According to the WHO recommendations, a BMI of 18.5–22 kg/m^2 is considered normal for Asian populations.[66]

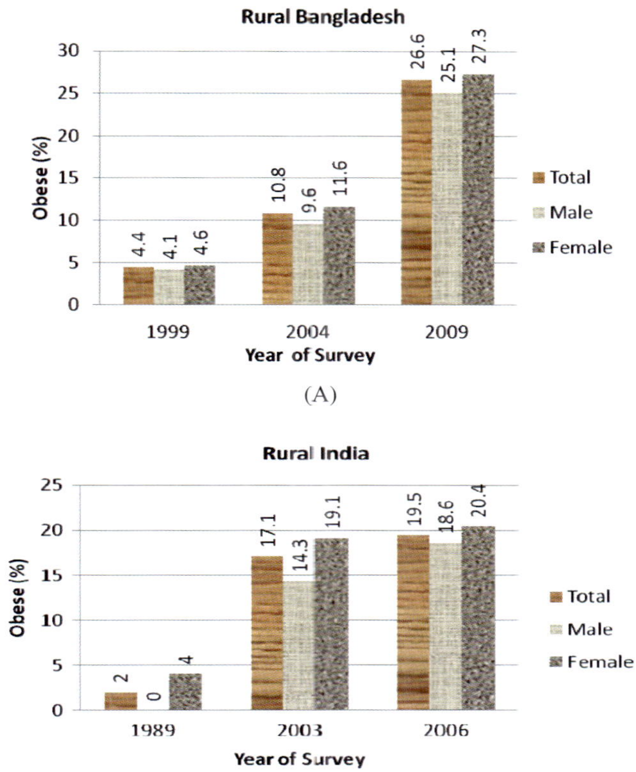

(A)

(B)

Fig. 1. Temporal changes in prevalence (%) of obesity ($\geq$25 kg/m^2) among (A) rural Bangladesh[19] and (B) rural Indian.[24]

Asian populations, especially those of SA descent, are more prone to abdominal obesity. Central obesity has been shown to play a vital role in the pathogenesis of insulin resistance,[67] increased plasma leptin, low plasma adiponectin[68] and stimulation of inflammatory cytokines.[62] All of these factors lead to development of diabetes and other cardiovascular diseases. Thus, WC and/or WHR reflecting central obesity are useful measures of obesity-related risk for T2DM, especially in individuals with normal BMI values.[69] In one study, we found that measures of central obesity, particularly WHR, WC, waist-to-height ratio (WHtR) and % body fat (BF%), showed a better association with obesity-related cardiometabolic risk factors for both sexes compared with BMI.[64]

The concept of different cut-offs for different ethnic groups has been proposed by the WHO[66] and IDF,[70] because some ethnic groups like SAs have higher cardiovascular and metabolic risks at lower cut-off levels for BMI, WC and WHR which may have been due to differences in body shape and fat distribution. For the same age, sex, and BMI, SAs had higher percentage body fat than Caucasians. In Caucasian men, a BMI of 30 kg/m^2 corresponds to 25% body fat[71] whereas in SA men, a BMI of <25 kg/m^2 corresponds to 33% body fat.[72] The data from the Health Survey for England[73] highlights the differences in central obesity among SA populations and the general population in the UK (total population of UK) (Table 3). The mean BMI of Bangladeshi, Indian and Pakistani men were lower than in the general population in the UK (27.1 kg/m^2). Indian women had similar BMI compared with the general population. Pakistani and Bangladeshi men and women had higher WHR and WC than the general population in the UK.

Despite having a lower body weight, Indian infants have higher subcutaneous fat, leptin, and insulin levels than Caucasian infants.[74] This "metabolically obese" phenotype (e.g., normal weight by conventional BMI standards but increased abdominal adiposity) has been associated with

Table 3. Comparison of BMI, WHR and WC in Asian populations and the general population aged 16 years and above in the UK.[73]

	Indian		Pakistani		Bangladeshi		UK	
	Men	**Women**	**Men**	**Women**	**Men**	**Women**	**Men**	**Women**
BMI (Kg/m^2)	25.8	26.2	25.9	27.1	24.7	25.7	27.1	26.8
Overweight and Obesity (%)*	53	55	55	62	44	51	67	57
WHR	0.92	0.82	0.92	0.84	0.91	0.85	0.92	0.82
Raised WHR (%)**	38	30	36	39	32	50	33	30
WC (cm)	93.0	83.9	95.0	87.7	88.7	85.7	96.5	86.4
Raised WC (%)***	20	38	30	48	12	43	31	41

*BMI ≥25 Kg/m^2; **≥0.95 for men and ≥0.85 for women; ***≥102 cm for men and ≥88 cm for women.

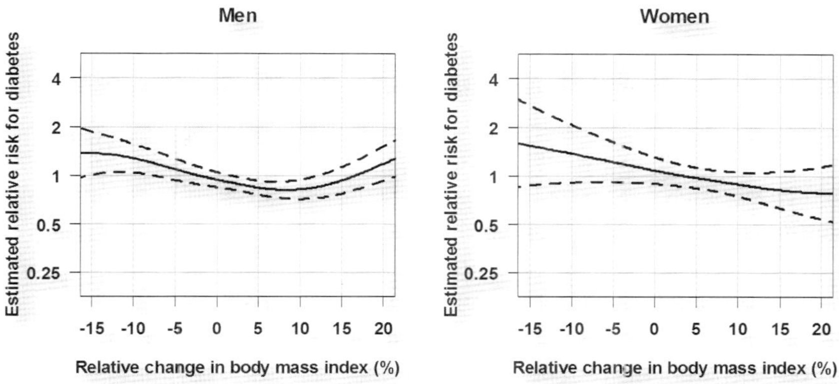

Fig. 2. Association between relative changes in BMI and the incidence of diabetes in rural Bangladesh.[76]

increased risk of insulin resistance and diabetes. Plasma adiponectin concentrations are lower in SAs compared with Caucasians that may contribute to the increased risk of T2DM and CVD in SAs.[75]

Despite the obesity epidemic, still one-fourth of individuals with T2DM in India and Bangladesh have a BMI below 19 Kg/m^2.[76] A rural Bangladesh study[76] found an inverse association between relative changes in BMI and the incidence of diabetes for those who reduced their BMI from baseline and those who gained excessive weight (Fig. 2). In general, those who maintained a stable BMI (–5% to +5%) had a lower risk of developing diabetes. This supports the observation that obesity alone may not explain the increased occurrence of diabetes in SA populations. Asian-Indian rural communities may be experiencing a dual burden of diabetes with obesity-related diabetes among the affluent and malnutrition-related diabetes in the poor.

4.2. Food Habits

Intake of dietary energy in excess of expenditure will result in weight gain and depending on the degree and type of weight gain, increased risk of T2DM. For each kg of weight gain it has been calculated that the risk for diabetes increases by about 4.5%.[77] A recent review has reported several dietary factors associated with insulin resistance among SAs, such as greater consumption of carbohydrate, saturated fatty acids, trans-fatty acids and *n*-6 poly unsaturated fatty acid (PUFA), and lower consumption of *n*-3 PUFA and fiber. Hence, the Asian diet may be an important contributoring factor to the increased disease prevalence.[78] SAs consume a smaller amount of protein and greater quantities of total fat, monounsaturated fatty acids, eggs, dairy products and carbohydrates (about 60–70% of energy intake) compared with Europeans.[79] In addition, frying was commonly used for food preparation method among SAs.[80]

Vegetable ghee, such as the Dalda commonly used for cooking in India and other SA countries, contains trans-fatty acid levels as high as 50%.[81] Greater intake of trans-fatty acids has been associated with weight gain, increased cardiometabolic risk, and insulin resistance.[82,83] Polished rice and refined wheat form the basis of most Asian diets with elevated glycemic index and load values, especially rice, which is associated with a 2-fold increased risk of T2DM, particularly in overweight and obese individuals.[62] Consumption of sugar-sweetened beverages, an important contributor of dietary glycemic load and excess calories, has increased rapidly worldwide, particularly in Asian Indian children. SAs have a lower consumption of *n*-3 PUFA that confer CVD protection than Europeans.[84] A recent Canadian study compared the consumption of carbohydrates with high density lipoprotein (HDL) cholesterol levels in four populations and concluded that SAs consumed the most carbohydrates, followed by Europeans, Aboriginals and Chinese, and that higher carbohydrate consumption was associated with lower HDL cholesterol levels.[85]

4.3. Physical Inactivity

Increased urbanization and use of automobiles have caused SAs to shift from a physically active, agrarian lifestyle marked by energy scarcity to a sedentary lifestyle marked by energy surplus. Physical inactivity represents an independent cardiometabolic risk factor with exercise recommended to control and also prevent diabetes. Regular physical activity reduces the risk of T2DM in adults by 20–60% in a dose response manner.[86] A recently conducted systematic review and meta-analysis reported physical inactivity as an independent risk factor for diabetes among

SAs.[23,55,56,58] Lower physical activity scores have been reported in SAs compared with Caucasian populations.[87,88] Levels of physical activity were inversely associated with BMI, WC, glucose and insulin levels in SAs.[88] SA women are especially prone to reduced physical activity.[89] Migration, unfamiliarity of surroundings and norms such as gender roles, religious modesty, mixed-gender activity, job participation levels among females and language difficulties are considered possible contributing factors.[90,91] Misra *et al.* has reported that resistance training decreased insulin resistance and subcutaneous fat in Asian Indians with T2DM, but has rarely been included in most exercise programs.[7] Recent consensus guidelines for physical activity in SAs includes 60 m of aerobic, work-related, and resistance exercise.[7]

4.4. Developmental Origins of Diabetes

Foetal under-nutrition and being born small for gestational age (SGA) have been identified as risk factors for T2DM among adults and youth.[92,93] Low birth weight (LBW; birth weight <2.5 kg) is a significant etiologic factor in the development of T2DM.[94] According to the "30 phenotype" hypothesis,[95,96] the combination of being undernourished *in utero* followed by a nutritionally overabundant environment later in life may unmask certain programmed predispositions in the fetus such as central adiposity, decreased pancreatic β-cell growth, sub-normal insulin secretory responses and insulin receptor functions, and activity of the hypothalamic–pituitary–adrenal axis. These abnormalities, in turn, may increase susceptibility to insulin resistance and T2DM.[97,98] Low birth weight and exposure to undernutrition *in utero* are common in some Asian populations, especially in the Indian subcontinent, where 30% of infants are underweight.[99] Prospective studies from India have shown the impact of foetal undernutrition (often manifested as LBW) as well as overnutrition (e.g., the infant of a mother with diabetes) on future risk for diabetes.[99] In India, leanness in infancy and overweight by the age of 12 or older were associated with increased risk of developing IGT or T2DM in young adulthood.[100]

The two-to three-fold greater risk of gestational diabetes (GDM) in Asian women than in their Caucasian counterparts may also contribute to the increasing epidemic of onset of diabetes in youth in Asia.[101] Asian women with a history of GDM have a substantially increased risk of T2DM, while their offspring exhibit early features of the metabolic syndrome, thus establishing a vicious cycle whereby "diabetes begets diabetes." The combination of GDM, *in utero* nutritional imbalance, childhood obesity, and overnutrition in adulthood will continue to fuel the epidemic in Asian countries undergoing rapid nutritional transition.[99]

4.5. Genetic Factors

T2DM is complex polygenic disorder in which common genetic variants interact with environmental factors to unmask the disease. Genetic factors thereby play an important part in the development of T2DM, as exemplified by rare monogenic subtypes, the high prevalence in particular ethnic groups and its modification by genetic admixture and the difference in concordance rates between monozygotic and dizygotic twins. However, the role of genetics in the development of diabetes is poorly understood. SAs are apparently genetically more prone to develop T2DM and insulin resistance than other ethnic populations. Moreover, SAs are more susceptible for developing truncal obesity, which might account for their tendency to insulin resistance referred to as the "Asian Indian phenotype". Most diabetes genetic variants identified so far, including *TCF7L2* and *KCNQ1*, appear to be associated with decreased insulin secretion in Caucasians as well as Asians.[101] In addition, among Asian adults diagnosed with diabetes before the age of 40 years, approximately 40% had a lean, non-autoimmune phenotype with rapid failure of oral medications.[102–105] Approximately 10% of these patients carried genetic variants encoding pancreatic β-cell pathways, including transcription factors and amylin, or mitochondrial polymorphisms. These findings provide further evidence that β-cell dysfunction plays a critical role in the development of diabetes in SAs.

4.6. Summary of Identified Risk Factors

Overweight is the most critical risk factor for developing diabetes, and should be targeted for prevention of T2DM especially among youths. Diet and physical activity, which mediate energy balance, are also clearly

Table 4. Modifiable and non-modifiable risk factors and associated disorders for T2DM.[1]

Modifiable risk factors	Non-modifiable risk factors
Overweight and obesity (central and total)	Ethnicity
Sedentary lifestyle	Family history of diabetes
Previously identified glucose intolerance (IGT and/or IFG)	Age
Metabolic syndrome:	Gender
Hypertension	History of gestational diabetes
Decreased HDL cholesterol	Polycystic ovary syndrome
Increased triglyceride	
Dietary factors	
Intrauterine environment	
Inflammation	

Notes: HDL — high-density lipoprotein; IFG — impaired fasting glucose; IGT — impaired glucose tolerance.

related to T2DM risk. Ethnicity and perinatal factors (i.e., being born either LGA or SGA or to a mother with diabetes during pregnancy) may also be risk factors. The risk appears to be of particular importance in certain ethnic groups. Perinatal factors include non-modifiable and modifiable risk factors for the development of T2DM and therefore should be included in preventive strategies. Non-modifiable risk factors useful in identifying high-risk youths include family history of T2DM. Risk factors for T2DM are summarized in Table 4.

5. PREVENTIVE STRATEGIES

There are a lack of randomised controlled trials elucidating to what extent risk factors for T2DM may be beneficially influenced by a culturally adapted approach especially among non-Western immigrants living in Western countries. The International Diabetes Federation (IDF) classifies diabetes prevention in three levels: primary, secondary and tertiary. Primary intervention includes activities that prevent diabetes from developing. Secondary prevention includes activities, such as early detection of diabetes, prompt and effective management of diabetes, and also measures to halt its progression. Tertiary prevention includes measures undertaken to prevent complications and physical disabilities due to diabetes. Diet, exercise, stress management, and weight control are important at any level of diabetes prevention and treatment. Public health efforts should be encouraged to implement education at the population level and encourage environmental changes to modify the impact of identifiable "diabesogenic" factors in "Western" societies.

To curb this epidemic, an integrated strategy combining population-wide preventive policies (e.g., changing foods and the physical environment to facilitate activities), early detection, and multidisciplinary care programs may reduce the risk of diabetes and associated complications in the general population and in high-risk individuals. On the basis of modifiable risk factors for T2DM, many prevention programs have focused on lifestyle modification although other strategies, including the use of pharmacological agents which target either β-cell function or insulin resistance, have also been used. The US Diabetes Prevention Program (DPP) had three arms, placebo, metformin and intensive life style changes. After an average follow-up of 2.8 years, there was a 58% relative risk reduction in the progression to diabetes in the lifestyle group compared with the control group. Within this group, 50% achieved the goal of more than 7% weight reduction and 74% maintained at least 150 min of moderately intense activity each week. Of note, the Indian Diabetes Prevention Programme (IDPP) demonstrated the significant role of moderate, lifestyle modification (LSM), even without significant weight reduction, on diabetes prevention. The Diabetes Prevention Program of Pakistan (DPPP) also showed that lifestyle intervention is important in preventing diabetes in subjects with IGT. However, the addition of metformin did not show any further improvement (Tables 5[106–115] and 6[110,111,113–123]). Nevertheless, the effectiveness of LSM in the SA population is almost half of that of Western population.

There appears to be a lack of intervention studies focusing both on the physiological and psychological aspects of blood glucose regulation.[124] Neither have there been any large scale lifestyle studies focused on immigrant populations.

Medications for diabetes have limited efficacy. On the other hand, there is consistent data demonstrating a positive relationship between changes

Table 5. Summary of studies involving lifestyle (diet and exercise) interventions.

Study	Number of people	Years of follow-up	Mean age and mean BMI	Type of intervention	Frequency of intervention	Targets	Effect of intervention
Malmo, Sweden (35, 36)	181 (men only)	6.0	48 years 26 kg/m^2	Diet, exercise	Monthly for 6/12, then every 12/12	Unspecified weight loss	Reduction in diabetes incidence in intervention group 37% 2.0–3.3 kg weight loss
Da Qing, China (37)	577	6.0	45 years 25.6 kg/m^2	Diet, exercise or both	7 sessions in 3/12, then every 3/12	BMI <23 kg/m^2, healthier diet	Reduction in diabetes incidence per group: 31%
DPS, Finland (38)	522	3.2	55 years 31 kg/m^2	Diet, exercise	7 sessions in 12/12, then every 3/12. Free gym membership and supervised activity sessions	5% weight loss, decrease fat intake, increase fibre intake >150 min exercise/week	Reduction in diabetes incidence in intervention group — 58% (63% in men and 54% in women) 3.5 kg weight loss after 2 years
New Zealand (39)	103	5.0	52 years 29 kg/m^2	Diet	Monthly for first 12/12	Unspecified weight loss, reduced fat intake	No benefit in progression to diabetes. No weight loss

(Continued)

Table 5. (*Continued*)

Study	Number of people	Years of follow-up	Mean age and mean BMI	Type of intervention	Frequency of intervention	Targets	Effect of intervention
Malmohus, Sweden (40)	267 (men only)	10.0	54.1 years (mean weight 76 kg)	Diet and exercise	Every 12/12		Reduction in diabetes — 13% diet group, 29% control, no weight loss
FHS (41)	188	6.0	50 years (mean weight 81.7 kg)	Diet, exercise	Every 3/12	Lose weight if BMI >22 kg/m^2, low fat diet, exercise 3–4 times/week	No benefit in progression to diabetes. No weight loss
DPP, US (42)	3234	2.8	51 years, 34 kg/m^2	Diet, exercise	16 diet sessions in 6/12, then monthly. Twice-weekly supervised exercise sessions	7% weight loss, low-fat diet, 150 min exercise/week	Decreased progression to diabetes per group 58% diet and exercise. 3.8 kg weight loss

(*Continued*)

Table 5. *(Continued)*

Study	Number of people	Years of follow-up	Mean age and mean BMI	Type of intervention	Frequency of intervention	Targets	Effect of intervention
Indian Diabetes Prevention Programme (IDPP) (43)	531	3.0	45.9 years 25.8 kg/m^2	Diet & exercise, Metfromin, Diet, Exercise & Metformin	6 months interval	Unspecified weight loss, reduce calorie and fat intake, moderate physical activity	Reduction in diabetes incidence in LSM – 28.5% Met Group – 26.4% LSM + Me – 28.2%
DPP, Japan (44)	304	3.0	51years 23 kg/m^2	Diet, exercise	Every 3/12 then 6/12	5% weight loss, increase leisure time physical activity — 700 kcal/week	Reduction in diabetes incidence -53%

Table 6. Summary of studies involving lifestyle interventions with oral antidiabetic agents.

Study	Number of people	Inclusion criteria	Years of follow up	Mean age and mean BMI	Oral antidiabetic agent	Type of intervention	Frequency of intervention	Specified targets other than to delay progression to diabetes	Effect of intervention
Malmohus, Sweden (45)	267 (men only)	IGT using a 30-g glucose/m² body surface area OGTT: 1-hr glu >8.9, 2-hr glu >6.7 or 3-hr glu >4.7 mmol/L	10	54.1 years (mean weight 76 kg)	Tolbutamide	Diet, exercise, weight loss	Every 12/12	—	Decreased progression to diabetes per group; 29%. No weight loss
Whitehall (46)	200	2-h glucose value after 50-g OGTT 6.7–11.0 mmol/L	5	56 years 26.2 kg/m²	Phenformin	Carbohydrate restricted diet	Once at start of study	Unspecified weight loss	No benefit in progression to diabetes, weight loss 1.2 kg
FHS (47)	188	Fasting glucose 5.5–7.7 mmol/L	6	50 years (mean weight 81.7 kg)	Gliclazide	Diet, exercise	Every 3/12	Lose weight if BMI >22 kg/m², low fat diet, exercise 3–4 times/week	No benefit in progression to diabetes, no weight loss

(*Continued*)

Table 6. *(Continued)*

Study	Number of people	Inclusion criteria	Years of follow up	Mean age and mean BMI	Oral antidiabetic agent	Type of intervention	Frequency of intervention	Specified targets other than to delay progression to diabetes	Effect of intervention
DPP, US (48–50)	3234	IGT + fasting glucose >5.3 mmol/L. 45% ethnic minority	2.8	51 years 34 kg/m²	Metformin	Diet, exercise	16 diet sessions in 6/12, then monthly. Twice weekly supervised exercise sessions	7% weight loss, low-fat diet, 150 min exercise/ week	Decreased progression to diabetes per group; 58% diet and exercise (71% in people aged >70) ">metformin. 3.8 kg weight loss diet + exercise. 1.8 kg weight loss metformin
STOP NIDDM (39, 40)	1429	IGT + fasting glucose > 5.6 mmol/L	3.3	55 years 31 kg/m²	Acarbose	General advice on diet, weight loss and activity.	Every 12/12	—	Acarbose decreased progression to diabetes by 25%. Weight loss 0.5 kg

(Continued)

Table 6. *(Continued)*

Study	Number of people	Inclusion criteria	Years of follow up	Mean age and mean BMI	Oral antidiabetic agent	Type of intervention	Frequency of intervention	Specified targets other than to delay progression to diabetes	Effect of intervention
EDIT (42, 51)	631	Fasting glucose 5.5–7.7 mmol/L	6	52 years 28.6 kg/m^2	Metformin, acarbose or both	None	Unspecified	—	In patients with IGT at baseline, decreased risk of progression to diabetes with acarbose, no weight loss
IDPP (43)	531	Fasting glucose <7.0 mmol/L 2 hr glucose 7.8 – 11.0 mmol/L	3	45.9 years 25.8 kg/m^2	Metformin	Diet, Exercise & Metformin	6 months interval	Unspecified weight loss Reduce calorie and fat intake Moderate physical activity	Reduction in diabetes incidence in LSM – 28.5% Met – 26.4% LSM + Met – 28.2%
DPPP (52)	317	Fasting glucose <7.0 mmol/L 2 hr glucose 7.8 – 11.0 mmol/L	18 m	43.6 years 27.1 kg/m^2	Metformin	Diet, Exercise & Metformin	2 months interval	5% weight loss, low-fat diet, 30 min/day	Reduction- LSM – 23.5% LSM + Met – 29%

in lifestyle including dietary habits, body weight and physical activity with the incidence of T2DM. While lifestyle intervention has been shown to prevent or postpone T2DM on an international scale in various native populations (Ref. [124], Tables 5 and 6), studies in immigrants are scarce.

Unfortunately, many immigrants are not accessed by national public health programs due to, amongst other factors, linguistic difficulties and different cultural perceptions regarding health and disease. Healthcare personnel tend to view the immigrant population as a particularly challenging group.[125] There are economic and ethical reasons for attempting to attenuate the burden of T2DM prevalence among immigrants, and reduce inequalities in health. Establishing a diabetes prevention program uniquely focused on the immigrant population would positively impact compliance, adherence, behavior modification, and would address the pathophysiological risk factors involved in the development of T2DM.

InnaDiab DE-PLAN study[126] has adopted a non-directive cultural approach in a randomized control trial (RCT) of Pakistani women living in Norway directed at post-meal blood glucose regulation for preventing T2DM in accordance with IDF recommendations. The non-directive support,[127] emphasizes an educational format rather than following directives. Instead of receiving specific, detailed dietary advice, participants were encouraged to customize their approach so as to achieve personal control of their life styles. Hawthorne *et al.*[128] also found cultural adaption to be valuable in a diabetes health education program for British Pakistani women. Kousar *et al.*[129] have shown that a culturally adopted lifestyle intervention in Pakistani women reduced risk factors for the metabolic syndrome.

6. CONCLUSION

In conclusion, the present overview highlighted the observation that that T2DM has become an epidemic among native and immigrant SAs. This epidemic is heterogeneous and is characterized by a rapid increase in a short timeframe with onset occurring at a relatively young age and at a low BMI. In parallel with economic development and nutritional transition, the incidence of overweight and obesity have also been increasing rapidly in this population. Abdominal or central adiposity is detrimental and is clearly associated with T2DM and other cardiometabolic risk factors in SAs. High rates of gestational diabetes, in combination with *in utero* exposure to poor nutrition, childhood obesity, and overnutrition in later life, may contribute substantially to the increasing diabetes epidemic in SAs.

Migration has become a key component of collective social and economic development. It is essential that the design of a prevention policy and training of healthcare practitioners take into account the health of migrants and the challenges posed by conditions such as diabetes. It is equally essential to work with migrants to ensure that they are aware of the possibilities for care and the risks they are exposed to. More research is needed to develop evidence-based guidelines relevant for Asian Indians with special focus on immigrant SAs.

To curb this epidemic, an integrated strategy combining population-based preventive policies (e.g., improving nutrition and the physical environment), early detection, and multidisciplinary care programs may reduce the risk of diabetes and other associated cardiometabolic risk factors in the general population and in high-risk individuals of this resource poor society.

REFERENCES

1. International Diabetes Federation. Diabetes Atlas. 5th edn. Brussels: International Diabetes Federation, 2011.
2. Gupta M, Singh N, Verma S. (2006) South Asians and cardiovascular risk: What clinicians should know. *Circulation* **113**: e924–e929.
3. Blackledge HM, Newton J, Squire IB. (2003) Prognosis for South Asian and white patients newly admitted to hospital with heart failure in the United Kingdom: Historical cohort study. *BMJ* **327**: 526–531.
4. Wild S, McKeigue P. (1997) Cross sectional analysis of mortality by country of birth in England and Wales, 1970–1992. *BMJ* **314**: 705–710.
5. Anand S, Yusuf S, Vuksan V *et al.* (2000) Differences in risk factors, atherosclerosis, and cardiovascular disease between ethnic groups in Canada: The study of health assessment and risk in ethnic groups. *Lancet* **356**: 279–284.
6. Hanif MW, Valsamakis G, Dixon A *et al.* (2008) Detection of impaired glucose tolerance and undiagnosed type 2 diabetes in UK South Asians: An effective screening strategy. *Diabet Obes Metab* **10**: 755–762.

7. Misra A, Khurana L. (2009) The metabolic syndrome in South Asians: Epidemiology, determinants, and prevention. *Metab Syndrome Relat Disord* **7**: 497–514.
8. Chandie Shaw PK, Vandenbroucke JP, Tjandra YI *et al.* (2002) Increased end-stage diabetic nephropathy in Indo-Asian immigrants living in the Netherlands. *Diabetologia* **45**: 337–341.
9. Mohanty SA, Woodhandler S, Himmelstein DU, Bor DH. (2005) Diabetes and cardiovascular disease among Asian Indians in the United States. *J Gen Intern Med* **20**: 474–478.
10. Mather HM, Chaturvedi N, Fuller J. (1998) Mortality and morbidity from diabetes in South Asians and Europeans: 11-year follow-up of the Southall Diabetes Survey, London, UK. *Diabet Med* **15**: 53–59.
11. Mather H, Keen H. (1985) The Southall Diabetes Survey: Prevalence of known diabetes in Asians and Europeans. *Br Med J* **291**: 1081–1084.
12. Simmons D, Williams DR, Powell MJ. (1989) Prevalence of diabetes in a predominantly Asian community: Preliminary findings of the Coventry diabetes study. *BMJ* **298**: 18–21.
13. Hussain A, Rahim M.A., Khan A.K., Ali SMK. (2005) T2DM in rural and urban population: Diverse prevalence and associated risk factors in Bangladesh. *Diabet Med* **22**: 931–937.
14. Mohan V, Mathur P, Deepa R *et al.* (2008) Urban-rural differences in prevalence of self-reported diabetes in India- The WHO-ICMR Indian NCD risk factor surveillance. *Diabet Res Clin Pract* **80**: 159–168.
15. Sadikot SM, Nigam A, Das Bajaj S *et al.* (2004) Comparing the ADA 1997 and the WHO 1999 criteria: Prevalence of diabetes in India Study. *Diabet Res Clin Pract* **66**: 309–315.
16. Shera AS, Rafique G, Khawaja IA, Baqai S, King H. (1999) Pakistan National Diabetes Survey: Prevalence of glucose intolerance and associated factors in Baluchistan province. *Diabet Res Clin Pract* **44**: 49–58.
17. Katulanda P, Constanttinet GR, Mahesh JG, Sheriff R *et al.* (2008) Prevalence and projections of diabetes and pre-diabetes in adults in Srilanka- Srilanka Diabetes, Cardiovascular Study (SLDCS). *Diabet Med* **25**: 1062–1069.
18. Mehta KD, Karki P, Lamsal M, Paudel M *et al.* (2011) Hyperglycemia, glucose intolerance, hypertension and socioeconomic position in eastern Nepal. *Southeast Asian J Trop Med Public Health* **42**: 197–207.
19. Bhowmik B, Afsana F, Diep LM, Munir SM, Wright E, Mahmood S, Azad Khan AK, Hussain A. (2013) Increasing Prevalence of Type 2 Diabetes in a Rural Bangladeshi Population: A Population Based Study for 10 Years. *Diabet Metab J* **37**: 46–53.

20. Rahim MA, Hussain A, Azad Khan AK, Sayeed MA, Keramat Ali SM, Vaaler S. (2007) Rising prevalence of type 2 diabetes in rural Bangladesh: A population based study. *Diabet Res Clin Pract* **77**: 300–305.
21. Mohan V, Deepa M, Deepa R, Shanthirani CS, Farooq S, Ganesan A, Datta M. (2006) Secular trends in the prevalence of diabetes and impaired glucose tolerance in urban South India–the Chennai Urban Rural Epidemiology Study (CURES-17). *Diabetologia* **49**: 1175–1178.
22. Ramachandran A, Snehalatha C, Vijay V. (2002) Temporal changes in prevalence of type 2 diabetes and impaired glucose tolerance in urban southern India. *Diabet Res Clin Pract* **58**: 55–60.
23. Ramachandran A, Snehalatha C, Latha E, Vijay V, Viswanathan M. (1997) Rising prevalence of NIDDM in an urban population in India. *Diabetologia* **40**: 232–237.
24. Ramachandran A, Snehalatha C, Baskar AD, Mary S, Kumar CK, Selvam S, Catherine S, Vijay V. (2004) Temporal changes in prevalence of diabetes and impaired glucose tolerance associated with lifestyle transition occurring in the rural population in India. *Diabetologia* **47**: 860–865.
25. Ramachandran A, Mary S, Yamuna A, Murugesan N, Snehalatha C. (2008) High prevalence of diabetes and cardiovascular risk factors associated with urbanization in India. *Diabet Care* **31**: 893–898.
26. Malavige G, de Alwis N, Weerasooriya N, Fernando D, Siribaddana S. (2002) Increasing diabetes and vascular risk factors in a sub-urban Sri Lankan population. *Diabet Res Clin Pract* **57**: 143–145.
27. Wijewardene K, Mohideen MR, Mendis S, Fernando DS, Kulathilaka T, Weerasekara D, Uluwitta P. (2005) Prevalence of hypertension, diabetes and obesity: Baseline findings of a population based survey in four provinces in Sri Lanka. *The Ceylon Med J* **50**: 62–70.
28. Illangasekera U, Rambodagalla S, Tennakoon S. (2004) Temporal trends in the prevalence of diabetes mellitus in a rural community in Sri Lanka. *J R Soc Promot Health* **124**: 92–94.
29. Fernando DJ, Siribaddana S, de Silva D. (1994) Impaired glucose tolerance and diabetes mellitus in a suburban Sri Lankan community. *Postgrad Med J* **70**: 347–349.
30. Mohan V, Deepa M, Anjana RM, Lanthorn H, Deepa R. (2008) Incidence of Diabetes and Pre-diabetes in a Selected Urban South Indian Population (Cups — 19). *J Assoc Phys India* **56**: 152–157.
31. Asgar S, Azad Khan AK, Keramot Ali SM, Sayeed MA, Bhowmik B, Diep ML, Shi Z, Hussain A. (2011) Incidence of diabetes in Asian-Indian

subjects: A five year follow-up study in Bangladesh. *Primary Care Diabet* **5**: 117–124.
32. World Migration Report 2010 (2010). The Future of Migration: Building Capacities for Change. International Organization for Migration. Retrieved 2010-11-30.
33. De Courten M, Bennett P, Tuomilehto J, Zimmet P. (1997) Epidemiology of NIDDM in non-Europids. In: Alberti KGMM, Zimmet P, DeFronzo RA (eds), *International Textbook of Diabetes Mellitus*, 2nd edn, pp. 143–170. Wiley, Chichester.
34. Dreyer G, Hull S, Aitken Z, Chesser A, Yaqoob MM. (2009) The effect of ethnicity on the prevalence of diabetes and associated chronic kidney disease. *Int J Med* **102**: 261–269.
35. Hanif MW, Valsamakis G, Dixon A *et al.* (2008) Detection of impaired glucose tolerance and undiagnosed T2DM in UK South Asians: An effective screening strategy. *Diabet Obesity Metab* **10**: 755–762.
36. Riste L, Khan F, Cruickshank K. (2001) High prevalence of T2DM in all ethnic groups, including Europeans, in a British inner city. *Diabet Care* **24**: 1377–1383.
37. Jenum AK, Holme I, Graff-Iversen S, Birkeland KI. (2005) Ethnicity and sex are strong determinants of diabetes in an urban Western society: Implications for prevention. *Diabetologia* **48**: 435–439.
38. Venkataraman R, Nanda NC, Baweja G, Parikh N, Bhatia V. (2004) Prevalence of diabetes mellitus and related conditions in Asian Indians living in the United States. *Am J Cardiol* **94**: 977.
39. Motala AA, Omar MAK, Pirie FJ. (2003) Epidemiology of type 1 and T2DM in Africa. *J Cardiovascular Risk* **10**: 77–83.
40. Yeo KK, Tai BC, Heng D *et al.* (2006) Ethnicity modifies the association between diabetes mellitus and ischaemic heart disease in Chinese, Malays and Asian Indians living in Singapore. *Diabetologia* **49**: 2866–2873.
41. Tan CE, Emmanuel SC, Tan BY, Jacob E. (1999) Prevalence of diabetes and ethnic differences in cardiovascular risk factors — The 1992 Singapore National Health Survey. *Diabet Care* **22**: 241–247.
42. Anand S, Yusuf S, Vuksan V *et al.* (2000) Differences in risk factors, atherosclerosis, and cardiovascular disease betweed ethnic groups in Canada: The study of health assessment and risk in ethnic groups. *Lancet* **356**: 279–284.
43. Scragg R, Baker J, Metcalf P, Dryson E. (1991) Prevalence of diabetes and impaired glucose tolerance in a New Zealand multi-racial workforce. *NZ Med J* **104**: 395–397.

44. Chan JC, Malik V, Jia W *et al.* (2009) Diabetes in Asia: Epidemiology, risk factors, and pathophysiology. *JAMA* **301**: 2129–2140.
45. Sara D, Garduno D, Santosh K. (2011) Prevalence, risk factors and complications associated with T2DM in migrant South Asians. *Diabet Metab Res Rev* **28**: 6–24.
46. Jonnalagadda SS, Diwan S. (2005) Health behaviors, chronic disease prevalence and self-rated health of older Asian Indian immigrants in the U.S. *J Immigrant Health* **7**: 75–83.
47. Mostafa SA, Davies MJ, Webb DR, Gray LJ, Srinivasan BT *et al.* (2010) The potential impact of using glycated haemoglobin as the preferred diagnostic tool for detecting type 2 diabetes mellitus. *Diabet Med* **27**: 762–769.
48. Mohanty SA., Woolhandler S, Himmelstein DU, Bor DH. (2005) Diabetes and cardiovascular disease among Asian Indians in the United States. *J General Internal Med* **20**: 474–478.
49. Srinivasan BT, Davies MJ, Webb D, Healey E, Farooqi A, Hiles S. (2007) Baseline characteristics and risk of progression from prediabetes to type 2 diabetes in a multiethnic, population based screening. *Diabet Med* **24**: 51.
50. Oldroyd JC, Yallop J, Fischbacher C, Bhopal R *et al.* (2007) Transient and persistent impaired glucose tolerance and progression to diabetes in South Asians and Europeans: New, large studies are a priority. *Diabet Med* **24**: 98–99.
51. Webb DR, Khunti K, Silverman R, Gray LJ, Srinivasan BT *et al.* (2010) Impact of metabolic indices on central artery stiffness: Independent association of insulin resistance and glucose with aortic pulse wave velocity. *Diabetologia* **53**: 1190–11198.
52. Wild SH, Fischbacher C, Brock A, Griffiths C, Bhopal R. (2007) Mortality from all causes and circulatory disease by country of birth in England and Wales 2001–2003. *J Public Health (Oxf)* **29**: 191–198.
53. Agyemang C, Bhopal RS. (2002) Is the blood pressure of South Asian adults in the UK higher or lower than that in European white adults? A review of cross-sectional data. *J Hum Hypertens* **16**: 739–51.
54. Jayawardena R, Ranasinghe P, Byrne MN, Soares JM, Katulanda P, Hills PA. (2012) Prevalence and trends of the diabetes epidemic in South Asia: A systemic review and meta-analysis. *BMC Public Health* **12**: 380.
55. Sayeed MA, Banu A, Haq JA, Khanam PA, Mahtab H, Azad Khan AK. (2002) Prevalence of hypertension in Bangladesh: Effect of socioeconomic risk factor on difference between rural and urban community. *Bangladesh Med Res Counc Bull* **28**: 7–18.

56. Ramachandran A, Snehalatha C, Kapur A, Vijay V, Mohan V, Das AK *et al.* (2001) High prevalence of diabetes and impaired glucose tolerance in India: National Urban Diabetes Survey. *Diabetologia* **44:** 1094–1101.
57. Vijayakumar G, Arun R, Kutty VR. (2009) High prevalence of type 2 diabetes mellitus and other metabolic disorders in rural Central Kerala. *J Assoc Phys India* **57**: 563–567.
58. Mohan V, Mathur P, Deepa R, Deepa M, Shukla DK, Menon GR, Anand K, Desai NG, Joshi PP, Mahanta J *et al.* (2008) Urban rural differences in prevalence of self-reported diabetes in India–the WHO-ICMR Indian NCD risk factor surveillance. *Diabet Res Clin Pract* **80**: 159–168.
59. Menon VU, Kumar KV, Gilchrist A, Sugathan TN, Sundaram KR, Nair V, Kumar H. (2006) Prevalence of known and undetected diabetes and associated risk factors in central Kerala–ADEPS. *Diabet Res Clin Pract* **74**: 289–294.
60. International Association for the Study of Obesity. www.iaso.org.
61. Yoon KH, Lee JH, Kim JW *et al.* (2006) Epidemic obesity and type 2 diabetes in Asia. *Lancet* **368**: 1681–1688.
62. Juliana CNC, Vasanti M, Weiping J *et al.* (2009) Diabetes in Asia: Epidemiology, Risk Factors, and Pathophysiology. *JAMA* **301**: 2129–2140.
63. Snehalatha C, Viswanathan V, Ramachandran A. (2003) Cutoff values for normal anthropometric variables in Asian Indian adults. *Diabet Care* **26**: 1380–1384.
64. Bhowmik B, Munir SB, Diep LM, Siddiquee T, Habib SH, Samad MA., Azad Khan AK, Hussain A. (2013) Anthropometric indicators of obesity for identifying cardiometabolic risk factors in a rural Bangladeshi population. *J Diabet Invest* **4**: 361–368.
65. Chandalia M, Abate N, Garg A, Stray-Gundersen J, Grundy SM. (1999) Relationship between generalized and upper body obesity to insulin resistance in Asian Indian men. *J Clin Endocrinol Metab* **84**: 2329–2335.
66. World Health Organization (2000) Western Pacific Region. The International Association for the Study of Obesity and the International Obesity Task Force. The Asia–Pacific Perspective: Redefining Obesity and its Treatment. Health Communications Australia Pty Limited, Sydney, Australia, 2000. Available at: www.diabetes.com.au/pdf/obesity_report.pdf (Last accessed August 23, 2006).
67. Abate N, Chandalia M. (2007) Ethnicity, type 2 diabetes & migrant Asian Indians. *Indian J Med Res* **125**: 251–258.
68. Abate N, Chandalia M, Snell PG *et al.* (2004) Adipose tissue metabolites and insulin resistance in nondiabetic Asian Indian men. *J Clin Endocrinol Metab* **89**: 2750–2755.

69. Balkau B, Deanfield JE, Despres JP, Bassand JP, Fox KA, Smith SC Jr, Barter P, Tan CE, Van Gaal L, Wittchen HU, Massien C, Haffner SM. (2007) International Day for the Evaluation of Abdominal Obesity (IDEA): A study of waist circumference, cardiovascular disease, and diabetes mellitus in 168,000 primary care patients in 63 countries. *Circulation* **116**: 1942–1951.
70. Alberti KG, Zimmet P, Shaw J. (2005) IDF Epidemiology Task Force Consensus Group. The metabolic syndrome: A new worldwide definition. *Lancet* **366**: 1059–1062.
71. Dudeja V, Misra A, Pandey RM, Devina G, Kumar G, Vikram NK. (2001) BMI does not accurately predict overweight in Asian Indians in northern India. *Br J Nutr* **86**: 105–112.
72. Banerji MA, Faridi N, Atluri R, Chaiken RL, Lebovitz HE. (1999) Body composition, visceral fat, leptin, and insulin resistance in Asian Indian men. *J Clin Endocrinol Metab* **84**: 137–144.
73. Hirani V, Stamatakis E. (2004) Anthropometric measures, overweight, and obesity, *The Scottish Health Survey* **6**: 163–203.
74. Yajnik CS, Lubree HG, Rege SS *et al.* (2002) Adiposity and hyperinsulinemia in Indians are present at birth. *J Clin Endocrinol Metab* **87**: 5575–5580.
75. Retnakaran R, Hanley AJ, Zinman B. (2006) Does hypoadiponectinemia explain the increased risk of diabetes and cardiovascular disease in South Asians? *Diabet Care* **29**: 1950–1954.
76. Asghar S, Hussain A, Khan AK, Ali SM, Sayeed MA, Bhowmik B *et al.* (2011) Incidence of diabetes in Asian-Indian subjects: A five year follow-up study from Bangladesh. *Prim Care Diabet* **5**: 117–124.
77. Mokdad AH, Bowman BA, Ford ES, Vinicor F, Marks JS, Koplan JP. (2001) The continuing epidemics of obesity and diabetes in the United States. *JAMA* **286**: 195–200.
78. Misra A, Khurana L, Isharwal S, Bhardwaj S. (2009) South Asian diets and insulin resistance. *Br J Nutr* **101**: 465–473.
79. Gilbert PA, Khokhar S. (2008) Changing dietary habits of ethnic groups in Europe and implications for health. *Nutr Rev* **66**: 203–215.
80. Khokhar S, Pandor A, Cade J. (2001) Eating habits: Food preparation and serving practices in ethnic populations: Critical review and assessment of dietary survey requirements. FSA project N08015. Report to the Food Standards Agency, London, UK.
81. Popkin BM, Horton S, Kim S, Mahal A, Shuigao J. (2001) Trends in diet, nutritional status, and diet-related noncommunicable diseases in China and India: The economic costs of the nutrition transition. *Nutr Rev* **59**: 379–390.

82. Haag M, Dippenaar NG. (2005) Dietary fats, fatty acids and insulin resistance: Short review of a multifaceted connection. *Med Sci Monit* **11**: 359–367.
83. Oh K, Hu FB, Manson JE, Stampfer MJ, Willett WC. (2005) Dietary fat intake and risk of coronary heart disease in women: 20 years of follow-up of the Nurses' Health Study. *Am J Epidemiol* **161**: 672–679.
84. Lovegrove JA, Lovegrove SS, Lesauvage SVM *et al.* (2004) Moderate fish oil supplementation reverses low-platelet, long-chain n-3 polyunsaturated fatty acid status and reduces plasma triacylglycerol concentrations in British Indo-Asians. *Am J Clin Nutr* **79**: 974–982.
85. Merchant AT, Anand SS, Kelemen LE, Vuksan V, Jacobs R, Davis B *et al.* (2007) Carbohydrate intake and HDL in a multiethnic population. *Am J Clin Nutr* **85**: 225–230.
86. Vuori I. (1995) Health benefits of physical activity with special reference to interaction with diet, *Diabetes* **44**: 1010–10.
87. Fischbacher CM, Hunt S, Alexander L. (2004) How physically active are South Asians in the United Kingdom? A literature review. *J Public Health* **26**: 250–258.
88. Hayes L, White M, Unwin N *et al.* (2002) Patterns of physical activity and relationship with risk markers for cardiovascular disease and diabetes in Indian, Pakistani, Bangladeshi and European adults in a UK population. *J Public Health Med* **24**: 170–178.
89. Sriskantharajah J, Kai J. (2007) Promoting physical activity among south Asian women with coronary heart disease and diabetes: What might help? *Family Practice* **24**: 71–76.
90. Eyler A. (2002) Correlates of physical activity among women from diverse racial/ethical groups. *J Women's Health Gender-Based Med* **11**: 239–252.
91. Jenum AK, Holme I, Graff-Iversen S, Birkeland KI. (2005) Ethnicity and sex are strong determinants of diabetes in an urban western society: Implications for prevention. *Diabetologia* **48**: 435–439.
92. Nemet D, Wang P, T. Funahashi T, Matsuzawa Y, Tanaka S, Engelman L *et al.* (2003) Adipocytokines, body composition and fitness in children. *Pediatr Res* **53**: 148–152.
93. McGarry JD. (2002) Banting Lecture 2001, Dysregulation of fatty acid metabolism in the etiology of type 2 diabetes. *Diabetes* **51**: 7–18.
94. International Diabetes Federation. (2002) Consensus on the Aetiology of Type 2 Diabetes Mellitus. Colombo, Sri Lanka, http://www. idf.org /home/ index.cfm?node=444.

95. Hales CN, Barker DJ. (2001) The thrifty phenotype hypothesis. *Br Med Bull* **60**: 5–20.
96. Neel JV. (1962) Diabetes mellitus: A "thrifty" genotype rendered detrimental by "progress"? *Am J Hum Genet* **14**: 353–362.
97. Eriksson J, Lindstrom J, Tuomiletho J. (2001) Potential for the prevention of type 2 diabetes. *Br Med Bull* **60**: 183–199.
98. Strauss RS. (1997) Effects of the intrauterine environment on childhood growth. *Br Med Bull* **53**: 81–95.
99. Yajnik CS. (2009) Nutrient-mediated teratogenesis and fuel-mediated teratogenesis: Two pathways of intrauterine programming of diabetes. *Int J Gynaecol Obstet* **104**: 27–31.
100. Bhargava SK, Sachdev HS, Fall CH *et al.* (2004) Relation of serial changes in childhood body-mass index to impaired glucose tolerance in young adulthood. *N Engl J Med* **350**: 865–875.
101. Chang YC, Chang TJ, Jiang YD *et al.* (2007) Association study of the genetic polymorphisms of the transcription factor 7-like 2 (TCF7L2) gene and T2DM in the Chinese population. *Diabetes* **56**: 2631–2637.
102. Yokoi N, Kanamori M, Horikawa Y *et al.* (2006) Association studies of variants in the genes involved in pancreatic beta-cell function in type 2 diabetes in Japanese subjects. *Diabetes* **55**: 2379–2386.
103. Ng MC, Lee SC, Ko GT *et al.* (2001) Familial early onset type 2 diabetes in Chinese patients: Obesity and genetics have more significant roles than autoimmunity. *Diabet Care* **24**: 663–671.
104. Chan JC, Ng MC. (2003) Lessons learned from youngonset diabetes in China. *Curr Diab Rep* **3**: 101–107.
105. Mohan V, Jaydip R, Deepa R. (2007) Type 2 diabetes in Asian Indian youth. *Pediatr Diabet* **8**: 28–34.
106. Dyson PA, Hammersley MS, Morris RJ, Holman RR, Turner RC. (1997) The Fasting Hyperglycaemia Study Group, The Fasting Hyperglycaemia Study: II. Randomized controlled trial of reinforced healthy-living advice in subjects with increased but not diabetic fasting plasma glucose. *Metabolism* **46**: 50–55.
107. The Diabetes Prevention Program Research Group (2000) The Diabetes Prevention Program, Baseline characteristics of the randomized cohort. *Diabet Care* **23**: 1619–1629.
108. The Diabetes Prevention Program Research Group (2003) Costs associated with the primary prevention of T2DM mellitus in the diabetes prevention program. *Diabet Care* **26**: 36–47.

109. Chiasson JL, Gomis R, Hanefeld M, Josse RG, Karasik A, Laakso M. (1998) The STOP-NIDDM Trial Research Group, The STOP-NIDDM Trial. An international study on the efficacy of an α-glucosidase inhibitor to prevent T2DM in a population with impaired glucose tolerance: Rationale, design, and preliminary data. *Diabet Care* **21**: 1720–1725.
110. Chiasson JL, Josse RG, Gomis R, Hanefeld M, Karasik A, Laakso M. (2002) Acarbose for prevention of T2DM mellitus: The STOP-NIDDM randomised trial. *Lancet* **359**: 2072–2077.
111. Hanefeld M, Josse RG, Gomis R, Karasik A, Laakso M, Chiasson JL. (2002) Efficacy of acarbose to prevent T2DM is different in subgroups of subjects with impaired glucose tolerance: The STOP-NIDDM trial. *Diabetologia* **45**: 104–105.
112. Chiasson J, Josse RG, Gomis R, Hanefeld M, Karasik A, Laakso M. (2002) Acarbose can prevent T2DM and cardiovascular disease in subjects with impaired glucose tolerance: The STOP-NIDDM trial. *Diabetologia* **45**: 104.
113. Holman RR, North BU, Tunbridge FKE. (2000) Possible prevention of T2DM with acarbose or metformin. *Diabet Med* **17**: 17.
114. Ramachandran A, Snehalatha C, Mary S, Mukesh B, Bhaskar AD, Vijay V. (2006) The Indian Diabetes Prevention Programme shows that lifestyle modification and metformin prevent T2DM in Asian Indian subjects with impaired glucose tolerance (IDPP-1). *Diabetologia* **49**: 289–297.
115. Sakane N, Sato J, Tsushita K, Tsujii S, Kotani K, Tsuzaki K *et al.* (2011) Prevention of T2DM in a primary healthcare setting: Three-year results of lifestyle intervention in Japanese subjects with impaired glucose tolerance. *BMC Public Health* **17**: 40.
116. Holman RR, Blackwell L, Stratton IM, Manley SE, Tucker L, Frighi V. (2003) Six-year results from the Early Diabetes Intervention Trial. *Diabet Med* **20**: 15.
117. Azen SP, Peters RK, Berkowitz K, Kjos S, Xiang A, Buchanan TA. (1998) TRIPOD (TRoglitazone In the Prevention of Diabetes): A randomized, placebo-controlled trial of troglitazone in women with prior gestational diabetes mellitus. *Control Clin Trials* **19**: 217–231.
118. Sjostrom L, Torgerson JS, Hauptman J, Boldrin M. (2002) XENDOS (XENical in the prevention of Diabetes in Obese Subjects): A landmark study. 9th International Congress on Obesity, Sao Paulo, Brazil.
119. Holman RR, North BU, Tunbridge FKE. (2000) Possible prevention of T2DM with acarbose or metformin. *Diabet Med* **17**:17.

120. Davies MJ, Tringham JR, Troughton J, Khunti KK. (2004) Prevention of T2DM mellitus. A review of the evidence and its application in a UK setting. **5**: 403–414.
121. Ritchie LD, Ganapathy S, Woodward-Lopez G, Gerstein DE, Fleming SE. (2003) Prevention of T2DM in youth: Etiology, promising interventions and recommendations. *Pediatric Diabet* **4**: 174–209.
122. Holman RR, Blackwell L, Stratton IM, Manley SE, Tucker L, Frighi V. (2003) Six-year results from the Early Diabetes Intervention Trial. *Diabet Med* **20**: S15.
123. Hydrie MZI, Basit A, Samad SA, Hussain A. (2012) Effect of Intervention in Subject with High Risk of Diabetes Mellitus in Pakistan. *J Nutrition Metab* **2012**: 867604.
124. Tuomilehto J. (2009) Nonpharmacologic therapy and exercise in the prevention of T2DM. *Diabetes Care* **32**: 189–193.
125. Hussain-Gambles M, Leese B, Atkin K, Brown J, Mason S, Tovey P. (2004) Involving South Asian patients in clinical trials. *Health Technol Assess* **8**: 109.
126. Hjellset VT. (2011) A culturally adapted lifestyle intervention with main focus on blood glucose regulation improved the risk profile for type 2 diabtes in pakistani immigrant women. They are not aliens. Faculty of medicine, University of Oslo.
127. Fisher EB, Jr., La Greca AM, Greco P, Arfken C, Schneiderman N. (1997) Directive and nondirective social support in diabetes management. *Int J Behav Med* **4**:131–144.
128. Hawthorne K. (2001) Effect of culturally appropriate health education on glycaemic control and knowledge of diabetes in British Pakistani women with T2DM mellitus. *Health Educ Res* **16**: 373–381.
129. Kousar R, Burns C, Lewandowski P. (2008) A culturally appropriate diet and lifestyle intervention can successfully treat the components of metabolic syndrome in female Pakistani immigrants residing in Melbourne, Australia. *Metabolism* **57**:1502–1508.

Chapter 10: European Initiatives in Diabetes Prevention: Policy Perspectives

Peter E. H. Schwarz,† and Jaakko Tuomilehto‡*

1. THE EUROPEAN PERSPECTIVES OF DIABETES PREVENTION

In the last decades, Europe like other parts of the world, has experienced a significant increase in the number of patients with diabetes mellitus (DM).[1,2] The International Diabetes Federation (IDF) global estimates show that 53 million people living in Europe aged 20–79 years had DM in 2011 and that the number will exceed 64 million by 2030. In addition, 63 million Europeans had impaired glucose tolerance (IGT) in 2011 (Table 1). The continuous increase in the prevalence of DM is not only due to a shift in the population age distribution, but also to changing lifestyles leading to an unhealthy diet, increased prevalence of overweight and physical inactivity.[1,2] Even though several European countries have the highest incidence of type 1 diabetes (T1D) in the world, which

*Corresponding author.
†Technical University Dresden, Germany.
Paul Langerhans Institute Dresden, German Center for Diabetes Research (DZD), Dresden, Germany.
Prevention and Care of Diabetes mellitus, Department of Medicine III, University of Dresden, Fetscherstrasse 74, 01307 Dresden, Germany. Email: peter.schwarz@uniklinikum-dresden.de
‡Centre for Vascular Prevention, Danube-University Krems, Krems, Austria.
Diabetes Prevention Unit, National Institute for Health and Welfare, Helsinki, Finland.
Instituto de Investigacion Sanitaria del Hospital Universario LaPaz (IdiPAZ), Madrid, Spain.
Diabetes Research Group, King Abdulaziz University, Jeddah, Saudi Arabia. Email: jaakko.tuomilehto@thl.fi

has steadily increased over last decades,[3] the increase in the number of people with diabetes is primarily due to type 2 diabetes (T2D). Parallel to this, the increase is mostly attributable to a significantly higher frequency of diabetes being diagnosed in those under 60, as well as below 35 years of age.[1]

The growing economic burden due to diabetes in complex socioeconomic structures becomes obvious. The development of the diabetes epidemic is predicted to have a significant impact on global economic growth[3] including Europe. Approximately 15% of all health care expenses in Europe are due to DM, and most of this is due to CVD complications.

This situation requires different approaches from national health planning and care systems regardless of national health care structures, medical, environmental, social and economic means. In order to respond rapidly in a coordinated fashion to the health threat posed by diabetes and its associated co-morbidities, it is necessary to standardize plans and prioritize the quality and structure of diabetes prevention and care. The goals, processes, responsibilities, availability and accessibility of diabetes care, are critical components of Chronic Care Management,[4] a segment of which is the National Diabetes Program (NDP).[5]

At the United Nations High Level Meeting for Non-Communicable Diseases (NCD) in September 2011 in New York, Ministers of Health requested international cooperation and policy decisions on diabetes according to the present context of globalization of health issues.[6,7] There was a consensus across countries that national programs for prevention and control of chronic diseases have to be developed and implemented and that strategies for monitoring progress on implementation needed to be established. In April 2012, the European Diabetes Leadership Forum[8] was held, hosted by the Organisation for Economic Cooperation and Development (OECD) and the Danish Diabetes Association, under the auspices of the Danish Presidency of the European Council. The focus of this Forum was to discuss developing strategies on political, medical and patient-centered approaches for improving diabetes prevention, early detection and management. Kofi Annan stated at the meeting *"There is no other option than to act — to improve quality of diabetes care."*

The most effective way to manage diabetes and its complications is to prevent its development in the first place.[9] Recent studies have conclusively demonstrated that preventive approaches delay the onset of diabetes or prevent its development.[10–13] Intervention strategies addressing diet and exercise may reduce the relative risk of developing diabetes by 50–60%. Economic evaluation has demonstrated the cost-effectiveness of primary prevention of T2D.[14] Despite the evidence of efficacy within randomized controlled trial (RCT) settings, it remains questionable to what extent diabetes prevention will be feasible at a population level. The challenge, therefore, is to establish a scientifically-based structural framework for efficiently managing nationwide prevention programs.

In 2008, the authors already defined actionable steps for diabetes prevention.[15] What is the situation today? What has been achieved? A number of large European and other initiatives have addressed the need for the prevention of T2D. These initiatives have enabled interaction among researchers, health care professionals, public health experts including involvement of lay persons in the development and recognition of activities for the prevention of diabetes.[16] It should be noted that before the year 2000, primary prevention of T2D was not listed among health priorities in any country in the world. Yet, WHO had recommended action to be taken in its member countries in the mid-1990s,[17] but none of the WHO member states initiated action to prevent diabetes at that time.

The first results from a RCT on prevention of T2D was published from Sweden in 1980[18] demonstrating that more than half of incident cases of T2D were prevented by either diet intervention or the sulfonylurea tolbutamide in people with IGT. The trial, however, had shortcomings and therefore did not receive much attention.

2. EUROPEAN ACTIVITIES

One of the first landmark projects has been the **DE-PLAN Project** ("Diabetes in Europe — Prevention using Lifestyle, Physical Activity and Nutritional intervention").[19] The project was led by the University of Helsinki, tried to translate the evidence and expertise derived from large clinical trials in the prevention of diabetes into clinical practice. The overall goal was to maintain scientific standards in their implementation while addressing needs defined by clinical and prevention practices. Most European partner institutions enabled the performance of screening for those at high-risk of T2D and implemented local projects for diabetes prevention whereas others cultivated the development of scientific and political milieus to increase awareness for diabetes prevention especially in Greece, Spain, Poland, Austria, Finland, Germany, Norway and Italy.[19–31] A large number of people have been included in the implementation trials showing various results. As DE-PLAN was an implementation study, and not an efficacy trial, it therefore did not employ RCT design. What is the reason for this? The translation from a structured RCT into public health and clinical practice is not simple and easy. The translation of trial results to routine practice in medicine depends on society values, available funds and political will to undertake necessary decisions, many of which need to include principal stakeholders that are mostly outside the health sector.[32] An important aspect of translation initiatives is that appropriate candidates are not as selective as those enrolled in clinical trials. Furthermore, scaling an intervention for public health practice will obviously loosen standardization of the intervention by gaining more practicability. Most of the DE-PLAN subprojects have been transitional, thus generating significant experience regarding barriers and gaps for the implementation of T2D prevention programs in Europe. DE-PLAN was the first to collate practice knowledge in order to establish diabetes prevention programs in "real life settings" that vary markedly even within Europe.

In parallel with DE-PLAN, the **DIAMAP** project,[33] initiated by the European Coalition for Diabetes, was a short European Union funded project to develop a roadmap for diabetes research in Europe. A substantial number of European scientists undertook specific focus groups in diabetes research to formulate research objectives needed to be in the forthcoming decade. One focus group addressing translational aspects in diabetes research identified diabetes prevention as a worthwhile objective for intervention. The DIAMAP Road Map was published in 2010 and currently serves as a consulting draft for the European Commission to formulate new research targets in the diabetes arena. Thus, DIAMAP continues to serve as an advocate for European diabetes research, including prevention.

The project "Better control in Pediatric and Adolescent diabete**S**: **W**orking to cr**E**ate c**E**n**T**ers of reference (**SWEET**) was not directly dedicated to primary prevention of T2D,[34] but was more focused on T1D diabetes aspects in children and adolescence. The landmark achievement of SWEET, which standardized therapeutic and preventive guidelines in the management of young patients with T1D, was in formulating clinical guidelines as one of the first steps for integrated individualized disease management in the diabetes sector. The SWEET projects offers an updated and continuous evaluation of diabetes treatment regimens for all children with diabetes in Europe. To support this goal, an appropriate and secure data management system has been created within the project.[35,36]

In parallel, the European Region of the IDF founded a working group — the **Diabetes Prevention Forum** — which aimed at building a platform to bring together researchers, politicians, health workers and health economists from Europe to enhance the capacity for developing public health and practice approaches for diabetes prevention.[15] The members of the steering committee of the Diabetes Prevention Forum formulated necessary action steps which have to be undertaken for implementing diabetes prevention programs within the health care system of European member states. Members of the Diabetes Prevention Forum together with the IDF described state of the art diabetes prevention and care policies with issuing the Policy Puzzle.[37–39] The latter included an assessment of national diabetes plans including disease management and prevention management strategies across all health policies in member states. This policy puzzle provided the first realistic picture of the existence of diabetes prevention policies, screening programs, prevention management concepts and educational activities for health care professionals in order to disseminate diabetes prevention expertise. Driven by this, the Diabetes Prevention Forum developed a robust platform to lobby for diabetes prevention activities at the political stakeholder level.

Based on European networks of diabetes prevention in 2006, the concept aims to combine existing evidence of diabetes prevention and to standardize this for translation into practice. This was started with the development of the **IMAGE** ("Development and Implementation of a European Guideline and Training Standards for Diabetes prevention")[40,41] project. IMAGE brought together more than 100 experts in diabetes prevention within the European Union and created a group of experts from science, public health, health insurance, health economists and politicians dedicated to the task of developing practical, relevant materials for a successful diabetes prevention initiative. The IMAGE Project Study Group collated information in a systematic manner based on clinical trials experience as well as from "real world" implementation programs, The IMAGE deliverables include an evidence-based guideline,[42] a practice toolkit,[43] a guideline for evaluation, quality indicators and management in T2D prevention.[44] Furthermore, a European training curriculum for prevention managers to perform T2D prevention intervention programs was developed.[45] Summarizing scientific and practical information in a condensed format for practice implementation is a key requirement for effective diabetes prevention. With this, IMAGE has developed the basis for diabetes prevention practice in Europe which has already spread internationally. The IMAGE Toolkit for prevention practice is translated into more than 20 languages and is available in more than 50 countries worldwide[43] and can be found on the IDF website. The curriculum for training prevention managers was used to train prevention experts in Europe, Asia and Latin America and is continuously gaining greater distribution.[45] Information regarding T2D prevention in Latin America is described in this text by Gabriel *et al.* (see Chapter 20). Some countries have started national projects to standardize and customize the training curriculum for prevention mangers to accommodate national circumstances. The Diabetes Prevention Forum currently collates all nationally running projects in order to build a European database for prevention management.

3. ONGOING EUROPEAN INITIATIVES

European activities have progressed from the initial planning period and targeted tasks for T2D prevention. It is now evident that European countries are by far the most advanced with regards to T2D prevention compared with other regions of the world. While Europeans can be proud of considerable achievements in advancing diabetes prevention, it is important to be humble and understand that there are still many questions left unanswered before T2D diminishes.

It is always important to study and comprehend history. Humanity has encountered numerous population-wide health problems or disasters. Many of these have been partially controlled while very few created by environmental exposure have been entirely eradicated. The effectiveness of interventions may vary. It is important to understand the extent to which lifestyle intervention alone or in combination with pharmacotherapy will be successful for prevention of NCD such as T2D and its complications. To address this, the **ePREDICE (Early Prevention of Diabetes Complications in Europe)** project has been initiated in Europe and Australia. This randomized, controlled, prospective trial will test the efficacy of lifestyle intervention compared with additional therapy using metformin, a DPP-4 inhibitor and the combination of both drugs over a 3 to 6-year period in the prevention of diabetes and its early complications in individuals with prediabetes.

Another question pertains to implementation of innovative disease management programs for effective prevention. Evidence from care-based and public health research suggests that disease management is only effective by including preventive activities as an integral part of modern, innovative chronic care management plans. This is being evaluated in a forthcoming large European public health funded project–**MANAGE-CARE**. The MANAGE-CARE ("Active Ageing with T2D as Model for the Development and Implementation of Innovative Chronic Care Management in Europe") project translates prevention management aspects into care of those with chronic diseases with T2D as a model. In this project, evidence from disease management will be translated back to prevention management with the aim of integrating prevention care and rehabilitation into a single, chronic care management concept. This project initiated in September 2013, may enhance the capability for addressing the burden of T2D and effective prevention management within Europe.

4. MONITORING WHAT HAS BEEN ACHIEVED — GLOBAL DIABETES SURVEY

Successful implementation of diabetes prevention programs must include a component of monitoring. Most of the political, public health and medical large-scale initiatives in the past such as the St. Vincent Declaration[46] and various diabetes education initiatives failed due to the lack of monitoring. A very recent initiative entitled **Global Diabetes Survey** addresses this need.[47] By using a standardized questionnaire which represents the essence of expertise from more than 700 experts in diabetes prevention and care globally, the Global Diabetes Survey assesses the quality of diabetes care and its prevention in several countries. This is achieved by inviting representative volunteers in each country from three core focus groups, and volunteers representing different diabetes management levels (affected persons, caretakers, stakeholders in 19 diabetes-related groups). The Global Diabetes Survey performs its assessment on a yearly basis in order to present a representative picture about the quality of diabetes care and T2D prevention for each country. With this tool, the aforementioned activities can be monitored and the effects relevant for achieving change on the primary care level can be observed. Initial results demonstrate considerable variability in the quality of diabetes care that is provided within the European Union (43% to 76% showing the highest quality of diabetes care). Patients rate all aspects of diabetes care much more critically than professional participants (more than a 25% difference).

5. NETWORK "WHO ARE ACTIVE IN DIABETES PREVENTION?"

An important current initiative is the start of an international network "Who are active in diabetes prevention?" The aim of which is to provide a single network for those interested in the prevention of T2D or who want to become active in the field. The network itself encourages exchanging knowledge, recent intervention materials as well as educational standards. The most important focus of the network is the exchange of experiences in diabetes prevention practices. It is also thought of as a platform to exchange scientific information or up-to-date study information among research groups and others active in diabetes prevention. Individuals from more than 140 countries have joined the network and, in particular, many participants come from low- and middle-income countries. The goal is to disseminate information about established diabetes prevention practices and newly initiated prevention programs which thereby will enhance the quality of interventions. Anyone interested in the prevention of diabetes is invited to register for free and benefit from this global network–www.activeindiabetesprevention.com.

6. WHAT ARE THE CHALLENGES FOR THE FUTURE?

To be effective in the prevention of T2D at the population level, political support at local and national levels is needed. Prevention plans help relevant stakeholders establish networks agreeing upon concerted actions involving resources from societal and individual sources. European experts, in 2008, identified the following challenges that have been addressed to achieve success in T2D prevention[15,33,35,36,39,41,47]: educational curricula are available for health care professionals,[45] the continued growth of evidence for feasibility of implementation of diabetes prevention programs[43] and achievement of an evidence-base for expertise in prevention management. Increased awareness on the political stakeholder level is needed to foster actions in T2D prevention and to specify individual interventions in order to increase their effectiveness. Attention should also be paid to disadvantaged groups in society. The risk of T2D and its complications are known to be particularly high in individuals with a lower socio-economic status in whom it may be more difficult to achieve lifestyle changes. Joint political action is needed to generate awareness for effective prevention and modern chronic care management. The European Coalition for Diabetes, the IDF — European Region, a number of other scientific, political and MANAGE-CARE stakeholders are engaged in this effort. It is obvious that one of the challenges which have to be addressed in the future is the personalized approach for T2D prevention.

7. FULFILLING THE DEVELOPMENT OF A NATIONAL DIABETES PREVENTION PROGRAM

Evolving from scientific discovery to broad population-wide implementation requires moving through a series of steps where each step builds on the achievements of the previous ones. T2D prevention provides an example of the necessity of moving from basic science to wide-spread distribution of proven public health and community-based interventions. In some countries, efforts to scale diabetes interventions for at-risk populations have begun,[48] but this presents challenges in achieving sizable regional and national programs. The scaling of regional or national programs requires a competent work force of lifestyle intervention providers as well as health services professionals, health economists, public health professionals, and community-based organizations capable of working with policymakers and gaining political support to develop national action plans and policies for the expansion of T2D prevention programs. A global stakeholder network can share experiences and build on knowledge gained from partnerships. There is a growing need for delivering effective and affordable prevention programs and to take urgent action to address the major public health challenge that T2D represents.

Within the European Union, only five of 27 countries have a national diabetes plan and only one has a national T2D prevention program.[15] In Asia, the situation is similar with a progressive increase in the number of countries including T2D prevention in their national policies.[49] The United States is at the forefront of governmental initiatives for developing a T2D prevention program with the CDC being the driving force for coordinating the national effort.[50] The existence of a national policy for supporting T2D prevention does not always equate with implementation of a real prevention program but it is a mandatory first step for a successful public health T2D prevention program. The European Coalition for Diabetes, together with the EU Diabetes Working Group, has created working groups which have elaborated recommendations for the EU institutions and local governments in order to address the need for delivering adequate diabetes care in Europe. These recommendations address prevention of T2D, provide an adequate scientific basis from basic research, efficacy studies in highly controlled environments, and effectiveness studies in real-world environments performed by clinical researchers and public health experts. To scale-up diabetes preventive actions to the population level, program strategies need to be adjusted to have the best effect for a relevant proportion of the population as well as for the supply and diffusion of interventions to the populace. Policy development is a necessary component of these steps. The development of national diabetes plans that are supported by local prevention management in conjunction with adequate networking and stakeholder involvement are necessary to address this challenge and guide implementation of T2D prevention.[5]

8. SUMMARY

8.1. The Evidence that T2D is a Preventable Disease is Excellent

A number of randomized, controlled, trials have shown that diabetes risk can be reduced by greater than 50%. Recent data also show that this effect is sustainable for more than a decade.[51] Programs that have attempted to translate scientific evidence into clinical and public health practice have proven that similar results are reachable in real life and that it is feasible to implement T2D prevention programs in different care processes and structures. Translation studies also have shown that health care policies and existing health care structures determine the formulation of a T2D prevention program and the outcome for those at high-risk. Over the last years, we have learned considerably about non-pharmacological lifestyle interventions and their documented effectiveness in clinical settings in preventing T2D. Furthermore, we have gained significant knowledge about policies that need to be developed[9] and effective strategies for identifying those with increased risk for T2D.[43]

Presently, we need to shift the focus of attention from the research arena into the political field. Political support is needed to build the framework for successful implementation of T2D prevention programs.[5] Together, with all relevant stakeholders, we have to build effective and sustainable prevention programs. There is no excuse for researchers and public health not to act–as Kofi Annan has stated: "We have not enough money to do nothing."

REFERENCES

1. Whiting DR, Guariguata L, Weil C, Shaw J. (2011) IDF diabetes atlas: Global estimates of the prevalence of diabetes for 2011 and 2030. *Diabetes Res Clin Pract* **94**: 311–321.
2. International Diabetes Federation. (2012) *IDF Diabetes Atlas*, 5th ed. International Diabetes Federation, Belgium, http://www.idf.org/diabetesatlas.
3. Zimmet P, Alberti KG, Shaw J. (2001) Global and societal implications of the diabetes epidemic. *Nature* **414**: 782–787.
4. Rothe U, Muller G, Schwarz PE, Seifert M, Kunath H *et al.* (2008) Evaluation of a diabetes management system based on practice guidelines, integrated care, and continuous quality management in a Federal State of Germany: A population-based approach to health care research. *Diabetes Care* **31**: 863–868.
5. Schwarz PE. (2011) Public health implications: Translation into diabetes prevention initiatives — four-level public health concept. *Med Clin North Am* **95**: 397–407.
6. Keeling A. (2011) The UN Summit and beyond: A new era for diabetes. *Diabetes Res Clin Pract* **94**: 163–165.
7. Keeling A. (2011) Anniversary of vote on UN Summit: Progress to date and challenges remaining. *Diabetes Res Clin Pract* **92**: 409–410.
8. Schwarz PE. (2012) Newsletter 6.2012 — European Diabetes Leadership Forum Report — 25–26 April 2012 in Copenhagen, Denmark. *Network Active in Diabetes Prevention* **3**: 5.
9. Schwarz PE, Greaves CJ, Lindstrom J, Yates T, Davies MJ. (2012) Nonpharmacological interventions for the prevention of type 2 diabetes mellitus. *Nat Rev Endocrinol* **8**: 363–373.
10. Knowler WC, Barrett-Connor E, Fowler SE, Hamman RF, Lachin JM *et al.* (2002) Reduction in the incidence of type 2 diabetes with lifestyle intervention or metformin. *N Engl J Med* **346**: 393–403.
11 Tuomilehto J, Lindstrom J, Eriksson JG, Valle TT, Hamalainen H *et al.* (2001) Prevention of type 2 diabetes mellitus by changes in lifestyle among subjects with impaired glucose tolerance. *N Engl J Med* **344**: 1343–1350.
12. Chiasson JL, Josse RG, Gomis R, Hanefeld M, Karasik A *et al.* (2002) Acarbose for prevention of type 2 diabetes mellitus: The STOP-NIDDM randomised trial. *Lancet* **359**: 2072–2077.
13. Pan XR, Li GW, Hu YH, Wang JX, Yang WY *et al.* (1997) Effects of diet and exercise in preventing NIDDM in people with impaired glucose tolerance. The Da Qing IGT and Diabetes Study. *Diabetes Care* **20**: 537–544.

14. Hernan WH, Brandle M, Zhang P, Williamson DF, Matulik MJ *et al.* (2003) Costs associated with the primary prevention of type 2 diabetes mellitus in the diabetes prevention program. *Diabetes Care* **26**: 36–47.
15. Schwarz PE, Muylle F, Valensi P, Hall M, Diabetes Prevention Forum IDFE. (2008) The European perspective of diabetes prevention. *Horm Metab Res* **40**: 511–514.
16. Halban PA, Boulton AJ, Smith U. (2012) A new paradigm for improved co-ordination and efficacy of European biomedical research: Taking diabetes as a model. *Diabetologia* **56**: 439–443.
17. World HealthOrganization. (1994) Prevention of Diabetes mellitus — Report of a WHO Study Group. WHO Technical Report Series WHO Technical Report Series 844.
18. Eriksson KF, Lindgarde F. (1991) Prevention of type 2 (non-insulin-dependent) diabetes mellitus by diet and physical exercise. The 6-year Malmo feasibility study. *Diabetologia* **34**: 891–898.
19. Schwarz PE, Lindstrom J, Kissimova-Scarbeck K, Szybinski Z, Barengo NC *et al.* (2008) The European perspective of type 2 diabetes prevention: Diabetes in Europe — prevention using lifestyle, physical activity and nutritional intervention (DE-PLAN) project. *Exp Clin Endocrinol Diabetes* **116**: 167–172.
20. Telle-Hjellset V, Raberg Kjollesdal MK, Bjorge B, Holmboe-Ottesen G, Wandel M *et al.* (2012) The InnvaDiab-DE-PLAN study: A randomised controlled trial with a culturally adapted education programme improved the risk profile for type 2 diabetes in Pakistani immigrant women. *Br J Nutr* **4**: 1–10.
21. Hjellset VT, Ihlebaek CM, Bjorge B, Eriksen HR, Hostmark AT. (2010) Health-related quality of life, subjective health complaints, psychological distress and coping in Pakistani immigrant women with and without the metabolic syndrome: The InnvaDiab-DEPLAN study on Pakistani immigrant women living in Oslo, Norway. *J Immigr Minor Health* **13**: 732–741.
22. Hjellset VT, Bjorge B, Eriksen HR, Hostmark AT. (2011) Risk factors for type 2 diabetes among female Pakistani immigrants: The InvaDiab-DEPLAN study on Pakistani immigrant women living in Oslo, Norway. *J Immigr Minor Health* **13**: 101–110.
23. Johansen KS, Bjorge B, Hjellset VT, Holmboe-Ottesen G, Raberg M *et al.* (2010) Changes in food habits and motivation for healthy eating among Pakistani women living in Norway: Results from the InnvaDiab-DEPLAN study. *Public Health Nutr* **13**: 858–867.
24. Kontogianni MD, Liatis S, Grammatikou S, Perrea D, Katsilambros N *et al.* (2012) Changes in dietary habits and their association with metabolic

markers after a non-intensive, community-based lifestyle intervention to prevent type 2 diabetes, in Greece. The DEPLAN study. *Diabetes Res Clin Pract* **95**: 207–214.
25. Makrilakis K, Liatis S, Grammatikou S, Perrea D, Stathi C *et al.* (2011) Validation of the Finnish diabetes risk score (FINDRISC) questionnaire for screening for undiagnosed type 2 diabetes, dysglycaemia and the metabolic syndrome in Greece. *Diabetes Metab* **37**: 144–151.
26. Makrilakis K, Liatis S, Grammatikou S, Perrea D, Katsilambros N. (2010) Implementation and effectiveness of the first community lifestyle intervention programme to prevent Type 2 diabetes in Greece. The DE-PLAN study. *Diabet Med* **27**: 459–465.
27. Sanchez A, Silvestre C, Sauto R, Martinez C, Grandes G. (2012) Feasibility and effectiveness of the implementation of a primary prevention programme for type 2 diabetes in routine primary care practice: A phase IV cluster randomised clinical trial. *BMC Fam Pract* **13**: 109.
28. Costa B, Barrio F, Cabre JJ, Pinol JL, Cos X *et al.* (2012) Delaying progression to type 2 diabetes among high-risk Spanish individuals is feasible in real-life primary healthcare settings using intensive lifestyle intervention. *Diabetologia* **55**: 1319–1328.
29. Esposito K, Maiorino MI, Ceriello A, Giugliano D. (2010) Prevention and control of type 2 diabetes by Mediterranean diet: A systematic review. *Diabetes Res Clin Pract* **89**: 97–102.
30. Schwarz PE, Li J, Reimann M, Schutte AE, Bergmann A *et al.* (2009) The Finnish Diabetes Risk Score Is Associated with Insulin Resistance and Progression towards Type 2 Diabetes. *J Clin Endocrinol Metab* **94**: 920–926.
31. Kulzer B, Hermanns N, Gorges D, Schwarz P, Haak T. (2009) Prevention of diabetes self-management program (PREDIAS): Effects on weight, metabolic risk factors, and behavioral outcomes. *Diabetes Care* **32**: 1143–1146.
32. Schwarz PEH, Albright AL. (2011) Prevention of type 2 diabetes: The strategic approach for implementation. *Horm Metab Res* **43**: 907–910.
33. Hills S, Halban PA. (2011) DIAMAP: A road map for diabetes research in Europe. *J Diabetes Sci Technol* **5**: 794–797.
34. Danne T, Aschemeier B, Perfetti R. (2012) SWEET — where are we heading with international type 1 diabetes registries? *Pediatr Diabetes* **13**: 1–4.
35. Danne T, Lion S, Madaczy L, Veeze H, Raposo F *et al.* (2012) Criteria for centers of reference for pediatric diabetes — a European perspective. *Pediatr Diabetes* **13**: 62–75.

36. Forsander G, Pellinat M, Volk M, Muller M, Pinelli L *et al.* (2012) Technical solution for data collection, data safety and data privacy legislation: Experiences from the SWEET study. *Pediatr Diabetes* **13**: 39–48.
37. Hall M, Felton AM, Henrichs HR, Barnett A. (2005) Diabetes, the policy puzzle: Towards benchmaking in the EU 25. International Diabetes Federation European Region and Federation of European Nurses in Diabetes. 103 p.
38. Felton AM, Henrichs HR, Barnett A, Hall M. (2008) Diabetes, the policy puzzle: is Europe making progress?: International Diabetes Federation European Region and Federation of European Nurses in Diabetes. 103 p.
39. Hall M, Felton A. (2011) The Policy Puzzle: The diabetes maze in Europe. *Br J Diabetes Vasc Dis* **12**: 97.
40. Schwarz PE, Gruhl U, Bornstein SR, Landgraf R, Hall M *et al.* (2007) The European perspective on diabetes prevention: Development and implementation of a European guideline and training standards for diabetes prevention (IMAGE). *Diab Vasc Dis Res* **4**: 353–357.
41. Schwarz PE, Lindstrom J. (2011) From evidence to practice — the IMAGE project — new standards in the prevention of type 2 diabetes. *Diabetes Res Clin Pract* **91**: 138–140.
42. Paulweber B, Valensi P, Lindström J, Lalic NM, Greaves CJ *et al.* (2010) A European evidence-based guideline for the prevention of type 2 diabetes. *Horm Metab Res* **42**: S3–S36.
43. Lindstrom J, Neumann A, Sheppard KE, Gilis-Januszewska A, Greaves CJ *et al.* (2010) Take action to prevent diabetes — the IMAGE toolkit for the prevention of type 2 diabetes in Europe. *Horm Metab Res* **42**: S37–55.
44. Pajunen P, Landgraf R, Muylle F, Neumann A, Lindstrom J *et al.* (2010) Quality indicators for the prevention of type 2 diabetes in Europe — IMAGE. *Horm Metab Res* **42**: S56–63.
45. Kronsbein P, Fischer MR, Tolks D, Greaves C, Puhl S *et al.* (2011) IMAGE — Development of a European curriculum for the training of prevention managers. *Br J Diabetes Vasc Dis* **11**: 163–167.
46. Cathelineau G. (1999) The St Vincent declaration. A long march for significant changes. *Diabetes Metab* **25**: 5–8.
47. Schwarz PE, Gallein G, Ebermann D, Muller A, Lindner A *et al.* (2013) Global diabetes survey — An annual report on quality of diabetes care. *Diabetes Res Clin Pract* **100**: 11–18.
48. Johnson M, Jones R, Freeman C, Woods HB, Gillett M *et al.* (2013) Can diabetes prevention programmes be translated effectively into real-world settings and still deliver improved outcomes? A synthesis of evidence. *Diabet Med* **30**: 3–15.

49. Onyegbutulem HC, PI HO, Reimann M, Li J, Bornstein SR *et al.* (2009) Metabolic syndrome in Africa: An emerging perspective. *Horm Metab Res* **41**: 75–78.
50. Albright A, Williamson DF. (2011) Community approaches to diabetes prevention. In: LeRoith D (ed), *Prevention of Type 2 diabetes; From Science to Therapies*. Springer, New York.
51. Tuomilehto J, Schwarz P, Lindstrom J. (2011) Long-term benefits from lifestyle interventions for type 2 diabetes prevention: Time to expand the efforts. *Diabetes Care* **34**: S210–214.

Chapter 11: Real Life Diabetes Prevention in Europe

*P.E.H. Schwarz and A. Gilis-Januszewska**

1. INTRODUCTION/BACKGROUND

The prevalence of type 2 diabetes (T2D) and associated co-morbidities are rising worldwide. Epidemiological evidence suggests that without effective prevention and control programs the prevalence will continue to increase globally.[1] In Europe, about 55 million people aged 20–79 have diabetes and the number is expected to rise to 66 million in 2030.[2]

More than half of the European population will acquire hyperglycemia and/or diabetes during their lifetimes.[3] Diabetes and impaired glucose tolerance are increasingly appearing amongst the elderly, and also in younger individuals, with a particularly rapid increase in those under 30–40 years of age.[4]

Individuals with T2D have a two to four time higher risk of cardiovascular disease (CVD) and their life expectancy is lower than the rest of the population. Premature mortality caused by diabetes results in an estimated 12 to 14 years of life lost.[5]

The dramatic increase in new cases of T2D has resulted in a major public health concern in the European Union (EU). Diabetes results in an economic burden to patients and society.[4] The escalating rates of micro- and macrovascular complications of diabetes dramatically increased the costs due to longer-term and intensified medical treatment.[6]

*Corresponding author: myjanusz@cyf-kr.edu.pl
Medical Faculty Carl Gustav Carus of the Technical University Dresden, Department of Medicine III, Dresden, Germany
Chair and Department of Endocrinology Collegium Medicum, Jagiellonian University

Most of the risk factors associated with T2D are preventable. There is evidence from several randomized control trials including the Finnish Diabetes Prevention Study (DPS), Diabetes Prevention Study (DPP), Indian Diabetes Prevention Study (IDPP), Japanese Prevention trial and others that through lifestyle intervention, mainly weight loss and physical activity and/or hypoglycemic drugs, an approximate 60% reduction in T2D incidence might be achieved.[7–12]

2. THE DE-PLAN STUDY

However, randomized control trials with individual counseling lasting usually several years are very expensive and their application in a "real life" setting is not always possible. In order to determine the feasibility and cost-effectiveness of translating current research evidence about preventive intervention program into clinical settings within existing health care systems in Europe, the "Diabetes in Europe — Prevention using Lifestyle, Physical Activity and Nutritional Intervention" (DE-PLAN) project, has been developed. The project, realized in 17 countries, is aimed at developing and testing models of efficient identification and site-specific intervention of individuals at high-risk of T2D in the community. A more detailed description of design, intervention strategy utilized in the DE-PLAN has been published elsewhere.[13]

The intervention was based on the model of lifestyle intervention developed by the DPS with the structure varying in different countries depending on the real life setting (Fig. 1).

3. DESIGN AND EDUCATION OF EDUCATORS

The DE-PLAN was carried out in both urban and rural populations, basically in primary health care and/or work place health care settings involving close cooperation among physicians, prevention managers, and other prevention-oriented staff.

The study curriculum consisted of written materials containing basic information about diabetes, diabetes prevention, diet, with diet examples booklets and information about physical activity. The added value of the DE-PLAN in Europe was training of future prevention managers and the

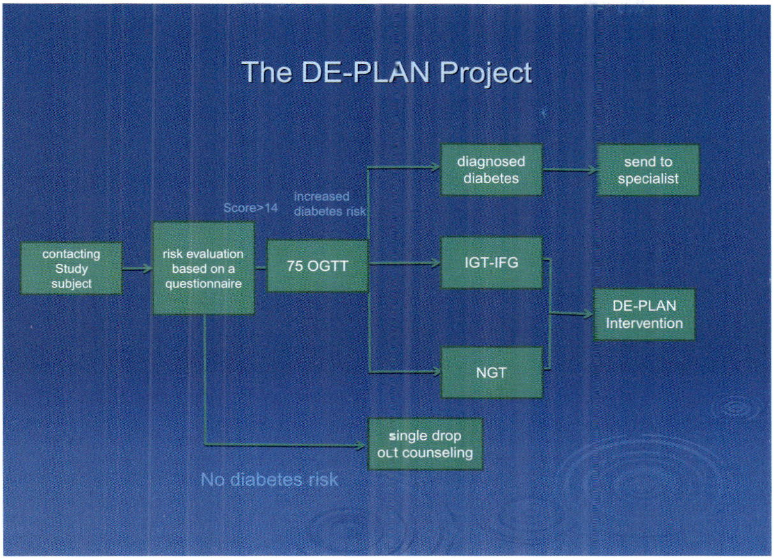

Fig. 1. The DE-PLAN core model of identification and intervention of individuals at high risk of T2D in the real life setting based on the DPS protocol.[14]

creation of local primary health care diabetes prevention networks. In several countries, these networks created for the study continue in prevention activities.

As it was assumed that the intervention needed to be administered by well-trained prevention managers having knowledge of the subject and practical skills in several centers, specially structured training conducted by physicians, dietitians, physical activity specialists and psychologists on diabetes prevention and motivation techniques was developed. As an example, in Poland, all nurses participated in 9 sessions, 6 hr each, led by a physician, dietitian, physical activity specialist and a psychologist. During the study intervention, there were organized meetings for prevention managers to discuss problems, share experiences, as well as for dietary, physical activity and motivation techniques consultations. There was also a quality control monitoring system established. Prevention managers had the opportunity for telephone consultations with dietitians and physical activity specialists, if required.[14,15]

4. RECRUITMENT OF PATIENTS

Recruitment in the DE-PLAN depended on the local setting but common principles were instituted for the entire study.

The study involved patients attending primary health centers/primary work place health care centers participating in the DE-PLAN project. The inclusion criteria was a Findrisc score over 14 and excluded those with known diabetes or diagnosed during an OGTT.[18]

Advertising was carried out by different media informing the public about the project including leaflets with the Findrisc questionnaire distributed in cooperating centers. Primary health care center patients known to have one or more diabetes or CVD risk factors were requested to complete the Findrisc questionnaire. Those with a Findrisc score over 14 were requested to have an OGTT. Those at high-risk for diabetes according to the FINDRISC, with normal glucose metabolism or impaired fasting glucose and/or impaired glucose metabolism were invited to participate in the lifestyle intervention.[13]

5. INTERVENTION

A core lifestyle intervention modified according to the country/local setting consisted of intensive and continuous segments and was based on reinforced behavior modification focusing on five goals of the DPS namely, weight loss, reduced intake of total and saturated fats, increased consumption of fruits, vegetables and fiber and increased physical activity.[18]

For example, in Poland, an intensive intervention segment consisted of 6–10 group sessions (10–14 people each) addressing lifestyle changes, diet and physical activity education and was followed by a 6 months continuous segment with telephone motivation sessions and letters sent to study participants using other motivation tools. The curriculum was created with written materials concerning basic information about diabetes, diabetes prevention, diet, with dietary example booklets and information about physical activity. During every session, printed educational materials related to the topic of the session were distributed. Social support was encouraged within the group settings and enhanced by their own social environments. Other family members could also participate in the sessions. In several countries, organized physical activity sessions such as water and gym aerobic sessions and Nordic walking were organized once or twice weekly.[14]

The design, recruitment and intervention of the study had very similar structures in many countries including Bulgaria, Lithuania, Italy, Spain and Serbia.[19]

6. RESULTS

The results of the DE-PLAN proved that prevention of diabetes through lifestyle intervention is feasible in primary/workplace health care settings and may produce beneficial changes in lifestyle, clinical and metabolic risk factors in high-risk individuals.[14,15,19]

As an example in Poland, at 12 months after initiation of the intervention, participants mean weight was reduced by 1.9 kg (SD = 5.01) (2.2%), BMI by 0.7 kg/m^2 (SD = 1.9) (2.2%) and waist circumference by 3.26 cm (SD = 6.11) (3.3%). About 24.6% of study participants lost 5% or more of their initial body weight (mean loss 7.76 kg SD = 5.7), 40% lost less than 5% of initial body weight (mean weight loss 1.95, SD = 1.22), 14.7% did not change their weight, 21.7% gained weight (mean weight gained 3.3 kg SD = 2.8). Mean fasting and post-load glucose levels showed a non-significant increase from 5.28 (95.0 mg/dL) and 5.86 mmol (105.5 mg/dL) to 5.39 (97.0 mg/dL) and 6.18 mmol/l (111.2 mg/dL), respectively. Total cholesterol decreased 4.2% from 5.56 (214.7 mg/dL) to 5.33 mmol/l (205.8 mg/dL) (p<0.05), TG decreased non-significantly from 1.75 (154 mg/dL) to 1.63 mmol/l (143.4 mg/dL) and HDL cholesterol did not change. Systolic and diastolic blood pressures decreased from baseline 133.18 mmHg and 82.98 mmHg to 130.41 mmHg and 81.02 mmHg (p<0.05) (by 1.6 and 2.4%), respectively (Table 1). Among those with baseline IGT (19.4%), 11% progressed to diabetes, and 40% reversed to normal glucose tolerance (NGT). Among those with baseline IFG (16%), 10.7% progressed to diabetes, and 35.7% reversed to NGT. The mean Findrisc score at baseline was 18.3 (SD = 2.84) indicating moderate to high diabetes risk (1 out of 3 person will develop diabetes within the next 10 years) and decreased to 15.8 (3.77) after intervention.[14]

There were also beneficial clinical and lifestyle changes observed, however, not surprisingly, these were more pronounced in those who reached the goal of losing more than 5% of weight (Table 2).[14]

Table 1. Changes in clinical outcome in baseline and after intervention: The DE-PLAN study.[14]

		Baseline		**After intervention**		**Change since baseline**		
	N	**Mean**	**Std. Deviation**	**Mean**	**Std. Deviation**	**Mean**	**SD**	**% Change**
Glycemia	175	5.28	0.75	5.39	0.65	–0.11	0.72	–2.1
Dttg	175	5.86	1.85	6.18	2.34	–0.31	2.35	–5.4
Cholesterol*	175	**5.56**	**1.00**	**5.33**	**0.98**	**0.23**	**1.16**	**4.2**
HDL	175	1.37	0.36	1.37	0.37	0.00	0.32	0.1
Triglycerides	175	1.76	1.18	1.63	0.80	0.13	1.14	7.2
WC*	175	**98.77**	**11.81**	**95.51**	**11.99**	**3.26**	**6.11**	**3.3**
Weight*	175	**85.65**	**16.12**	**83.73**	**15.97**	**1.92**	**5.01**	**2.2**
BMI*	175	**31.76**	**5.01**	**31.07**	**4.98**	**0.69**	**1.90**	**2.2**
SBP*	175	**133.22**	**14.41**	**131.15**	**12.64**	**2.07**	**14.40**	**1.6**
DBP*	175	**82.98**	**8.52**	**81.02**	**8.96**	**1.96**	**9.01**	**2,4**

*$p<0.05$

Table 2. Diet and physical activity at baseline and after intervention.[14]

	Baseline (%)	**After intervention (%)**
I have increased consumption of vegetables, fruits during the past year*	**24.0**	**51.4**
I have changed the saturated fat to unsaturated fat used during the past year*	**29.1**	**61.7**
I have decreased the amount of fat in your diet during the past year*	**25.1**	**52.6**
I think I exercise enough to maintain your physical condition or health*	**9.7**	**20.0**
I have increased physical activity during the past year*	**7.4**	**25.7**

*$p < 0.05$

Significant improvements were also found in lifestyle risk factors. In Poland, 51.4% of study participants have increased fruit and vegetable consumption during the past year compared to baseline ($p<0.05$). 52.6% and 61.7% of study participants have decreased total dietary fat and changed to unsaturated fat (baseline 25.1% and 29.1%, respectively; $p<0.05$).

25.7% of study participants have increased physical activity during the past year compared to 7% at baseline ($p<0.05$). The percentage of those who "think, that they have enough exercise to maintain their own physical condition or health" increased to from 9.7% at baseline to 20.0% ($p<0.05$).[14,19] Very similar results were obtained in the Greek arm of the DE-PLAN which was performed successfully in the workplace.[15] Among participants who completed the program, average weight loss was 4.7 kg (SD=1.0; $p = 0.022$). Greater adherence to the intervention sessions resulted in more significant weight loss. The percentage of those with any type of dysglycemia (IFG/IGT) was lower after the intervention (68% at baseline and 53.6% 1 year later, $p = 0.009$).[15] In Catalonian DE-PLAN study, during a 4.2-year median follow-up, the incidence of diabetes was 7.2 cases per 100 person-years in the standard treatment group and 4.6 in the intensive lifestyle intervention group with a 36.5% relative risk reduction ($p < 0.005$). The number of participants needed to be treated by intensive intervention for 4 years to reduce one case of diabetes was 9.5.[20]

In Catalonia at the end of the first year of follow-up, 24.7% of individuals in the intensive group and 18.8% of those in the standard care group reduced their weight by at least 3%. These percentages were 20.4% and 20.3% at the end of the second year, 20.5% and 17.6% at the end of the third, and 19.6% and 14.7% at the end of the fourth year of the study, respectively.[20]

In another arm of the DE-PLAN study performed in 4 provinces in central Spain, after 12 months of intervention, a significantly important decrease in body weight ($p<0.03$), triglycerides ($p<0.001$), and systolic ($p = 0.039$) and diastolic ($p = 0.002$) blood pressures were observed.[19]

7. THE DE-PLAN DIABETES PREVENTION IN IMMIGRANTS

The majority of immigrants to Western Europe originate from the developing world where the most rapid increase in the prevalence of diabetes mellitus is occurring. Recent immigrants, particularly women and immigrants of South Asian and African origins, are at high risk for diabetes compared with long-term residents of Western countries.[21] In Oslo, Norway, the age-adjusted prevalence of T2D among 40 to 59-year-old immigrant women from South Asia was 27.5%, with an OR of 11.0 for developing diabetes compared with Western women.[21] Therefore, the InnvaDiab study as a part of the DE-PLAN study was performed to explore whether a culturally adapted lifestyle education program would improve the risk factor profile for T2D and the metabolic syndrome (MetS) among Pakistani immigrant women in Oslo, Norway.

The randomized controlled trial, lasting 7.1 months, comprised six educational sessions about blood glucose, physical activity and diet. Participants (age 25–62 years) were randomized to either a control ($n = 97$) or an intervention ($n = 101$) group. The methodology and results of the study were published elsewhere and are summarized below.[22]

8. THE INTERVENTION SPECIFICITY IN IMMIGRANTS

The main focus in the intervention in immigrants was a cultural adaptation of the education program. The education was concentrated on the physiological importance of blood glucose and its regulation by diet and physical activity and on knowledge about Pakistani lifestyle in Pakistan and Norway. Due to low levels of literacy, mainly culturally adapted pictures and figures were used during the educational sessions. Printed materials were not handed out during the intervention. All communication in the intervention group was conducted in the preferred language either with multilingual personnel or an interpreter. All research personnel were female.

The education approach was based on the principles of empowerment including participation and cooperation without assuming responsibility for the other person's performance, and accepting without judgment the other's feelings and choices.[23] After the first group session, participants were given brief individual feedback concerning diet and physical activity based on blood test result. Education was focused on diet and about the beneficial effect of mild physical activity on blood glucose especially the effect of post-meal walking. Women were encouraged to walk for 1 hr twice per week throughout the trial period. Sub-groups were organized practicing 1 hr per day of walking. Child care was offered, and walking paths where baby carriages could be brought were chosen. Furthermore, good walking shoes were provided since many participants did not have footwear suitable for outdoor walking.

9. RESULTS

During the intervention period, the mean fasting and post-glucose load blood glucose as well as fasting insulin levels decreased in the intervention group compared to the control group. Among individuals who attended four or more of the educational sessions ($n = 59$), there was a more pronounced decrease in serum triglycerides and BMI compared with the control group. During the intervention period, there was a significant increase in participants having the MetS in the control group (from 41 to 57%; $p = 0.011$), which was not seen in the intervention group (from 44% to 42%; p = NS).[22] The study demonstrated that participation in a culturally adapted education program may improve risk factors for T2D and prevent the development of the MetS in Pakistani immigrant women.[22]

10. THE IMPLEMENTATION OF A EUROPEAN GUIDELINE (IMAGE) PROJECT

There are many steps involved in order to create a prevention program for people with increased risk of T2D extending from the methods for selecting those at risk, design of the study, training of educators, to quality control. In the DE-PLAN study, primary health care nurses received structured training on diabetes prevention and motivation techniques conducted by specialists experienced in diabetes prevention. However, jointly developed prevention strategies were lacking in Europe. Therefore, the IMAGE project was developed by the Technical University Dresden in response to diabetes as the major public health concern of the EU (www.image-project.eu).This three-year-project began in June 2007; the IMAGE study group comprised a Europe-wide consortium of health care professionals and behavioral and health scientists with experience in diabetes prevention. The IMAGE project has collated available information in a systematic manner and developed practical relevant standards for diabetes prevention. These include an evidence-based guideline,[23] a practice guideline "Toolkit" for the prevention of diabetes[24] and guidelines on quality indicators in diabetes prevention[25] as well as a training curriculum for diabetes prevention intervention programs.[26]

The evidence-based and practical guidelines represent a major step in making T2D prevention a reality. The major output of the IMAGE project relevant for diabetes prevention practice is the practical guideline "Toolkit for the prevention of T2D". This Toolkit was designed for people who would like to implement a diabetes prevention program, including those working in primary and specialized health care services, physicians, physical activity experts, dieticians, nurses, and also others planning or already involved in diabetes prevention interventions (e.g., teachers, business partners), but also stakeholders and politicians. The IMAGE Toolkit for diabetes prevention provides practical information for preventive intervention for adults at risk of developing diabetes. The Toolkit includes all that is necessary for a diabetes prevention program covering management, financial, interventional and quality assurance aspects. It refers to the latest evidence in the science of diabetes prevention and allows translating this knowledge into practice. It contains practical examples and worksheets which facilitate the implementation of a prevention program. The Toolkit addresses the need for change, how to budget and finance a prevention program and how to identify people at risk. A process model for supporting lifestyle behavior change is presented and described in its phases from motivation to action and to maintenance. The Toolkit concludes with an overview on how to evaluate intervention programs and how to establish a quality assurance program.[24]

As part of the IMAGE project, a curriculum for the training of prevention managers was also developed.[26] The rationale behind this was to propose common European learning goals, teaching methods and content as well as teaching materials for the training of certified prevention managers. For the first time, a standardized state-of-the-art training curriculum was offered.

In several countries, a pilot study of acceptability and practicability with about 100 medical professionals in Europe was performed. The added value of the pilot study was education of certified and ready-to-act prevention managers.[26–28]

11. FINNISH EXPERIENCE

Finland has considerable experience with T2D prevention presenting as a pioneer in the prevention of diabetes with the DPS. Finland is also one of the first countries in the world to create a national program for prevention and better care of patients with T2D, DEHKO.[29] The DPS results and prevention design was the basis for practical implementation of T2D prevention in several initiatives in Finland. These included three different prevention programs: FIN-D2D,[30] involving risk-screening and repeated consultation in primary health care, FINNAIR, a workplace-targeted intervention project involving airline employees, and the good ageing in Lahti (GOAL) region[32] program, a community-based prevention program. Almost all other diabetes prevention programs in Europe were also based on the experience and methodology established in the DPS.

12. DPS

The DPS was started in 1993 and completed in five centers in Finland. 522 middle-aged, overweight men and women at high-risk for T2D and IGT were recruited and randomly allocated to a control group with standard care or to an intensive lifestyle intervention group.[1]

The intervention goals were to reduce body weight (5% or greater reduction from baseline weight), limit dietary fat (30% of total energy consumed) and saturated fat (10% of total energy consumed), and to increase both dietary fiber intake (15 g/1000 kcal)) and physical activity (30 min/d). The lifestyle intervention was delivered by study nutritionists through individual counseling sessions. Participants were individually instructed with diet and methods for increasing physical activity. Endurance exercise was recommended. Supervised, progressive, individually tailored, circuit-type moderate intensity resistance training sessions were also offered to participants.[1]

13. RESULTS OF THE DPS

The intervention group showed significantly greater improvement in each intervention goal. After 1 and 3 years, mean weight reductions were, respectively, 4.5 and 3.5 kg in the intervention group, and 1.0 and 0.9 kg in the control group. Cardiovascular risk factors improved more in the intervention group.[18,33]

After a mean follow-up period of 3.2 years, the risk of diabetes was reduced by 58% in the intervention group compared with the control group.[1]

The reduction in incidence of diabetes was associated with the number of achieved lifestyle goals. Among those who achieved four or all five of the goals at year 1, there were no diabetes cases diagnosed during the entire intervention period. Increasing physical activity was an independent predictor of diabetes risk reduction.[34]

Patients consuming a moderate fat, high-fiber diet achieved the largest weight reduction and the lowest diabetes risk during the intervention period even after adjustment for weight reduction.[35]

During the post-intervention follow-up period of 3 years, the risk of diabetes was still 36% lower among the former intervention group participants compared with former control group participants.[36]

14. THE IMPLEMENTATION PROJECT FOR THE PREVENTION OF T2D IN FINLAND: THE FIN-D2D, DEHKO PROGRAM

Finland was one of the first countries to set up a national program for the prevention and better care of patients with T2D (**DEHKO**) to address the emerging diabetes epidemic.[29]

The program for the prevention of T2D in Finland was launched in 2003, focusing not only on the population at high-risk of developing T2D but also the general population and on the early diagnosis and management of T2D. An implementation project, FIN-D2D, was carried out in five hospital districts in Finland during 2003–2007.[30]

The project was a common initiative of hospital districts, the Finnish Diabetes Association and the National Public Health Institute. The main objective of the implementation project was to establish prevention models that would be feasible within the regular primary and occupational healthcare system. The principal screening tool to identify individuals with high T2D risk was the Finnish diabetes risk score. High-risk individuals underwent an oral glucose tolerance test and were referred for lifestyle intervention, delivered primarily by public health nurses in collaboration with local multiprofessional teams. Weight management and physical activity were the basis for prevention and prevention counseling occurred through group intervention.[30]

15. RESULTS OF THE FIN-D2D

The implementation project proved that large-scale screening was possible; 10,000 high-risk individuals and 10,000 moderate-risk individuals were identified.[30]

According to preliminary results after 1-year follow-up, there were desirable changes in CVD risk factors and glucose tolerance in the high-risk cohort in both sexes. In high-risk women, a modest but statistically significant weight loss was achieved and associated with a decrease in the incidence of diabetes. It was demonstrated that implementation of large-scale lifestyle interventions in primary health care is possible and effective.[30]

16. FINNAIR: SCREENING AND PREVENTION OF T2D IN AN AIRLINE COMPANY

The aim of the Finnair project was to assess the risk for T2D and CVD among employees of a Finnish airline, to study the association of shift work with T2D and CVD risk and to implement prevention in occupational primary health service.[31] During the years 2006–2008, 4,169 employees were invited for a health check-up and 2,312 participated in the study. The check-up included physical examinations, questionnaires on working hours, sleep and lifestyle, diabetes risk score FINDRISC assessment, and blood tests. Lifestyle counseling by an occupational health nurse or physician was offered for those with increased T2D risk (assessed with the FINDRISC diabetes risk score, fasting blood glucose and/or oral glucose tolerance test).[31] Altogether, 15% of participants were at high-risk for T2D (FINDRISC score ≥15 and/or elevated blood glucose but not diagnostic of diabetes), and a further 15% had moderate risk (FINDRISC score 10–14 and normal blood glucose). Of those, 60% agreed to attend lifestyle counseling. Group counseling was not the best option due to the specificity of shift work, therefore individual counseling was offered.[31]

17. THE GOAL REGION

The GOAL Lifestyle Implementation trial was designed for the primary health care setting with lifestyle and risk reduction objectives based on the DPS.[32,38]

This trial, in addition to components from the DPS program, focused on targeted effectiveness of self-regulation in changing diet and physical activity using information provision, group discussions, self-monitoring of behavior, goal setting and planning. The GOAL trial was delivered by public health nurses. Facilitators received two days of training with a standardized program, training manuals and practical exercises. Participants were also offered local sports facilities and guided exercise training (e.g., gym, aquatic exercise, Nordic walking). The program extended over eight months with the first five sessions held at 2-week intervals and one booster session after a 6-months break.

A total of 352 middle-aged participants with elevated risk for T2D were recruited from health care centers. Measurements were performed at baseline and at 12 months. Clinical risk factors were measured by study nurses and lifestyle outcomes were analyzed from self-reports. Lifestyle outcomes were compared with outcomes achieved in relevant efficacy trials and within-subject changes were tested for risk reduction. At 12 months, 20% of participants achieved at least four of five key lifestyle outcomes comparable with the DPS. However, physical activity and weight loss goals were achieved significantly less frequently (65 vs 86% and 12 vs 43%, respectively). Several clinical risk factors decreased more so among men than women.[32,38]

This trial demonstrated that lifestyle counseling can be effective and is feasible in real-world settings for individuals with elevated risk of T2D. It was concluded that to increase program impact program exposure and treatment intensity needed to be increased.

18. OTHER EUROPEAN INITIATIVES IN DIABETES PREVENTION

There are several other initiatives across Europe to prevent T2D.

The Prevention of Diabetes Self-Management Program (PREDIAS) was developed as a group program for the prevention of T2D based on the Diabetes Prevention Program (Fig. 2).[9]

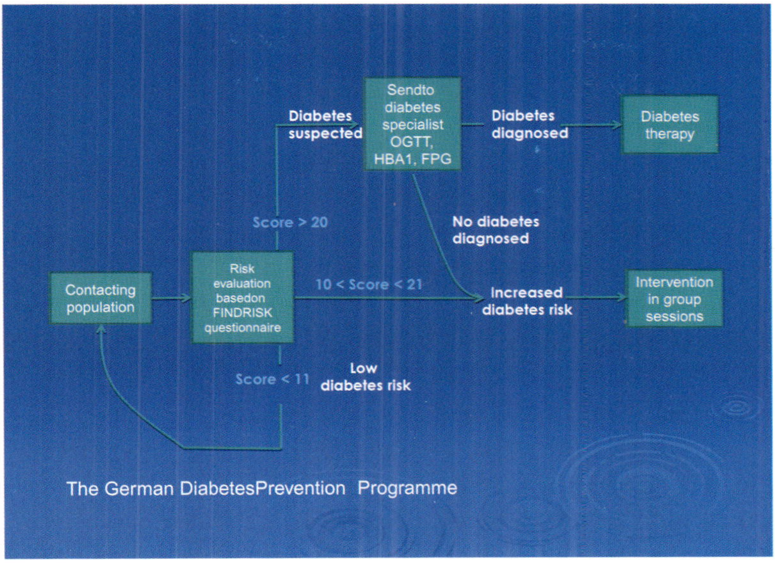

Fig. 2. The German National Diabetes Prevention Program model of identification and intervention of individuals at high risk of T2D in the real life setting based on the DPP protocol.[39]

The prevention program consisted of 12 lessons lasting ~90 min each. During the first eight weeks, eight core lessons were given, one per week; the last four lessons were bimonthly booster lessons. The program was based on self-management theory conducted in small groups (median size of seven people) and was delivered by either diabetes educators or psychologists. The program comprised a set of educational materials and a curriculum for the prevention manager. Each participant received an exercise book, which contained information about diabetes prevention and resources for participants such as a table of caloric values and worksheets (e.g., eating diaries and logbooks for physical activity). The control group received written information about diabetes prevention. A total of 182 persons with elevated risk for diabetes participated (aged 56.3 ± 10.1 years, 43% female, and BMI 31.5 ± 5.3 kg/m^2).

After 12 months, weight loss was significantly greater ($p = 0.001$) in the intervention than in the control group (−3.8 ± 5.2 vs −1.4 ± 4.09 kg). There were also significant effects ($p = 0.001$) on fasting glucose (control group 1.8 ± 13.1 mg/dl vs intervention −4.3 ± 11.3 mg/dl), duration of physical activity per week (control group 17.9 ± 63.8 min vs intervention 46.6 ± 95.5 min; $p = 0.03$), and eating behavior.[39] The PREDIAS prevention program proved that lifestyle intervention could significantly reduce weight and modify eating behavior and physical activity thus, decrease diabetes risk. In the PREDIAS study, the magnitude of these effects and the observed metabolic changes were similar to results from previously performed diabetes prevention programs.[39]

The APHRODITE study, a 2.5-year lifestyle intervention for the prevention of T2D, was performed in 14 general practices in the Netherlands among 479 individuals at high-risk for T2D and was compared to 446 individuals receiving usual care.[40] Intervention consisted of individual lifestyle counseling by nurse practitioners and GPs and group consultations.

After the intervention, satisfaction with the program and perceived implementation barriers were assessed with questionnaires.

Attendance at individual consultations was high (intervention: 80–97%; usual care: 86–94%). Providers were confident about diabetes prevention by lifestyle intervention in primary care. Participants were more satisfied with counseling from nurse practitioners than from GPs. A majority of GPs reported low self-assessment regarding knowledge of dietary guidance. Lack of counseling time (60%), participant motivation (12%), and financial reimbursement (11%) were regarded by providers as important barriers for intervention implementation.[40]

It was observed that high participant compliance and a positive attitude of providers make primary care a suitable setting for diabetes prevention by lifestyle counseling. Results from the Dutch study support a role for the nurse practitioner as the key player in guiding lifestyle modification.[40] Within the United Kingdom, there are several on-going initiatives investigating optimal methods of translating diabetes prevention programs based on promotion of a healthy lifestyle into routine primary care.

The "Walking away from T2D" study, in the 2010–2014 time frame, aims to establish the behavioral and clinical effectiveness of a structured educational program designed to target perceptions and knowledge of diabetes risk and promote a healthy lifestyle, particularly increased walking activity, in a multi-ethnic population at a high-risk of developing T2D.[41] This study is a clustered, randomized controlled trial undertaken at the level of primary care practices. Follow-up will be conducted at 12, 24 and 36 months. The primary outcome is change in objectively measured ambulatory activity. Secondary outcomes include progression to T2D, biochemical variables (including fasting glucose, 2-hr glucose, HbA_{1c} and lipids), anthropometric variables, quality of life and depression. The study will be performed in 10 primary care practices (5 interventional, 5 control). Within each practice, individuals at high-risk of impaired glucose regulation will be identified using an automated version of the Leicester Risk Assessment tool. Practices will be assigned to either the control group (advice leaflet) or the intervention group in which participants will be invited to attend a 3 hr structured educational program designed to promote physical activity and a healthy lifestyle. Participants in the intervention practices will also be invited to attend annual group-based maintenance workshops and will receive telephone contact halfway between annual sessions. This study will provide new evidence surrounding the long-term effectiveness of a diabetes prevention program conducted within routine primary care in the United Kingdom.[41]

19. DISCUSSION

Evidence from randomized control trials has shown that through lifestyle intervention, including dietary modification, weight loss and physical activity, an approximate 60% reduction in T2D incidence could be achieved.[7–12]

In order to determine the feasibility of translating research findings from preventive intervention programs into clinical settings within existing health care systems, several implementation programs have been performed worldwide. Results from studies undertaken in Europe show that prevention of T2D, through lifestyle intervention, is feasible in primary health care and workplace settings may produce improvement in lifestyle and clinical risk factors in high-risk individuals.

Similar conclusions regarding the feasibility of intervention programs in T2D prevention in primary health care settings were drawn by Laatikainen and colleagues.[42]

In their study (GGT Diabetes Project), a structured group program with six 90-min sessions was delivered to 237 middle-aged individuals during an eight months period by trained nurses in an Australian primary health care setting and resulted in a reduction in weight, waist circumference and in risk factors. In this study, significant improvements in most psychological measures were also found.[42]

In the US, the Montana Diabetes Control Program in 2008, working collaboratively with four health care facilities, implemented an adapted DPP lifestyle intervention based on group sessions.[43]

355 adults at high-risk for diabetes and CVD enrolled. About 70% of participants achieved the physical activity goal of ≥150 m per week. There was a significant decrease in weight from baseline (mean difference, 4.0 kg +/− 6.7; $p < 0.001$). About 40% of participants achieved the 7% weight loss goal and 67% achieved at least a 5% weight loss.[43]

However, although the implementation trials described above have been reasonably successful, we still need to learn more about the implementation of effective diabetes prevention programs in different settings, cultures, regions and age groups. Furthermore, cost-effectiveness of applied intervention strategies need to be assessed in addition to their feasibility and efficacy.

In the implementation studies in real life settings, the beneficial clinical and lifestyle changes were observed with all interventions, however, not surprisingly, they were more pronounced in those who reached the goal of more than 5% of weight loss.[14]

According to the review by Johnson *et al.* addressing translational lifestyle interventions, effectiveness could not be easily demonstrated with clinical parameters such as blood glucose or diabetes risk. Given the relatively short follow-up and small sample size, real life prevention studies have sufficient statistical power to measure change in weight rather than in diabetes incidence. Therefore, weight loss in these studies can be regarded as a marker for efficacy potential prevention in the long-term.[44] In the DPP study, weight loss was reported to be the dominant factor in diabetes prevention with a loss of 5 kg explaining the 55% reduction in the incidence of diabetes during the three years of follow-up.[45] The other question that arises is whether the efficacy results from randomized controlled trials can be replicated or improved upon in future diabetes prevention projects in real life settings.

In most of the presented studies, the percentage of people who lost > 5% of initial weight was substantially lower than in the DPS or DPP studies. The DPS demonstrated that diabetes had not developed in any of the subjects who reached four or five of the study goals indicating that effectiveness in goal-reaching by study participants is very important.

Johnson *et al.* analyzed 17 real-world diabetes prevention studies based on either or both DPP and DPS protocols.[44] The main modification of the original trial's protocol was in the number of sessions provided and mode of delivery (group sessions rather than individual counseling). An important finding is that most of the analyzed studies attracted predominantly women, highlighting the well-known need to address lifestyle prevention studies also in men.[44]

However, the general rules for diabetes prevention studies are identical regarding the need for customization for each country, health care system, culture and work place. The important issue involves the cultural modification of an intervention such as that described in the InnvaDiab-DE-PLAN study by TelleHjellset *et al.*[22] among South Asia immigrants in Oslo, Norway based on the DE-PLAN study. Also, the US church-based interventions were culturally adapted and tailored to the needs of the mainly Afro-American population. The latter highlights the need for increasing applicability of interventions to real-life settings to meet requirements of local populations.[46]

In recent years, several EU supported initiatives were established to support "real-life" diabetes prevention programs. The European training program for health care professionals to deliver preventive interventions was created within the IMAGE project.[27,28] Also, evidence-based and practice-oriented European step-by-step guidelines for diabetes prevention and quality assessment guidelines have been published and are available on-line and can serve as a practical tool for new prevention initiatives.[23–26]

20. CONCLUSIONS

Diabetes prevention initiatives provide evidence that diabetes prevention, through lifestyle intervention, is feasible in real life settings and may produce beneficial changes in terms of lifestyle, clinical and metabolic improvements in high-risk individuals.

The results of many programs implementing intervention studies performed in Europe and the world suggest that group lifestyle counseling can be effective and that lifestyle intervention is feasible in the primary health care setting.

REFERENCES

1. Alberti KG, Zimmet P, Shaw J. (2007) International Diabetes Federation: a consensus on Type 2 diabetes prevention. *Diabet Med* **24**: 451–463.
2. Wild S, Roglic G, Green A, Sicree R, King H. (2004) Global prevalence of diabetes: estimates for the year 2000 and projections for 2030. *Diabetes Care* **27**: 1047–1053.
3. Decode Study Group (2003) Age- and sex-specific prevalences of diabetes and impaired glucose regulation in 13 European cohorts. *Diabetes Care* **26**: 61–69.
4. Lammi N, Taskinen O, Molchanova E *et al.* (2007) A high incidence of type 1 diabetes and an alarming increase in the incidence of type 2 diabetes among young adults in Finland between 1992 and 1996. *Diabetologia* **50**: 1393–1400.
5. Manuel DG, Schultz SE. (2004) Health-related quality of life and health-adjusted life expectancy of people with diabetes in Ontario, Canada, 1996–1997. *Diabetes Care* **27**: 407–414.
6. Gillies CL, Lambert PC, Abrams KR, Sutton AJ, Cooper NJ, Su RT *et al.* (2008) Different strategies for screening and prevention of type 2 diabetes in adults: cost effectiveness analysis. *BMJ* **336**: 1180–1185.
7. Tuomilehto J, Lindström J, Eriksson JG *et al.* (2001) Prevention of type 2 diabetes mellitus by changes in lifestyle among subjects with impaired glucose tolerance. *N Engl J Med* **344**: 1343–1350.
8. Lindström J, Ilanne-Parikka P, Peltonen M *et al.* (2006) Finnish Diabetes Prevention Study Group. Sustained reduction in the incidence of type 2 diabetes by lifestyle intervention: follow-up of the Finnish Diabetes Prevention Study. *Lancet* **368**: 1673–1679.
9. Knowler WC, Barrett-Connor E, Fowler SE *et al.* (2002) Reduction in the incidence of type 2 diabetes with lifestyle intervention or metformin. *N Engl J Med* **346**: 393–403.
10. Knowler WC, Fowler SE, Hamman RF *et al.* (2009) Diabetes Prevention Program Research Group. 10-year follow-up of diabetes incidence and weight loss in the Diabetes Prevention Program Outcomes Study. *Lancet* **374**: 1677–1686.

11. Kosaka K, Noda M, Kuzuya T. (2005) Prevention of type 2 diabetes by lifestyle intervention: a Japanese trial in IGT males. *Diabetes Res Clin Pract* **67**: 152–162.
12. Ramachandran A, Snehalatha C, Mary S *et al.* (2006) The Indian Diabetes Prevention Programme shows that lifestyle modification and metformin prevent type 2 diabetes in Asian Indian subjects with impaired glucose tolerance (IDPP-1). *Diabetologia* **49**: 289–297.
13. Schwarz PE, Lindström J, Kissimova-Scarbeck K *et al.* (2008) DE-PLAN project. The European perspective of type 2 diabetes prevention: diabetes in Europe — prevention using lifestyle, physical activity and nutritional intervention (DE-PLAN) project. *Exp Clin Endocrinol Diabetes* **116**: 167–172.
14. Aleksandra Gilis-Januszewska, Zbigniew Szybinski, Katarzyna Kissimova-Skarbek, Beata Piwonska-Solska, Dorota Pach, Roman Topor-Madry, Jaakko Tuomilehto, Jaana Lindström, Markku Peltonen, Peter Eh Schwarz and Alicja, Hubalewska-Dydejczyk (2011) Prevention of type 2 diabetes by lifestyle intervention in primary health care setting in Poland: Diabetes in Europe Prevention using Lifestyle, Physical Activity and Nutritional intervention (DE-PLAN) project, *Brit J Diabet Vas Dis* **11**: 198.
15. Makrilakis K, Liatis S, Grammatikou S, Perrea D, Katsilambros N. (2010) Implementation and effectiveness of the first community lifestyle intervention programme to prevent Type 2 diabetes in Greece. The DE-PLAN study. *Diabet Med* **27**: 459–465.
16. Lindström J, Tuomilehto J. (2003) The diabetes risk score: a practical tool to predict type 2 diabetes risk. *Diabetes Care* **26**: 725–731.
17. Schwarz PE, Lindström J, Kissimova-Scarbeck K *et al.* (2008) DE-PLAN project. The European perspective of type 2 diabetes prevention: diabetes in Europe — prevention using lifestyle, physical activity and nutritional intervention (DE-PLAN) project. *Exp Clin Endocrinol Diabetes* **116**: 167–172.
18. Lindström J, Louheranta A, Mannelin M *et al.* (2003) Finnish Diabetes Prevention Study Group. The Finnish Diabetes Prevention Study (DPS): Lifestyle intervention and 3-year results on diet and physical activity. *Diabetes Care* **26**: 3230–3636.
19. Schwarz PE, Reddy P, Greaves C, Dunbar J, Schwarz J (Eds.). (2010) *Diabetes Prevention in Practice*. Dresden, Germany, TUMAINI Institute for Prevention Management.
20. Costa B, Barrio F, Cabré JJ, Piñol JL, Cos X, Solé C, Bolíbar B, Basora J, Castell C, Solà-Morales O, Salas-Salvadó J, Lindström J, Tuomilehto J. (2012) Delaying progression to type 2 diabetes among high-risk Spanish individuals

is feasible in real-life primary healthcare settings using intensive lifestyle intervention. DE-PLAN-CAT Research Group. *Diabetologia* **5**: 1319–1328.

21. Jenum AK, Holme I, Graff-Iversen S *et al.* (2005) Ethnicity and sex are strong determinants of diabetes in an urban Western society: implications for prevention. *Diabetologia* **48**: 435–439.
22. Telle-Hjellset V, Råberg Kjøllesdal MK, Bjørge B, Holmboe-Ottesen G, Wandel M, Birkeland KI, Eriksen HR, Høstmark AT. (2012) The InnvaDiab-DE-PLAN study: a randomised controlled trial with a culturally adapted education programme improved the risk profile for type 2 diabetes in Pakistani immigrant women. *Br J Nutr* **4**: 1–10.
23. Fisher Jr EB, La Greca AM, Greco P *et al.* (1997) Directive and nondirective social support in diabetes management. *Int J Behav Med* **4**: 131–144.
23. Paulweber B, Valensi P, Lindström J *et al.* (2010) A European evidence-based guideline for the prevention of type 2 diabetes. *Horm Metab Res* **42**: S3–36, a practice guideline "Toolkit" for the prevention of diabetes.
24. Lindström J, Neumann A, Sheppard KE *et al.* (2010) Take action to prevent diabetes: the IMAGE toolkit for the prevention of type 2 diabetes in Europe. *Horm Metab Res* **42**: S37–55.
25. Pajunen P, Landgraf R, Muylle F, *et al.* (2010) Quality indicators for the prevention of type 2 diabetes in Europe-IMAGE. *Horm Metab Res* **42**: S56–63.
26. Kronsbein P *et al.* for the IMAGE Study Group. (2011) IMAGE: Development of a European curriculum for the training of prevention managers. *Br J Diabetes Vasc Dis* **11**: 163.
27. Schwarz PE, Gruhl U, Bornstein SR, Landgraf R, Hall M, Tuomilehto J. (2007) The European perspective on diabetes prevention: development and Implementation of A European Guideline and training standards for diabetes prevention (IMAGE). *Diab Vasc Dis Res* **4**: 353–357.
28. Schwarz PE, Lindström J. (2011) From evidence to practice — the IMAGE project — new standards in the prevention of type 2 diabetes. *Diabetes Res Clin Pract* **91**: 138–140. Epub 2010 Dec 30.
29. http://www.diabetes.fi/files/1108/Programme_for_the_Prevention_of_Type_2_Diabetes_in_Finland_2003–2010.
30. Saaristo T, Peltonen M, Keinänen-Kiukaanniemi S, Vanhala M, Saltevo J, Niskanen L, Oksa H, Korpi-Hyövälti E, Tuomilehto J; FIN-D2D Study Group. (2007) National type 2 diabetes prevention programme in Finland: FIN-D2D. *Int J Circumpolar Health* **66**: 101–112.
31. Viitasalo K, Lindström J, Hemiö K, Puttonen S, Koho A, Härmä M, Peltonen M. (2012) Occupational health care identifies risk for type 2 diabetes and cardiovascular disease. *Prim Care Diabetes* **6**: 95–102.

32. Absetz P, Valve R, Oldenburg B *et al.* (2007) Type 2 diabetes prevention in the 'real world': one-year results of the GOAL Implementation Trial. *Diabetes Care* **30**: 2465–2470.
33. Ilanne-Parikka P, Eriksson JG, Lindström J *et al.* (2008) Effect of lifestyle intervention on the occurrence of metabolic syndrome and its components in the Finnish diabetes prevention study. *Diabetes Care* **31**: 805–807.
34. Laaksonen DE, Lindström J, Lakka TA *et al.* (2005) Physical activity in the prevention of type 2 diabetes: the Finnish diabetes prevention study. *Diabetes* **54**: 158–165.
35. Lindstrom J, Peltonen M, Eriksson JG *et al.* (2006) Highfibre, low-fat diet predicts long-term weight loss and decreased type 2 diabetes risk: the Finnish diabetes prevention study. *Diabetologia* **49**: 912–920.
36. Lindstrom J, Ilanne-Parikka P, Peltonen M *et al.* (2006) Sustained reduction in the incidence of type 2 diabetes by lifestyle intervention: the follow-up results of the Finnish diabetes prevention study. *Lancet* **368**: 1673–1679.
37. Timo Saaristo, Leena Moilanen, Jari Jokelainen, Eeva Korpi-Hyövälti, Mauno Vanhala, Juha Saltevo, Leo Niskanen, Markku Peltonen, Heikki Oksa, Henna Cederberg, Jaakko Tuomilehto, Matti Uusitupa (2010) Sirkka Keinänen-KiukaanniemiCardiometabolic profile of people screened for high risk of type 2 diabetes in a national diabetes prevention programme (FIN-D2D) Primary Care Diabetes **4**: 231–239.
38. Absetz P, Oldenburg B, Hankonen N *et al.* (2009) Type 2 diabetes prevention in the real world: three-year results of the GOAL lifestyle implementation trial. *Diabetes Care* **32**: 1418–1420.
39. Kutze *et al.* (2009) Prevention of Diabetes Self-Management Program (PREDIAS): Effects on Weight, Metabolic Risk Factors, and Behavioral Outcomes. *Diabetes Care* **32**: 1143–1146.
40. Vermunt *et al.* (2012) Implementation of a lifestyle intervention for type 2 diabetes prevention in Dutch primary care: opportunities for intervention delivery. *BMC Fam Pract* **13**: 79.
41. Yates T, Davies MJ, Henson J, Troughton J, Edwardson C, Gray LJ, Khunti K. (2012) Walking away from type 2 diabetes: trial protocol of a cluster randomised controlled trial evaluating a structured education programme in those at high risk of developing type 2 diabetes. *BMC Fam Pract* **13**: 46.
42. Laatikainen T, Dunbar JA, Chapman A *et al.* (2007) Prevention of type 2 diabetes by lifestyle intervention in an Australian primary health care setting: Greater Green Triangle (GGT) Diabetes Prevention Project. *BMC Public Health* **7**: 249.

43. Helen A. Amundson, Marcene K. Butcher, Dorothy Gohdes, Taryn O. Hall, Todd S. Harwell, Steven D. Helgerson, Karl K. Vanderwood (2009) Translating the Diabetes Prevention Program Into Practice in the General Community: Findings From the Montana Cardiovascular Disease and Diabetes Prevention Program. *Diabetes Educ* **35**: 209

44. Johnson M, Jones R, Freeman C, Woods HB, Gillett M, Goyder E, Payne N. (2013) Can diabetes prevention programmes be translated effectively into real-world settings and still deliver improved outcomes? A synthesis of evidence. *Diabet Med* **30**: 632.

45. Hamman RF, Wing RR, Edelstein SL, Lachin JM, Bray GA, Delahanty L, Hoskin M, Kriska AM, Mayer-Davis EJ, Pi-Sunyer X, Regensteiner J, Venditti B, Wylie-Rosett J. (2006) Effect of weight loss with lifestyle intervention on risk of diabetes. *Diabetes Care* **29**: 2102–2107.

46. Boltri JM, Davis-Smith YM, Seale JP, Shellenberger S, Okosun IS, Cornelius ME. (2008) Diabetes prevention in a faith-based setting: results of translational research. *J Public Health Manag Pract* **14**: 29–32.

Chapter 12: Characteristics of Prediabetes/ Diabetes and Prevention Initiatives in East Asia

*Hirohito Sone**

1. DIABETES EPIDEMICS IN EAST ASIA

As in the rest of the world, there is also an epidemic of diabetes in East Asia, which is typically comprised of China (including Hong Kong), Taiwan, Korea, Mongolia and Japan. According to the *Diabetes Atlas* (the sixth edition) of the International Diabetes Federations, these countries have approximately 112 million people with diabetes, which accounts for approximately 30% of the world diabetes population. Because of the much lower incidence of type 1 diabetes than in most parts of the world, the majority of the diabetes population in this region has type 2 diabetes.

The *Atlas* indicated that the comparative prevalence of diabetes, which is calculated by assuming that each country has the same age profile (i.e., that of the world population), in these countries ranges from 5.1% (Japan) to 9.0% (China), a range that is comparable to that of the world average which is 8.3%. However, because of the marked ageing of the population in this region, the crude prevalence of diabetes is much higher. The National Health and Nutrition Survey 2012 in Japan showed that 10.9% (15.7% of men and 7.6% of women) of the population 20 years and older had diabetes, which is defined by $HbA_{1c} \geq 6.5\%$ and/or currently receiving

* E-mail: sone@med.niigata-u.ac.jp

diabetes care. Survey of a nationally representative sample of nearly 100,000 Chinese adults also revealed a similar diabetes prevalence of 11.6% (12.1% of men, 11.0% of women) based on the 2010 American Diabetes Association (ADA) criteria (Xu Y).

In terms of prediabetes, its prevalence is strongly affected by the definitions used. A study of another nationally representative sample of 46,239 subjects in China during 2007–2008 showed that 15.5% (16.1% of men, 14.9% of women) had prediabetes based on the World Health Organization diagnostic criteria, which is either impaired fasting glucose (IFG) [110–125 mg/dL (6.1–7.0 mmol/L)] or impaired glucose tolerance (IGT) [2-hr glucose, 140–199 mg/dL (7.8–11.1 mmol/L)] (Yang W). On the other hand, the Chinese group (Xu Y) that used the 2010 ADA criteria for diagnosing prediabetes by adding HbA_{1c} between 5.7% and 6.4% to the WHO criteria and modifying the WHO definition of IFG from 110–125 mg/dl to 100–125 mg/dL (5.6–7.0 mmol/L) employed in the US, showed a dramatic increase in prediabetes prevalence to as high as 50.1% (52.1% of men, 48.1% of women) in 2010. Although progress in rapid industrialization during the few years between these two survey periods could have affected this marked increase in prevalence, the pathophysiological background and clinical significance of these changes in definition on prevalent prediabetes is a focus of interest and should be further investigated in East Asian populations.

2. CHARACTERISTICS OF (PRE)DIABETES IN EAST ASIA

Compared with individuals with type 2 diabetes in other parts of the world, those in East Asia have several characteristic phenotypes that also affect the natural course of the disease. In particular, it has long been a focus of interest that people in this area have a relatively high prevalence of diabetes in spite of the lower prevalence of obesity compared to other regions, including Western countries. In other words, type 2 diabetes develops at a lower mean body mass index (BMI) in East Asian individuals compared with those of European descent. These differences should affect strategies for diabetes prevention specific to this ethnic group.

2.1. Degree of Obesity

East Asians in general have an apparently lower mean BMI and lower rate of obesity than persons in Western countries. In Western countries, it has been well-known that patients with diabetes are generally obese and are more obese than those without diabetes, a belief that is typified in the study using data from the US National Health and Nutrition Survey III evaluated between 1988 and 1994 that concluded that *'The majority of individuals with type 2 diabetes were overweight'*. In fact, according to that report, almost half of patients with diabetes had a BMI > 30 kg/m^2 and only 18% had a BMI < 25 kg/m^2 (Nelson). The situation has not changed to the present time according to data from a survey conducted in 1999–2006, which indicated that 80.3% of subjects with diabetes had a BMI > 25 kg/m^2 and 49.1% of these had a BMI > 30 kg/m^2 (Nguyen).

Table 1 compares clinical characteristics of representative patients with diabetes in East Asia, Europe and the United States of similar ages and duration of diabetes. Despite similar glycemic and other parameters, compared with patients in the United States (US) and the United Kingdom (UK), Japanese patients had a much lower BMI approximating 23 kg/m^2. Moreover, the difference in BMI between patients with diabetes and the

Table 1. Comparison of characteristics of patients with established type 2 diabetes in typical cohorts in Japan, the United Kingdom (UK) and the United States (US). (modified from Sone 2003, Saydah).

	JDCS (Japan)	UKPDS (UK)	NHANES (US)
Number of patients	2,033	2,015	441
Age (y)	59	62	59
Diabetes duration (y)	11	9	13
Blood pressure (mmHg)	132/77	140/80	135/72
Fasting glucose (mg/dL)(mmol/L)	158 (8.75)	147 (8.14)	n.d.
HbA_{1c} (%)	8.1	7.9	7.8
Total cholesterol (mg/dL) (mmol/L)	201 (5.2)	205 (5.3)	209 (5.4)
BMI (kg/m^2)	23.1	29.4	32.3
Mean BMI of total population (kg/m^2)	22.7	24.1	28.5

total population was much larger for the US and the UK population than for Japanese (Sone 2003, Saydah). This simple comparison suggests that pancreatic reserve permitting insulin secretion is still well-preserved in Western patients despite a lengthy duration of diabetes about 10 years while Japanese patients experienced an earlier decline supported by a detailed analysis of the same patients (Sone 2007).

The cross-sectional relationships between BMI and diabetes prevalence in different regions of the world determined by the DECODA and DECODE studies also demonstrated higher diabetes prevalence at any given BMI in Japanese and Chinese than in Europeans (Nyamdorj).

2.2. Even Slight Obesity Could Greatly Enhance Diabetes Risk

Also, as speculated from lower BMI levels in East Asian patients with established type 2 diabetes, even slight obesity is known to greatly enhance the risk of type 2 diabetes in East Asians (Chan). Because of the limited pancreatic reserve for insulin secretion, type 2 diabetes develops at a relatively younger age with many patients tending to require early insulin treatment even though their mean BMIs are almost identical to those in the non-diabetic population in the same region. Onset of type 2 diabetes in the young represents an increased risk for diabetic complications. In a 7-year prospective study of 16,829 men and 8,370 women in Japan, although the subjects were on average non-obese (mean BMI 23.1 kg/m^2 for men, 22.3 kg/m^2 for women), a dose-dependent risk for diabetes even within the non-obese level was observed; even a 1 kg/m^2 increase in BMI, which corresponds to a 2.4–2.9 kg weight gain, was significantly associated with an approximate 25% increase in diabetes risk (Nagaya).

2.3. Higher Abdominal and Visceral Adiposity

Visceral adiposity is a well-known predictor of type 2 diabetes. East Asians have a greater amount of body fat and a tendency toward visceral adiposity at any given BMI (Deurenberg, Lear). In Japanese–Americans, baseline intra-abdominal fat as well as change at 5-year follow-up were shown to be independent predictors of the development of type 2 diabetes. An increase of 1 standard deviation in intra-abdominal fat was associated with a 1.65-fold (95% CI 1.21–2.25) increase in the odds of diabetes over 10 years after adjustment for confounders, including thoracic, thigh, and abdominal subcutaneous fat as well as changes in weight (Wander).

3. PATHOPHYSIOLOGY OF (PRE)DIABETES IN EAST ASIA

3.1. Low Pancreatic Reserve for Insulin Secretion

Several studies including meta-analyses demonstrated that East Asians had a clearly lower insulin response to glucose although their insulin sensitivity was higher than subjects in other ethnic groups. According to a meta-analysis of 74 cohorts in which the insulin sensitivity index and acute insulin response to glucose were determined in three major ethnic groups, East Asians were shown to have a lower acute insulin response to glucose but a higher insulin sensitivity index than African or Caucasian populations. This could, at least in part, explain the greater susceptibility to type 2 diabetes in East Asians despite demonstrating a lower mean BMI than Caucasians or Africans (Kodama K). This relationship was preserved in the continuum extending from normal glucose tolerance to type 2 diabetes which strongly implies ethnicity-specific mechanisms of diabetes development. A direct comparison between 120 Japanese and 150 Caucasians also confirmed lower β-cell response to glucose as well as higher insulin sensitivity in Japanese than in Caucasians which could largely be explained by differences in BMI (Møller). Further investigations involving a larger cohort are expected by taking into account both visceral adiposity and genetic background.

As can be speculated from these results, impaired insulin secretion was shown to have a greater impact on the incidence of type 2 diabetes compared with insulin resistance in East Asians, but both are synergistic. In a Japanese prospective study, 3,059 subjects aged 30–69 years without baseline diabetes were classified into four categories according to the results of an oral glucose tolerance test (OGTT): normal (50.7%); isolated impaired insulin secretion (i-IIS) (29.4%); isolated insulin resistance (i-IR) (16.5%); and IIS plus IR (3.4%) (Morimoto). The multivariable-adjusted HRs (95% CI) for type 2 diabetes in the i-IIS, i-IR and IIS plus IR groups compared to the normal group as a reference were 8.27 (5.33–12.83), 4.90 (2.94–8.17) and 16.93 (9.80–29.25), respectively. A further larger influence of IIS was observed at the population level; the population-attributable fractions of type 2 diabetes onset due to i-IIS, i-IR, and IIS plus IR were 50.6%, 14.2% and 12.9%, respectively (Morimoto).

3.2. Genetic Background of Diabetes in East Asia

Along with recent rapid progress in genetic epidemiology, the identification of new diabetes susceptibility loci through a genome-wide association study (GWAS) has been promoted vigorously. The latter was initiated in populations of European origin and resulted in discovering a number of loci associated with the development of type 2 diabetes including *TCF7L2*, which has one of the most prominent impacts. However, it was discovered that the frequency of the *TCF7L2* risk allele, identified in approximately one-quarter of the Caucasian population, was found in only 4–5% of East Asians such as Japanese. Therefore, the same strategy was applied to identifying the genetic background explaining different phenotypes between Caucasians and East Asians. Two Japanese groups independently found the same cluster of common variants within the KCNQ1 (potassium voltage-gated channel, KQT-like subfamily, member 1) gene to be a strong and significant candidate for conferring susceptibility to the disease in a Japanese population, which increased individual odds of type 2 diabetes by 30–40% (Yasuda, Unoki). The association of KCNQ1 with type 2 diabetes was replicated in populations of Koreans, Chinese, and Singaporeans but also in Europeans even though the frequency of the risk allele was lower than in East Asians.

A meta-analysis of GWASs identified eight new loci significantly associated with type 2 diabetes risk in East Asian populations some of which are speculated to be involved in pancreatic β-cell development or insulin gene expression (Cho). Although substantially large variations in the frequencies of risk alleles for type 2 diabetes were reported between East Asians and Caucasians, the majority of these loci showed a similar effect size for the development of type 2 diabetes in both populations (Ma RC).

Moreover, most of these genes are thought to be related to β-cell dysfunction rather than insulin resistance. Therefore, further investigations are required to explain phenotypic differences between these two populations.

4. INFLUENCE OF LIFESTYLES

Before the last war, diabetes was relatively rare in this region but afterward evolved into a rapidly growing epidemic. For example, in Japan the prevalence of diabetes is said to become approximately 40 times higher associated with rapid Westernization of lifestyles symbolized by the penetration rate of automobiles. Westernization of diet, which is typically measured by fat intake, is also considered to be one of the main causes of the diabetes epidemic in East Asians (Fig. 1). In Chinese Singaporeans, those with a relatively frequent (≥2 times per week) intake of Western-style fast food items had a significant 1.27-fold increased risk of developing type 2 diabetes and a 1.56 times higher risk of mortality from coronary heart disease compared to those with little or no reported fast food consumption; these findings were independent of the overall dietary pattern,

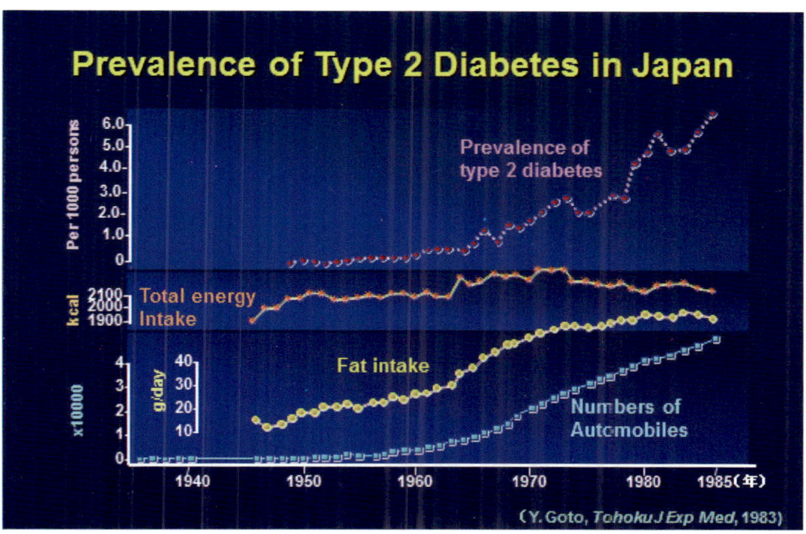

Fig. 1. Crude prevalence of type 2 diabetes in Japan along with other parameters. (Modified from Goto).

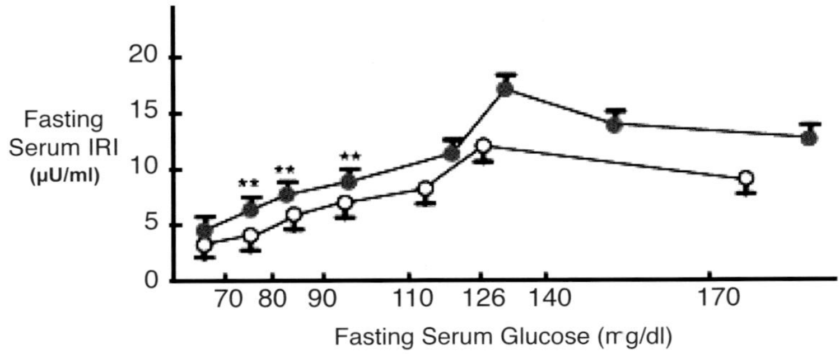

Fig. 2. Relationship between fasting glucose and insulin levels among Japanese-Americans and native Japanese people. The open and dark circles indicate native Japanese ($N = 1284$) and Japanese-Americans ($N = 1255$), respectively. *$P < 0.01$ adjusted for gender, age, BMI and glucose tolerance status. (Nakanishi) (adapted with permissions of authors and publisher).

energy intake, and BMI (Odeqaard, 2012). The effects of these environmental changes in lifestyle factors are also typically observed in US immigrants of East Asian origin. In the Hawaii-Los Angeles-Hiroshima Study, Japanese-Americans, whose genetic background is Japanese but whose lifestyle is American, had significantly higher insulin levels than Japanese living in Japan (Fig. 2) (Nakanishi), suggesting that lifestyle or the environment also affects the development of insulin resistance.

4.1. Diet and Dietary Patterns

The aforementioned observations suggest that high-fat Western diets are known to be a risk factor for type 2 diabetes and prediabetes in East Asians. In Chinese adults without known diabetes, four dietary patterns identified by factor analysis, i.e., the Western, high-wheat, traditional and hedonic patterns, were used to investigate their effects on insulin resistance defined by the homeostasis model assessment of insulin resistance (HOMA-IR) (Zuo). After adjustment for potential confounders, the Western pattern was significantly associated with greater odds for insulin resistance, and the highest quartile of the Western pattern had a higher odds ratio of 1.89 for insulin resistance compared with the lowest quartile.

HOMA-IR levels as a continuous variable also increased across quartiles of the Western pattern (Zuo). The Singapore Chinese Health Study, including 43,176 Chinese men and women (aged 45–74 years), also showed that a dietary pattern with higher intake of dim sum, meat and processed meat, sweetened foods and beverages, and fried foods was associated with a significantly increased risk of type 2 diabetes while higher intake of vegetables, fruits, and soy foods was inversely associated with this risk (Odegaard 2011).

However, it should be mentioned that even among East Asian subjects, there still exists a substantially wide variation in the relationship between the amount of food consumed and degree of obesity. Figure 3 demonstrates the relationship between overeating and obesity in Japanese patients with type 2 diabetes. Although patients who overate or were obese each accounted for approximately 20–25% of the total number, only 5% manifested both over-eating behavior and obesity. This suggests that just a small proportion of overeating patients were obese and, likewise, just a few obese patients overate (Sone 2004). In other words, over-eating behavior and obesity do not significantly overlap.

Although the rapid Westernization of diet is seen especially in younger generations, the eating habit of Asia, including East Asian countries, has been well-characterized by the rice diet. White rice is especially the common staple across this area in spite of some regional variations in the

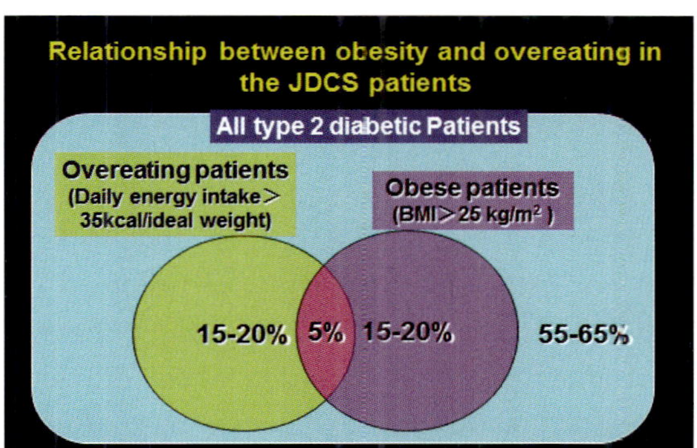

Fig. 3. Relationship between obesity and overeating in Japanese patients with type 2 diabetes from the Japan Diabetes Complications Study (made from the data of Sone 2004).

types of side dishes. A meta-analysis of prospective studies demonstrated that Chinese and Japanese populations had much higher white rice consumption than did Western populations (average intake levels were three to four servings per day versus one to two servings per week). The pooled relative risk was 1.55 (95% CI 1.20–2.01) comparing the highest with the lowest category of white rice intake among Asian populations. With a dose response for each increment in servings per day of white rice, the relative risk of type 2 diabetes was 1.11 (1.08–1.14) in all subjects including Asians and Western populations (Hu). In the United States, a large-scale ($n = 197{,}228$) prospective study revealed that substitution of brown rice for white rice might lower the risk of type 2 diabetes (Sun). After multivariate adjustment for confounders, a higher intake of white rice (≥5 servings per week vs <1 per month) was associated with a 1.17 (1.02 – 1.36) fold higher risk of type 2 diabetes while high brown rice intake (≥2 servings per week vs <1 per month) was associated with a lower risk of type 2 diabetes with a pooled relative risk of 0.89 (0.81–0.97). It was also estimated that replacing 50 grams per day (cooked, equivalent to one-third serving per day) intake of white rice with the same amount of brown rice was associated with a 16% (9–21%) lower risk of type 2 diabetes. Substituting brown for white rice would be expected to have a larger effect in East Asians who usually consume much more white rice than individuals in the US.

4.2. Role and Potential Effect of Exercise

The dietary pattern was not shown to be associated with type 2 diabetes risk in a Japanese population where there was greater and earlier industrialization than in other East Asian countries. In the Japan Public Health Center-based prospective study, 27,816 men and 36,889 women aged 45–74 years with no history of diabetes were followed over 5 years for incident type 2 diabetes (Nanri). In this study, three dietary patterns, prudent, Westernized and traditional Japanese, were utilized but none was significantly associated with type 2 diabetes risk after adjustment for covariates in both men and women although a small protective effect of the prudent dietary pattern was observed. As was observed previously (Fig. 1), the number of individuals with diabetes in Japan continued to increase even though mean energy intake remained almost constant. Exercise possibly had a stronger impact than diet in this country which was the most economically developed in East Asia. In Japanese patients with type 2 diabetes, participants in the top tertile of exercise amount had approximately one- third the risk of mortality compared to those in the bottom tertile (Sone 2013).

In general, few intervention studies focusing strictly on exercise (i.e., without diet) have demonstrated successful results in preventing diabetes or its complications. The independent and combined associations of physical activity and obesity with incident type 2 diabetes were investigated in 675,496 Korean men (Lee). During a mean follow-up of 7.5 years, men classified as overweight, obese I, and obese II had 1.47, 2.05, and 3.69 times higher risk of type 2 diabetes, respectively, compared with those who were normal weight. Men with low, medium, and high activity levels had a 5%, 10%, and 9% lower risk of type 2 diabetes, respectively, compared with inactive men after adjustment for confounders. Not being overweight or obese and having higher levels of physical activity were both independently associated with a lower risk of type 2 diabetes.

4.2.1. *Smoking*

Active smoking is an established risk factor for increased risk of type 2 diabetes (Willi). Exposure to passive smoke was also reportedly associated with an increased risk of diabetes after adjustment for a large number of possible confounders (Hayashino). East Asia is notorious as one of the regions having the largest epidemic of tobacco use in the world with 37–53% of adult men identified as current smokers and a smoking prevalence among middle-aged men of 63%. Forty-six percent or more of men and 20% or more of women were exposed to passive smoking at workplaces and at home (Katanoda). The considerable tobacco exposure, including passive smoking, may have intensified diabetes incidence and prevalence in this region. Policies are urgently required to address this issue. It was also demonstrated that smoking in Japanese patients with type 2 diabetes, was a risk factor for early nephropathy (Saito) and current smoking doubled the risk of overt nephropathy (Katayama).

5. PREDIABETES AS A RISK OF INCIDENT TYPE 2 DIABETES

An additional prediabetes criterion of HbA1c 5.7–6.4% was proposed by the American Diabetes Association in 2010 (American Diabetes Association). The relevance of diagnostic criteria of prediabetes for predicting incident diabetes was studied in a Japanese population (Heianza 2011). Subjects with a baseline diagnosis of prediabetes according to impaired fasting glucose (IFG) of 5.6–6.9 mmol/L (100–125 mg/dl) or HbA1c 5.7–6.4%, or both, were divided into four groups on the basis of the baseline diagnosis of prediabetes. During a mean follow-up period of 4.7 years, multivariate-adjusted hazard ratios for incident diabetes were 6.16 (95% CI 4.33–8.77) for those diagnosed with prediabetes by IFG alone and 6.00 (3.76–9.56) for a diagnosis by HbA1c alone, and were substantially increased to 31.9 (22.6–45.0) for diagnosis by both IFG and HbA1c compared with normoglycemic individuals. Therefore, the two tests combined could effectively target those most likely to develop diabetes which would allow for early intervention. A risk score based on this finding was developed to identify individuals at risk of incident diabetes in East Asians (Heianza 2012).

The addition of the OGTT was suggested to further improve the predictive ability in a population-based, cross-sectional study of 6,989 participants (mean age 52 years) who had an OGTT and HbA1c measurement in southern China. The area under the receiver operating characteristic curve of HbA1c was 0.903 (95% CI 0.883–0.922) and the optimal cut-off value was 6.25% (sensitivity 75.6% and specificity 91.9%). When either HbA1c or OGTT was used, prevalence of newly-diagnosed diabetes increased by 117.4% (Huang).

6. INTERVENTION AND INITIATIVES FOR DIABETES PREVENTION

6.1. Lifestyle Intervention

As shown in Western populations, group-based diet and/or exercise interventions were also shown to lead to a significant decrease in the incidence of diabetes in East Asian subjects. One of the earliest of these was the DaQing study, which followed Chinese subjects with IGT over a six-year period and demonstrated that diet, exercise, and diet-plus-exercise interventions were associated with significant 31%, 46%, and 42% reductions, respectively, in the risk of developing diabetes (Pan). Extended observations revealed that lifestyle interventions over 5 years could prevent or delay diabetes for up to 14 years after the active intervention (Li). Participants in the combined lifestyle intervention groups experienced a 51% lower incidence of diabetes (HR 0.49 95% CI 0.33–0.73) during the active intervention period and a 43% lower incidence (HR 0.57 0.41–0.81) over the 20-year period compared with control participants. This was associated with a 47% reduction in the incidence of severe, vision-threatening retinopathy over a 20-year interval, primarily due to the reduced incidence of diabetes in the intervention group (Gong). However, it remains unclear whether lifestyle intervention, especially focusing on weight loss, also leads to reduced cardiovascular disease and mortality. These findings were similar to those observed in Western subjects with newly diagnosed type 2 diabetes (Look AHEAD, Peters).

Intensive lifestyle intervention aiming to achieve and maintain ideal body weight was shown to be effective in prevention of type 2 diabetes in Japanese men with IGT (Kosaka). In this study, participants in the control and the intervention groups were advised to maintain BMI of <24.0 kg/m^2 and of <22.0 kg/m^2, respectively, by diet and exercise. Body weight decreased by 0.39 kg in the control group and by 2.18 kg in the intervention group and, as a result, the cumulative 4-year incidence of diabetes was 9.3% in the control group versus 3.0% in the intervention group representing a significant 67% reduction with intervention. These investigators also compared BMI with incidence of diabetes in five diabetes prevention studies of lifestyle interventions and generally found a linear correlation between these variables (Kosaka).

Results of another randomized controlled trial of 304 middle-aged Japanese with IGT and mean BMI of 24.5 kg/m^2 showed that a 3-year lifestyle intervention program administered by public health nurses in a primary healthcare setting was beneficial in preventing diabetes (Sakane). Insulin sensitivity assessed by the Matsuda index was improved by the intervention during this period. The 3-year cumulative incidence of type 2 diabetes tended to be lower in the intervention group (14.8% vs 8.2%). A significant reduction in the cumulative incidence was found in a subanalysis of subjects with a BMI > 22.5 kg/m^2.

6.2. Pharmacological Intervention to Prevent Diabetes

The alpha-glucosidase inhibitors, a class of oral hypoglycemic agents, are less commonly used in Western countries compared to East Asia. Voglibose, in addition to lifestyle modification, was shown to reduce the development of type 2 diabetes in high-risk Japanese individuals with IGT. 1,780 eligible patients with IGT who were on a standard diet and engaging in regular exercise were randomly assigned to oral voglibose, 0.2 mg three times a day, or placebo in a multicenter, double-blind, parallel group trial. During the three-year period, patients treated with voglibose had a lower risk of progression to type 2 diabetes than those on placebo (50 of 897 vs 106 of 881; hazard ratio 0.60, 95% CI 0.43–0.82) (Kawamori). Long-term cost-effectiveness analysis of voglibose for prevention of type 2 diabetes is required.

6.3. Regional Situations

6.3.1. *Japan*

Due to enormous economic growth after World War II as well as universal coverage by well-organized public health insurance that allows citizens free access to medical facilities along with healthy traditional foods and dietary lifestyles, considered as an intangible cultural heritage by the United Nations Educational, Scientific and Cultural Organization (UNESCO), the average life expectancy for men and women in Japan was 80 and 86, respectively, in 2010. This represents amongst the longest life expectancies in the world. The latter in conjunction with having one of the world's lowest birthrates, has resulted in Japan being one of the most aged societies in the world. The proportion of Japanese citizens aged 65 or older of the total population was 25% in 2013 and is expected to reach 33.4% in 2023.

Having experienced both an aging population and an economic boom earlier than any other Asian country, Japan has become a good predictive model for other East Asian countries that share similar genetic and cultural backgrounds and have experienced subsequent economic growth. As mentioned previously, the proportion of individuals with diabetes and prediabetes in the total population is very high. Results of the National

Health and Nutrition Survey showed that approximately one-third of the Japanese population over the age of 40 is estimated to have diabetes or prediabetes. Every year, approximately 15,000 individuals receive dialysis for the first time resulting from diabetic nephropathy and 2,500–3,000 people experience vision loss as a result of diabetic retinopathy. Figures for both complications have not decreased for years despite progress in diabetes management and availability of medications. Accordingly, medical costs for diabetes have also increased rapidly despite the current modest economic growth.

Undiagnosed diabetes remains a serious issue in Japan in spite of widespread health screening system. A significantly large percentage of Japanese patients with acute coronary syndrome (Hashimoto) or ischemic stroke (Urabe) without previously known diabetes were found to have diabetes or prediabetes during an OGTT. IGT and diabetes were found in 37% and 10%, respectively, of patients with acute coronary syndrome who were not previously diagnosed to have diabetes and did not have a fasting glucose concentration of $\geq$ 7.0 mmol/L (126 mg/dL) or HbA1c >6.0% (Hashimoto). Likewise, IGT and diabetes were found in 34.5% and 24.8%, respectively, of patients with ischemic stroke without previously diagnosed diabetes (Urabe). Scoring systems for effective screening of undiagnosed diabetes, with and without laboratory testing such as fasting plasma glucose and HbA1c, were developed for Japanese individuals (Heianza 2013).

In aiming to improve this situation, a government-based nationwide program, the Specific Health Checkup and Specific Counseling Guidance ("Tokutei-Kensin"), targeting those between 40 and 74 years of age, was started in 2008. Its main purpose is to specifically screen for the metabolic syndrome and to offer these individuals instruction and guidance regarding lifestyle modification and management that will lead to the reduction in type 2 diabetes and related end-stage renal and cardiovascular diseases. The outcome of this program is now being assessed.

The government also launched a project, with a national fund of 4 billion yen (Yazaki), with the aim of preventing type 2 diabetes and its complications, consisting of three research programs: (i) a program aimed at a 50% reduction in the conversion rate of IGT to diabetes by intensive education and lifestyle modification, (ii) a program aimed at a 50%

reduction in the dropout rate from diabetes treatment, and (iii) a program aimed at a 30% reduction in the development and exacerbation of complications from diabetes by combining intensive drug therapy with highly aggressive modification of lifestyle. These three programs have been designated as the Japan Diabetes Outcome Intervention Trial (J-DOIT) 1, 2 and 3, respectively. Government-supported genome-wide scanning to identify genes related to the disease using a database of single-nucleotide polymorphisms is now also being undertaken.

One concern regarding future diabetes in Japan is the recent increase in low birth weight infants which is speculated to be closely associated with the increase in emaciation of young women, a phenomenon characteristic of this country (Sugawara). Low birth weight and subsequent large catch-up growth are becoming established predictors for future adiposity and diabetes in adulthood, known as the concept of developmental origins of health and disease (DOHaD) based on epigenetics.

6.3.2. *China, Taiwan and Hong Kong*

Although many minority races exist, especially in Mainland China, the majority of individuals in these areas are of the Han race, which is the world's largest ethnic group and comprises approximately 20% of the global population. In Mainland China, which has the world's largest population, an ongoing economic boom and associated lifestyle changes have resulted in a serious issue regarding the global epidemic burden of type 2 diabetes. A nationally representative cross-sectional survey of 98,658 Chinese adults in 2010 by the China Non-Communicable Disease Surveillance Group defining diabetes according to the 2010 American Diabetes Association criteria (American Diabetes Association) demonstrated that the overall prevalence of diabetes was estimated to be 11.6%, similar between men and women. The prevalence of diagnosed and undiagnosed diabetes was 3.5% and 8.1%, respectively, in the Chinese population. In addition, the prevalence of prediabetes was estimated to be 50.1% in Chinese adults: 52.1% in men and 48.1% in women as mentioned earlier (Xu). Projections, based on sample weighting, suggest this may represent up to 114 million Chinese adults with diabetes and 493 million with prediabetes. Among those with diabetes, only 25.8% received treatment for diabetes and only 39.7% of those treated had adequate glycemic control.

China experiences vast domestic economic disparities due to geographic and cultural differences, typically seen between coastal areas that are rapidly developing and interior provinces in which many ethnic minorities live. Accordingly, regional differences in diabetes prevalence between coastal and interior provinces have been noted, with the prevalence higher in coastal than in interior provinces. For example, in a study comparing Fujian and Shaanxi provinces representing coastal and interior provinces, respectively, age-standardized prevalent diabetes among those 20 years of age in Fujian vs. Shaanxi were 11.5% vs 8.0%, differences remaining significant even after adjustment for known risk factors (Xu). Lifestyle risk factors contributed differently to diabetes prevalence in the two provinces; cigarette smoking was significantly associated with prevalence in Fujian and physical activity was significantly associated with prevalence in Shaanxi.

The prevalence of diabetes is even higher in Taiwan and Hong Kong, which share the same ethnicity but have experienced an economic growth spurt earlier than on the mainland (Wong). Between 1995 and 2003, Hong Kong and Taiwan had significantly higher prevalence rates of diabetes than their mainland counterparts with odds ratios of 1.5 and 2.0, respectively. The situation is similar regarding a larger proportion of those with undiagnosed diabetes, i.e., 53%, remained undiagnosed in Hong Kong and Taiwan compared to 68.6% in Mainland China.

6.3.3. *Korea*

Korea is ranked 21st among the 30 Organization for Economic Co-operation and Development (OECD) member countries in terms of adult (aged 20–79) diabetes prevalence estimated at 5.45 million (10.85%). Korea may have the highest prevalence of diabetes among the OECD countries by 2030. The Korean Diabetes Association collaborated with the Health Insurance Review & Assessment Service and estimated that the prevalence of diabetes in 2003 was 5.92%, representing 2.86 million individuals,

5.33% and 6.52% in men and women, respectively. The prevalence was 1.22 times higher in women. Among those individuals, only 52.9% used healthcare services for diabetes at least once a year. The total medical cost in patients with diabetes increased by as much as 7.99-fold, and now accounts for about one-fifth (19.2%) of the total medical costs for the entire adult population. The total medical cost per each patient with diabetes was 4.6 times higher than that in the general population (Task Force).

7. CONCLUSIONS

The greater susceptibility to type 2 diabetes in East Asians, despite lower mean BMI compared with those in Western countries, is characterized by early β-cell dysfunction. More research is needed to explain these interethnic differences. In the face of an economic boom as well as the rapid aging of the largest population in this region, urgent and effective initiatives are required to prevent type 2 diabetes and its complications.

This chapter has adopted the 'Harvard style (modified)' citation at the request of the author.

REFERENCES

American Diabetes Association (2010). Diagnosis and classification of diabetes mellitus. *Diabetes Care* **33**: S62–S69.

Chan JC, Malik V, Jia W, Kadowaki T, Yajnik CS, Yoon KH, Hu FB. (2009) Diabetes in Asia: Epidemiology, risk factors, and pathophysiology. *JAMA* **301**: 2129–2140.

Cho YS, Chen CH, Hu C, Long J, Ong RT, Sim X, Takeuchi F, Wu Y, Go MJ, Yamauchi T, Chang YC, Kwak SH, Ma RC, Yamamoto K, Adair LS, Aung T, Cai Q, Chang LC, Chen YT, Gao Y, Hu FB, Kim HL, Kim S, Kim YJ, Lee JJ, Lee NR, Li Y, Liu JJ, Lu W, Nakamura J, Nakashima E, Ng DP, Tay WT, Tsai FJ, Wong TY, Yokota M, Zheng W, Zhang R, Wang C, So WY, Ohnaka K, Ikegami H, Hara K, Cho YM, Cho NH, Chang TJ, Bao Y, Hedman ÅK, Morris AP, McCarthy MI; DIAGRAM Consortium; MuTHER Consortium, Takayanagi R, Park KS, Jia W, Chuang LM, Chan JC, Maeda S, Kadowaki T, Lee JY, Wu JY, Teo YY, Tai ES, Shu XO, Mohlke KL, Kato N, Han BG, Seielstad M. (2011) Meta-analysis of genome-wide association studies identifies eight new loci for type 2 diabetes in East Asians. *Nat Genet* **44**: 67–72.

Deurenberg P, Deurenberg-Yap M, Guricci S. (2002) Asians are different from Caucasians and from each other in their body mass index/body fat per cent relationship. *Obes Rev* **3**: 141–146.

Gong Q, Gregg EW, Wang J, An Y, Zhang P, Yang W, Li H, Li H, Jiang Y, Shuai Y, Zhang B, Zhang J, Gerzoff RB, Roglic G, Hu Y, Li G, Bennett PH. (2011) Long-term effects of a randomised trial of a 6-year lifestyle intervention in impaired glucose tolerance on diabetes-related microvascular complications: The China Da Qing Diabetes Prevention Outcome Study. *Diabetologia* **54**: 300–307.

Goto Y. Prevalence of diabetes in Japan. In Diabetes Network http://www.dm-net.co.jp/gotoh/43/ (in Japanese).

Hashimoto K, Ikewaki K, Yagi H, Nagasawa H, Imamoto S, Shibata T, Mochizuki S. (2005) Glucose intolerance is common in Japanese patients with acute coronary syndrome who were not previously diagnosed with diabetes. *Diabetes Care* **28**: 1182–1186.

Hayashino Y, Fukuhara S, Okamura T, Yamato H, Tanaka H, Tanaka T, Kadowaki T, Ueshima H, HIPOP-OHP Research Group (2008) A prospective study of passive smoking and risk of diabetes in a cohort of workers: The High-Risk and Population Strategy for Occupational Health Promotion (HIPOP-OHP) study. *Diabetes Care* **31**: 732–734.

Heianza Y, Hara S, Arase Y, Saito K, Fujiwara K, Tsuji H, Kodama S, Hsieh SD, Mori Y, Shimano H, Yamada N, Kosaka K, Sone H. (2011) HbA1c 5.7–6.4% and impaired fasting plasma glucose for diagnosis of prediabetes and risk of progression to diabetes in Japan (TOPICS 3): A longitudinal cohort study. *Lancet* **378**: 147–155.

Heianza Y, Arase Y, Hsieh SD, Saito K, Tsuji H, Kodama S, Tanaka S, Ohashi Y, Shimano H, Yamada N, Hara S, Sone H. (2012) Development of a new scoring system for predicting the 5 year incidence of type 2 diabetes in Japan: The Toranomon Hospital Health Management Center Study 6 (TOPICS 6). *Diabetologia* **55**: 3213–3223.

Heianza Y, Arase Y, Saito K, Hsieh SD, Tsuji H, Kodama S, Tanaka S, Ohashi Y, Shimano H, Yamada N, Hara S, Sone H. (2013) Development of a screening score for undiagnosed diabetes and its application in estimating absolute risk of future type 2 diabetes in Japan: Toranomon Hospital Health Management Center Study 10 (TOPICS 10). *J Clin Endocrinol Metab* **98**: 1051–1060.

Hu EA, Pan A, Malik V, Sun Q. (2012) White rice consumption and risk of type 2 diabetes: Meta-analysis and systematic review. *BMJ* **344**: e1454.

Huang H, Peng G, Lin M, Zhang K, Wang Y, Yang Y, Zuo Z, Chen R, Wang J. (2013) The diagnostic threshold of HbA1c and impact of its use on diabetes prevalence-A population-based survey of 6898 Han participants from southern China. *Prev Med* **57**: 345–350.

Katanoda K, Jiang Y, Park S, Lim MK, Qiao YL, Inoue M. (2013) Tobacco control challenges in East Asia: Proposals for change in the world's largest epidemic region. *Tob Control* [Epub ahead of print] PubMed PMID: 23596197.

Katayama S, Moriya T, Tanaka S, Tanaka S, Yajima Y, Sone H, Iimuro S, Ohashi Y, Akanuma Y, Yamada N. (2011) Japan Diabetes Complications Study Group. Low transition rate from normo- and low microalbuminuria to proteinuria in Japanese type 2 diabetic individuals: The Japan Diabetes Complications Study (JDCS). *Diabetologia* **54**: 1025–1031.

Kawamori R, Tajima N, Iwamoto Y, Kashiwagi A, Shimamoto K, Kaku K. (2009) Voglibose Ph-3 Study Group. Voglibose for prevention of type 2 diabetes mellitus: A randomised, double-blind trial in Japanese individuals with impaired glucose tolerance. *Lancet* **373**: 1607–1014.

Kodama K, Tojjar D, Yamada S, Toda K, Patel CJ, Butte AJ. (2013) Ethnic differences in the relationship between insulin sensitivity and insulin response: A systematic review and meta-analysis. *Diabetes Care* **36**: 1789–1796.

Kosaka K, Noda M, Kuzuya T. (2005) Prevention of type 2 diabetes by lifestyle intervention: A Japanese trial in IGT males. *Diabetes Res Clin Pract* **67**: 152–162.

Lear SA, Humphries KH, Kohli S, Chockalingam A, Frohlich JJ, Birmingham CL. (2007) Visceral adipose tissue accumulation differs according to ethnic background: Results of the Multicultural Community Health Assessment Trial (M-CHAT). *Am J Clin Nutr* **86**: 353–359.

Lee DC, Park I, Jun TW, Nam BH, Cho SI, Blair SN, Kim YS. (2012) Physical activity and body mass index and their associations with the development of type 2 diabetes in korean men. *Am J Epidemiol* **176**: 43–51.

Li G, Zhang P, Wang J, Gregg EW, Yang W, Gong Q, Li H, Li H, Jiang Y, An Y, Shuai Y, Zhang B, Zhang J, Thompson TJ, Gerzoff RB, Roglic G, Hu Y, Bennett PH. (2008) The long-term effect of lifestyle interventions to prevent diabetes in the China. Da Qing Diabetes Prevention Study: A 20-year follow-up study. *Lancet* **371**: 1783–1789.

Look AHEAD Research Group, Wing RR, Bolin P, Brancati FL, Bray GA, Clark JM, Coday M, Crow RS, Curtis JM, Egan CM, Espeland MA, Evans M, Foreyt JP, Ghazarian S, Gregg EW, Harrison B, Hazuda HP, Hill JO, Horton ES, Hubbard VS, Jakicic JM, Jeffery RW, Johnson KC, Kahn SE, Kitabchi AE, Knowler WC, Lewis CE, Maschak-Carey BJ, Montez mg, Murillo A, Nathan DM, Patricio J, Morimoto A, Tatsumi Y, Deura K, Mizuno S, Ohno Y, Miyamatsu N, Watanabe S. (2013) Impact of impaired insulin secretion and insulin resistance on the incidence of type 2 diabetes mellitus in a Japanese population: The Saku study. *Diabetologia* **56**: 1671–1679.

Ma RC, Chan JC. (2013) Type 2 diabetes in East Asians: similarities and differences with populations in Europe and the United States. *Ann N Y Acad Sci* **1281**: 64–91.

Møller JB, Pedersen M, Tanaka H, Ohsugi M, Overgaard RV, Lynge J, Almind K, Vasconcelos NM, Poulsen P, Keller C, Ueki K, Ingwersen SH, Pedersen BK, Kadowaki T. (in press) Body composition is main determinant for the difference in type 2 diabetes pathophysiology between japanese and caucasians. *Diabetes Care*.

Morimoto A, Tatsumi Y, Deura K, Mizuno S, Ohno Y, Miyamatsu N, Watanabe S. (2013) Impact of impaired insulin secretion and insulin resistance on the incidence of type 2 diabetes mellitus in a Japanese population: The Saku study. *Diabetologia* **56**: 1671–1679.

Nakanishi S, Okubo M, Yoneda M, Jitsuiki K, Yamane K, Kohno N. (2004) A comparison between Japanese-Americans living in Hawaii and Los Angeles and native Japanese: The impact of lifestyle westernization on diabetes mellitus. *Biomed Pharmacother* **58**: 571–577.

Nagaya T, Yoshida H, Takahashi H, Kawai M. (2005) Increases in body mass index, even within non-obese levels, raise the risk for Type 2 diabetes mellitus: A follow-up study in a Japanese population. *Diabetes Med* **22**: 1107–1111.

Nanri A, Shimazu T, Takachi R, Ishihara J, Mizoue T, Noda M, Inoue M, Tsugane S. (2013) Japan Public Health Center-based Prospective Study Group. Dietary patterns and type 2 diabetes in Japanese men and women: the Japan Public Health Center-based Prospective Study. *Eur J Clin Nutr* **67**: 18–24.

Nelson KM, Reiber G, Boyko EJ. (2002) NHANES III. Diet and exercise among adults with type 2 diabetes: Findings from the third national health and nutrition examination survey (NHANES III). *Diabetes Care* **25**: 1722–1728.

Nguyen NT, Nguyen XM, Lane J, Wang P. (2011) Relationship between obesity and diabetes in a US adult population: Findings from the National Health and Nutrition Examination Survey, 1999–2006. *Obes Surg* **21**: 351–355.

Nyamdorj R, Pitkäniemi J, Tuomilehto J, Hammar N, Stehouwer CD, Lam TH, Ramachandran A, Janus ED, Mohan V, Söderberg S, Laatikainen T, Gabriel R, Qiao Q, DECODA and DECODE Study Groups (2010) Ethnic comparison of the association of undiagnosed diabetes with obesity. *Int J Obes* **34**: 332–339.

Odegaard AO, Koh WP, Butler LM, Duval S, Gross MD, Yu MC, Yuan JM, Pereira MA. (2011) Dietary patterns and incident type 2 diabetes in chinese men and women: The singapore chinese health study. *Diabetes Care* **34**: 880–885.

Odegaard AO, Koh WP, Yuan JM, Gross MD, Pereira MA. (2012) Western-style fast food intake and cardiometabolic risk in an Eastern country. *Circulation* **126**: 182–188.

Pan XR, Li GW, Hu YH, Wang JX, Yang WY, An ZX, Hu ZX, Lin J, Xiao JZ, Cao HB, Liu PA, Jiang XG, Jiang YY, Wang JP, Zheng H, Zhang H, Bennett PH, Howard BV. (1997) Effects of diet and exercise in preventing NIDDM in people with impaired glucose tolerance. The Da Qing IGT and Diabetes Study. *Diabetes Care* **20**: 537–544.

Peters A, Pi-Sunyer X, Pownall H, Reboussin D, Regensteiner JG, Rickman AD, Ryan DH, Safford M, Wadden TA, Wagenknecht LE, West DS, Williamson DF, Yanovski SZ. (2013) Cardiovascular effects of intensive lifestyle intervention in type 2 diabetes. *N Engl J Med* **369**: 145–154.

Saito K, Sone H, Kawai K, Tanaka S, Kodama S, Shu M, Suzuki E, Kondo K, Yamamoto S, Shimano H, Ohashi Y, Yamada N. (2007) Risk imparted by various parameters of smoking in Japanese men with type 2 diabetes on their development of microalbuminuria: Analysis from the Tsukuba Kawai Diabetes Registry. *Diabetes Care* **30**: 1286–1288.

Sakane N, Sato J, Tsushita K, Tsujii S, Kotani K, Tsuzaki K, Tominaga M, Kawazu S, Sato Y, Usui T, Kamae I, Yoshida T, Kiyohara Y, Sato S, Kuzuya H. (2011) Japan Diabetes Prevention Program (JDPP) Research Group. Prevention of type 2 diabetes in a primary healthcare setting: Three-year results of lifestyle intervention in Japanese subjects with impaired glucose tolerance. *BMC Public Health* **11**: 40.

Saydah SH, Fradkin J, Cowie CC. (2004) Poor control of risk factors for vascular disease among adults with previously diagnosed diabetes. *JAMA* **291**: 335–342.

Sone H, Ito H, Ohashi Y, Akanuma Y, Yamada N. (2003) Japan Diabetes Complication Study Group. Obesity and type 2 diabetes in Japanese patients. *Lancet* **361**: 85.

Sone H, Yoshimura Y, Ito H, Ohashi Y, Yamada N. (2004) Japan Diabetes Complications Study Group. Energy intake and obesity in Japanese patients with type 2 diabetes. *Lancet* **363**: 248–249.

Sone H, Yoshimura Y, Tanaka S, Iimuro S, Ohashi Y, Ito H, Seino H, Ishibashi S, Akanuma Y, Yamada N. (2007) Japan Diabetes Complications Study (JDCS) Group. Cross-sectional association between BMI, glycemic control and energy intake in Japanese patients with type 2 diabetes. Analysis from the Japan Diabetes Complications Study. *Diabetes Res Clin Pract* **77**: S23–S29.

Sone H, Tanaka S, Tanaka S, Suzuki S, Seino H, Hanyu O, Sato A, Toyonaga T, Okita K, Ishibashi S, Kodama S, Akanuma Y, Yamada N. (2013) Leisure-Time

Physical Activity Is a Significant Predictor of Stroke and Total Mortality in Japanese Patients with Type 2 Diabetes. Analysis from the Japan Diabetes Complications Study (JDCS). *Diabetologia* **56**: 1021–1030.

Sugawara A, Saito K, Sato M, Kodama S, Sone H. (2009) Thinness in Japanese young women. *Epidemiology* **20**: 464–465.

Sun Q, Spiegelman D, van Dam RM, Holmes MD, Malik VS, Willett WC, Hu FB. (2010) White rice, brown rice, and risk of type 2 diabetes in US men and women. *Arch Intern Med* **170**: 961–969. Erratum in: *Arch Intern Med* **170**: 1479.

Saydah SH, Fradkin J, Cowie CC. (2004) Poor control of risk factors for vascular disease among adults with previously diagnosed diabetes. *JAMA* **291**: 335–342.

Task Force Team for Basic Statistical Study of Korean Diabetes Mellitus of Korean Diabetes Association, Park IeB, Kim J, Kim DJ, Chung CH, Oh JY, Park SW, Lee J, Choi KM, Min KW, Park JH, Son HS, Ahn CW, Kim H, Lee S, Lee IB, Choi I, Baik SH. (2013) Diabetes epidemics in Korea: Reappraise nationwide survey of diabetes "diabetes in Korea 2007". *Diabetes Metab J* **37**: 233–239.

Unoki H, Takahashi A, Kawaguchi T, Hara K, Horikoshi M, Andersen G, Ng DP, Holmkvist J, Borch-Johnsen K, Jørgensen T, Sandbaek A, Lauritzen T, Hansen T, Nurbaya S, Tsunoda T, Kubo M, Babazono T, Hirose H, Hayashi M, Iwamoto Y, Kashiwagi A, Kaku K, Kawamori R, Tai ES, Pedersen O, Kamatani N, Kadowaki T, Kikkawa R, Nakamura Y, Maeda S. (2008) SNPs in KCNQ1 are associated with susceptibility to type 2 diabetes in East Asian and European populations. *Nat Genet* **40**: 1098–1102.

Urabe T, Watada H, Okuma Y, Tanaka R, Ueno Y, Miyamoto N, Tanaka Y, Hattori N, Kawamori R. (2009) Prevalence of abnormal glucose metabolism and insulin resistance among subtypes of ischemic stroke in Japanese patients. *Stroke* **40**: 1289–1295.

Wander PL, Boyko EJ, Leonetti DL, McNeely MJ, Kahn SE, Fujimoto WY. (2013) Change in visceral adiposity independently predicts a greater risk of developing type 2 diabetes over 10 years in Japanese Americans. *Diabetes Care* **36**: 289–293.

Willi C, Bodenmann P, Ghali WA, Faris PD, Cornuz J. (2007) Active smoking and the risk of type 2 diabetes: A systematic review and meta-analysis. *JAMA* **298**: 2654–2664.

Wong KC, Wang Z. (2006) Prevalence of type 2 diabetes mellitus of Chinese populations in Mainland China, Hong Kong, and Taiwan. *Diabetes Res Clin Pract* **73**: 126–134.

Xu S, Ming J, Xing Y, Gao B, Yang C, Ji Q, Chen G. (2013) Regional differences in diabetes prevalence and awareness between coastal and interior provinces in China: A population-based cross-sectional study. *BMC Public Health* **13**: 299.

Xu Y, Wang L, He J, Bi Y, Li M, Wang T, Wang L, Jiang Y, Dai M, Lu J, Xu M, Li Y, Hu N, Li J, Mi S, Chen CS, Li G, Mu Y, Zhao J, Kong L, Chen J, Lai S, Wang W, Zhao W, Ning G. (2013) 2010 China Noncommunicable Disease Surveillance Group. Prevalence and control of diabetes in Chinese adults. *JAMA* **310**: 948–959.

Yang W, Lu J, Weng J, Jia W, Ji L, Xiao J, Shan Z, Liu J, Tian H, Ji Q, Zhu D, Ge J, Lin L, Chen L, Guo X, Zhao Z, Li Q, Zhou Z, Shan G, He J. (2010) China National Diabetes and Metabolic Disorders Study Group. Prevalence of diabetes among men and women in China. *N Engl J Med* **362**: 1090–1101.

Yasuda K, Miyake K, Horikawa Y, Hara K, Osawa H, Furuta H, Hirota Y, Mori H, Jonsson A, Sato Y, Yamagata K, Hinokio Y, Wang HY, Tanahashi T, Nakamura N, Oka Y, Iwasaki N, Iwamoto Y, Yamada Y, Seino Y, Maegawa H, Kashiwagi A, Takeda J, Maeda E, Shin HD, Cho YM, Park KS, Lee HK, Ng MC, Ma RC, So WY, Chan JC, Lyssenko V, Tuomi T, Nilsson P, Groop L, Kamatani N, Sekine A, Nakamura Y, Yamamoto K, Yoshida T, Tokunaga K, Itakura M, Makino H, Nanjo K, Kadowaki T, Kasuga M. (2008) Variants in KCNQ1 are associated with susceptibility to type 2 diabetes mellitus. *Nat Genet*; **40**: 1092–1097.

Yazaki Y, Kadowaki T. (2006) Combating diabetes and obesity in Japan. *Nat Med* **12**: 73–74.

Zuo H, Shi Z, Yuan B, Dai Y, Pan X, Wu G, Hussain A. (2013) Dietary patterns are associated with insulin resistance in Chinese adults without known diabetes. *Br J Nutr* **109**: 1662–1669.

Chapter 13: Real Life Diabetes Prevention Initiatives in India

Harish Ranjani[†], *Mary Beth Weber*[‡], *KM Venkat Narayan*[‡] *and Viswanathan Mohan*[*,†]

1. PREVALENCE IN INDIA

Diabetes is a global public health epidemic and is growing at an alarming rate in developing countries like India with a resultant increase in morbidity and mortality.[1] India ranks second in the world in total number for people with diabetes in any given country, next only to China. According to the recent Indian Council of Medical Research — India Diabetes (ICMR-INDIAB) national diabetes survey there were 62.4 million individuals with diabetes and a further 77 million at high-risk of developing diabetes with pre-diabetes in India in 2011.[2] The International Diabetes Federation (IDF) Diabetes Atlas estimates that the number of people with diabetes in India (aged 20–79 years) will rise to 101 million by 2030 unless urgent preventive steps are taken.[3]

The diabetes epidemic in low- and middle-income countries (LMIC) like India is growing in all populations, in both rural and urban settings,

*Corresponding author. Madras Diabetes Research Foundation & Dr. Mohan's Diabetes Specialities Centre, WHO Collaborating Center for Non-Communicable Disease Prevention and Control & IDF Centre for Education, 4, Conran Smith Road, Gopalapuram, Chennai 600 086, India. Email: drmohans@diabetes.ind.in

†Madras Diabetes Research Foundation & Dr. Mohan's Diabetes Specialities Centre, WHO Collaboroting Centre for Non-communicable Diseases Prevention and Control, IDF Centre of Education, Gopalapuram, Chennai, India.

‡Hubert Department of Global Health, Rollins School of Public Health, Emory University, Atlanta, GA, USA.

among the affluent and the less privileged, and in all age groups.[2,4,5] A particularly disturbing trend is the shift in onset of diabetes to younger ages.[6,7] As LMIC develop and people start to live longer, the morbidity and mortality due to diabetes will only increase unless effective prevention and management measures are put in place. In India, the number of diabetes-related deaths among 20–79-year olds is estimated to be 1 million; however, estimating deaths from diabetes is difficult because it is rarely reported as the cause of death in medical records. Studies using the risk of death due to diabetes in different populations allow researchers to generate more realistic estimates of the true mortality burden. These estimates are almost certainly an underestimate but show that a substantial proportion of deaths occur in people under the age of 60. This is well below the life expectancy in many countries and could be a result of the serious complications that can develop in untreated diabetes and could have long lasting adverse effects on a nation's health and economy.[1]

1.1. Economic Consequences of Diabetes

The mean diabetes-related expenditure per person with diabetes is estimated to be US$68 in India.[3] An Indian study[8] showed that the total annual expenditure by patients on diabetes care was, on average, Rs. 10,000 (US$156) in urban areas and Rs. 6,260 (US$96) in rural areas (using an exchange rate of Rs. 65/US$). A secular increase of 113% was observed in the total expenditure between 1998 and 2005 in the urban population. The cost of treatment further increased dramatically if there were associated diabetes complications. Individuals belonging to the low-income group spent a high proportion of their income on diabetes care (34% and 27% for urban poor versus rural poor, respectively). The medical costs incurred by a person with diabetes were two to five times higher than those without diabetes. The cost of diabetes care annually could approximate 130 billion rupees (US$2 billion at Rs. 65/US$1).

The Cost of Diabetes in India (CODI) study showed that college-educated people were on average diagnosed 7 years before illiterate people and despite having diabetes for a longer period of time, had lower rates of complications (55%) compared to those with little or no education (80%).[9]

Hence, the most socioeconomically disadvantaged groups in Indian society are at a higher risk of developing diabetes-related complications because of delays in diagnosis. Furthermore, these complications often require expensive therapies and prolonged hospitalizations, thereby contributing to increasing direct costs and indirect costs in terms of productivity loss and absenteeism. One Indian study revealed that those with high income spent 12% of their total income on treatment as compared to 59% by the low-income group.[10] A recent study from our group (unpublished data) highlighted direct and indirect costs (e.g., preseentism and excess cost burden due to diabetes) across government, private, and rural clinics in India compared to age-, sex-, and socioeconomic status (SES)-matched persons without diabetes. Excess direct costs were highest among those attending a private clinic (INR 19,552, US$425) and lowest among those attending a government clinic (INR 1,204, US$26.17). Private clinic attendees had the lowest incremental absenteeism (2.36 work days/year) and highest presenteeism (0.06 work days/year) whereas those attending the government clinic reported the highest absenteeism (7.48 work days/year) and lowest presenteeism (–0.31 work days/year).

1.2. Levels of Diabetes Prevention

The natural history of diabetes is characterized by gradual progression from normal glucose tolerance through a stage of pre-diabetes defined as impaired glucose tolerance (IGT) or impaired fasting glucose (IFG), then to clinical diabetes and finally to the stage of complications. However, not all individuals go through these stages in a linear manner.

Prevention of diabetes can be done at every stage in the natural history of diabetes resulting in four levels of diabetes prevention (Fig. 1).[11] *Primordial prevention* refers to efforts to prevent the development of diabetes risk factors (e.g., prevention of obesity or pre-diabetes by individual or mass media education programs). *Primary prevention* is prevention of diabetes before the onset of the condition (e.g., diabetes prevention through lifestyle or drug interventions).[12] *Secondary prevention* is the prevention of complications in those with established diabetes by good control of blood sugars, blood pressure and lipids. *Tertiary*

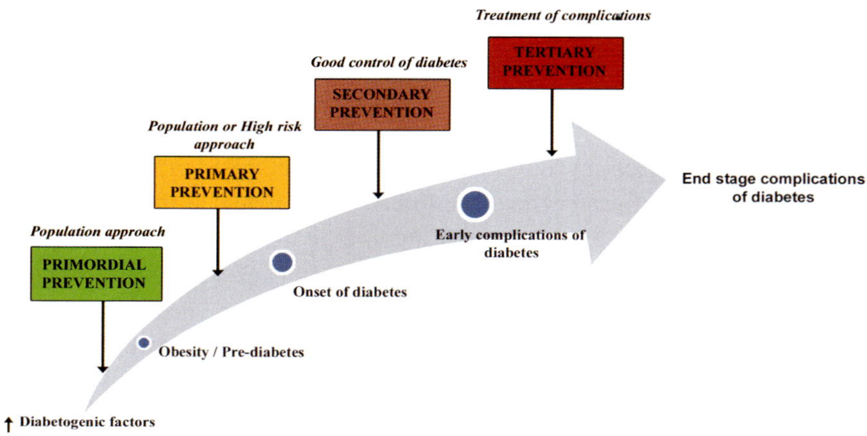

Fig. 1. Levels of diabetes prevention.

prevention focuses on limiting disability and impairment in people who already have developed some early complications of diabetes. All the levels of prevention are important and complementary. Primordial and primary prevention contribute most to the health of the whole population by preventing the onset of the disease and its risk factors, while secondary and tertiary prevention are focused on restoring the health of individuals with disease.

1.3. What is Translational Research?

Translational research takes the data, programs, and products from controlled research trials and transforms them into practical tools for public health and clinical practice.[13] The ability to study effectiveness and efficiency, rather than efficacy alone, comes as a result of translational research.[14]

1.4. Phases of Translation Research

The primary goal of translational research is to determine how to apply advances in basic science or efficacy research findings from the bench-to-bedside-to-community so that it ultimately benefits mankind. The different types of translational research are described below.

- *Bench to bed side*: this involves translating molecular level, drug development research in a controlled laboratory setting to clinical research in a select number of patients afflicted with a disease or condition. This stage includes the 'T1 & T2' translational blocks.
- *Bedside to practice*: this examines how the efficient and safe treatment findings from laboratory research or small in-patient trials function when applied to real patients in real life situations. Phase IV clinical trials and post-marketing surveillance come under this approach. This stage includes the 'T3' translational block.
- *Clinical practice or controlled trial to community, public health and health policy*: this involves translating evidence-based research from a clinical research setting to real world practice. It helps to translate treatment and prevention strategies developed in 'T2 & T3' translation blocks into sustainable solutions. This represents the "practice to community" definition of translational research. This stage includes the 'T4' translational block and is associated with the challenge of moving scientific knowledge into the public sector and thereby changing everyday lives of people.[15,16]

1.5. Challenges in Real Life Diabetes Translation Research

A major challenge in health promotion and prevention of chronic diseases like diabetes is translating the research findings from an ideal setting of a RCT to a less than optimal real world environment. This difficulty is reflected in the lag between scientific discovery and community implementation; it takes approximately 17 years for basic science findings to reach the public and actually improve health.[17] Furthermore, the size of benefits demonstrated in efficacy trials under idealized condition are generally not obtained when interventions are delivered in real-life situations.[18] Hence, targeting individuals at high-risk is at most likely to have a moderate impact on the incidence of diabetes. The real challenge is to tackle the underlying determinants of diabetes globally, which, basically implies modifying environments to make them less obesogenic. This challenge is as great if not greater than reducing tobacco consumption. Modifying the obesogenic environment will require a broad range of multi-sectoral policy measures (e.g., reform in agriculture and food production; urban planning; changes in transportation; school curricula; worksite policies) and need to involve the community.[1]

1.6. Community-Based Diabetes Prevention Initiatives in India

This chapter will report some translational, community-based research studies and programs in India. Because most (90–95%) of all diabetes is type 2 diabetes mellitus (T2DM), the examples selected for this chapter focus on primary prevention of T2DM, with some examples of programs aimed at secondary and tertiary prevention described in Sec. 2 (Community-based Diabetes Management Programs). Programs focusing on gestational diabetes are outside the scope of this chapter, but there are several examples of gestational diabetes prevention programs in India.[19,20]

This section will focus first on research studies of primary prevention, then describe some of the community-based programs, which although sometimes lacking in data and formal program assessments, still provide important information about diabetes prevention efforts in India. Finally, the section will conclude by describing a few programs that focus on secondary and tertiary prevention, and include tools for diabetes and prediabetes screening.

2. RANDOMIZED TRIALS OF PRIMARY PREVENTION OF DIABETES IN INDIA (ALSO REFER TO CHAPTER 5)

RCTs provide the strongest scientific evidence for the effectiveness of prevention programs. The studies described here include both efficacy trials (the IDPP-1 and IDPP-3) of diabetes prevention in India and translational research trials (an IDPP-3 translations being conducted in the UK and India, D-CLIP, and K-DPP), which test the effectiveness of utilizing proven diabetes prevention programs in the Indian context.

2.1. The Indian Diabetes Prevention Program (IDPP-1)[21]

The Indian Diabetes Prevention Program (IDPP-1) was the first trial diabetes primary prevention trial conducted in India. In a prospective community-based study, IDPP-1 tested whether the progression to diabetes could be influenced by interventions in Asian Indians with IGT. The research team randomised 531 (421 men, 110 women) subjects with IGT (mean age 45.9 ± 5.7 years, BMI 25.8 ± 3.5 kg/m^2) into four groups. Group 1 was the control, Group 2 was given advice on lifestyle modification (LSM), Group 3 was treated with metformin (MET) and Group 4 was given LSM plus MET.

The IDPP-1 study showed that LSM and MET could be effective means to prevent diabetes in Asian Indians. The primary outcome measure was incidence of T2DM. The 3-year cumulative incidences of diabetes were 55.0%, 39.3%, 40.5% and 39.5% in Groups 1–4, respectively, and, compared to the control arm, the relative risk reduction was 28.5% with LSM (95% CI 20.5–37.3, $p = 0.018$), 26.4% with MET (95% CI 19.1–35.1, $p = 0.029$) and 28.2% with LSM + MET (95% CI 20.3–37.0, $p = 0.022$). Although the relative risk reduction in the IDDP-1 study was smaller than what was found in the US Diabetes Prevention Program (DPP) or Finnish Diabetes Prevention Study trials, the absolute risk reductions in the Indian trial was much larger. This is reflected in the low numbers needed to treat to prevent one incident case of diabetes was 6.4 for LSM, 6.9 for MET and 6.5 for LSM + MET. This was because the IDDP-1 recruited people with prediabetes at very high baseline risk.

2.2. Effectiveness of Mobile Phone Messaging in Prevention of Type 2 Diabetes by Lifestyle Modification in Men in India: A Prospective, Parallel Group, Randomized Controlled Trial-Indian Diabetes Prevention Program-3 (IDPP-3)[22]

As traditional lifestyle intervention programs can be labor intensive, mobile phone messaging may be an inexpensive alternative way to deliver educational and motivational advice about lifestyle modification. A pilot study conducted by Shetty *et al.* in 2011 showed that frequent communication via SMS was acceptable to patients with diabetes, and it helped to improve health outcomes.[23] IDPP-3 was a RCT conducted at ten sites in southeast India to assess whether mobile phone messaging that encouraged lifestyle changes could reduce incident T2DM in Indian Asian men with IGT (NCT00819455). Participants (aged 35–55 years) were randomly assigned (1:1) to a mobile phone messaging intervention with frequent SMS text messages or standard care (control group receiving standard lifestyle advice at baseline).

The primary outcome was incidence of T2DM, analysed by intention to treat. Five hundred thirty-seven patients were randomly assigned to either the mobile phone messaging intervention ($n = 271$) or standard care ($n = 266$). The cumulative incidence of T2DM was significantly lower in those who received mobile phone messages than in controls: 50 (18%) participants in the intervention group developed T2DM compared with 73 (27%) in the control group [hazard ratio 0.64, 95% confidence interval (CI) 0.45–0.92]. The number needed to treat with the intervention to prevent one case of T2DM was 11 (95% CI 6–55). The study concluded that interpretive mobile phone messaging can be an effective and acceptable method to deliver advice and support on LSM to prevent T2DM in men.

Such studies form the basis for future prevention programs using cheaper modes of communication to educate and motivate large number of people. For example, the IDPP-3 researchers initiated *A Pragmatic and Scalable Strategy Using Mobile Technology to Promote Sustained Lifestyle Changes to Prevent Type 2 Diabetes in India and the UK*[24] in January 2012 in India and the UK. This on-going study proposes a similar prevention strategy as that used in the IDPP-3 trial, namely a lifestyle modification program delivered by text messaging. Subjects will be invited to participate and once recruited, will be randomised to usual care or the SMS intervention group. Usual care will consist of a one-to-one 30 minute interview, conducted by the research team, delivering personalised diet and exercise advice. The intervention group will undergo the same initial interview and in addition, will receive 3 times weekly text messaging with education, advice, support and motivation. The messages will be personalised to individual targets set at the initial interview. The researchers are including tools to ease the translation of the mobile program into the community. For example, this trial will identify subjects based on HbA1c measurement, instead of the more invasive oral glucose tolerance test, and the trial will include measurements of efficacy, program acceptibility and cost-effectiveness of the intervention in both study settings (UK and India).

2.3. D-CLIP: Diabetes Community Lifestyle Improvement Program[25]

The D-CLIP study is an on-going translational research study testing the effectiveness, cost-effectiveness, and acceptability of a stepwise model of diabetes prevention with lifestyle as a continuous approach and MET added when needed. In the D-CLIP study, individuals with pre-diabetes were randomized into two arms — an intervention and a control arm. The control arm received standard care. The intervention consisted of aggressive LSM through sixteen once weekly classes regarding diet and exercise followed by eight maintenance classes. The classes were modeled after the lesson plans developed for the highly successful diabetes prevention program and were culturally modified for the Indian setting. Each class was paired with one or many community volunteers also called as Dia-ambassadors). Participants were divided into peer support groups to increase social support for lifestyle change. This strategy also enhanced the sustainability of the program by empowering and educating community members to teach diabetes prevention to their peers. Unlike other published diabetes prevention trials that have included only individuals with IGT or individuals with both IGT and IFG, the D-CLIP study includes participants with either IGT, IFG, or both IGT and IFG (including those with FPG between 100–110 mg/dL, a group previously excluding from diabetes prevention trials). By recruiting people with IGT, IFG, or both, interventions like D-CLIP advance the ability to generalize diabetes prevention to a much wider population. Early results of the D-CLIP trial are promising, with improvements shown in metabolic, nutritional and biochemical parameters in the intervention group compared to control group participants.[26]

2.4. K-DPP: Kerala Diabetes Prevention Program, Kerala, South India[27]

K-DPP was planned and developed based on the results of a need assessment survey that highlighted the need to develop and implement a group-based peer support program that would address cultural and family determinants of lifestyle risks, including family decision-making regarding adoption of healthy dietary and physical activity patterns using a community approach.[28] The K-DPP in collaboration with Monash University, Australia, is a cluster RCT of a culturally tailored and group-based lifestyle intervention program. K-DPP targets individuals at high risk of developing T2DM in 60 neighborhoods from a rural area of Thiruvananthapuram district in Kerala State, India. The study aims to: (i) implement and evaluate the K-DPP and its impact on T2DM incidence at 36 months compared with a standard care control group; (ii) identify individual, household, and local factors likely to affect the wider system-wide uptake of K-DPP in India and other developing countries in the future; and (iii) estimate the population health impact and cost-effectiveness of screening and intervention in reducing the incidence of T2DM. The intervention involves twelve, 90-m group educational sessions (providing simple, practical and culturally appropriate lifestyle advice) over an 8-month period. Each group will consist of 12–15 participants accompanied by family members or friends. These groups will be jointly delivered by a group facilitator and a peer leader and will address three linked themes: (1) how to prevent T2DM and the importance of modest but appreciable lifestyle change to accomplish this goal; (2) how best to provide emotional/social and environmental support for lifestyle change and a healthy lifestyle; and (3) how to access and link with community resources/supports for change, maintenance and sustainability. These group sessions will be supplemented by peer support sessions. This project is currently ongoing.

3. TARGETED COMMUNITY EDUCATION PROGRAMS FOR PRIMARY PREVENTION OF DIABETES IN INDIA

Targeted community projects exist to address the specific needs of a community and often serve as proof of concept studies for implementing different prevention techniques (e.g., use of Community-Based Participatory research to design programs or applying social marketing techniques in a rural setting). Successful programs applied to target communities can be used to inform the development and design of programs with a broader reach.

3.1. The Asiad Colony Project[29,30]

The Chennai Urban Population Study (CUPS) was an epidemiological study carried out in two urban residential colonies (a cluster of buildings surrounded by a common boundary), one representing a middle-income group and the other representing the low-income group in Chennai India.[31] CUPS showed a significantly higher prevalence of diabetes in the middle-income colony (12.4%) as compared to the lower income group (6.5%).[32] Because the rate of diabetes was relatively low in the low-income group, this colony was offered only a single class providing standard lifestyle advice (e.g., increasing physical activity and improving diet), whereas the middle-income group with the higher diabetes prevalence were provided with a variety of health promotion activities (for example, several awareness lectures and distribution of educational material on healthy food options and the need for increasing physical activity). Independently, as a result of the educational program, residents in the middle-income community raised funds to build a neighborhood park to promote physical activity.

The program in the middle-income colony significantly improved knowledge and physical activity levels (the percentage of residents who exercised increased from 14.2% to 58.7%, representing a 300% increase in physical activity).[29] A follow-up study was conducted 10 years after the diabetes education program to assess the new diabetes prevalence rates in the same two colonies (Fig. 2). As seen in Fig. 2, during this period, in the lower income group, the prevalence of diabetes increased from 6.5% to 15.3% (a 135% increase) whereas in the middle-income group, the prevalence increased from 12.4% to 15.4% (24% increase).[30] This project indicates that a moderate investment of time and effort might arrest the rapid rise in the prevalence of diabetes. This phenomenon is referred to as 'prevention of excess gain'.[33] This study has been cited as a potential model for prevention of diabetes through community action in developing countries in the WHO publication 'Preventing chronic disease — a vital investment'.[34]

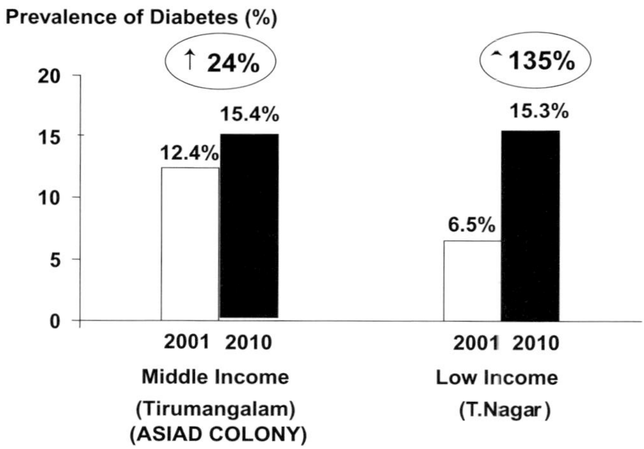

Fig. 2. Changes in prevalence rates of diabetes in middle and lower income groups in Chennai (2001–2010) (Deepa *et al.*, 2011).

3.2. A Community-Based Diabetes Prevention and Management Education Program in a Rural Village in Tamilnadu, South India[35]

This study evaluated a 7-month community-based non-pharmacological lifestyle intervention to prevent/reduce the risk of developing diabetes and its complications in the village of Alamarathupatti in Tamil Nadu. A total of 703 village inhabitants aged 10–92 years were provided an educational intervention using trained trainers. The trainers were science graduates trained at Gandhigram Rural Institute and were housed in the village for the duration of the intervention. Culturally and linguistically appropriate health education messages addressed diet, physical activity, simple relaxing breathing techniques and knowledge improvement. Ten face-to-face encounters were provided to all respondents with health messages tailored for sex, age and socioeconomic differences. Reinforcement of these messages was supported by group events. The prevalence of diabetes and the effectiveness of the intervention were assessed using select parameters. The intervention reduced levels of fasting blood glucose by 11% in adults with prediabetes, 17% in youth with prediabetes, and 25% in adults with

T2DM. Improvements in obesity parameters and dietary intake were also seen.

3.3. A Community-Based Participatory Diabetes Prevention and Management Intervention in Rural India using Community Health Workers[36]

The purpose of this study was to test the effectiveness of a 6-month community-based diabetes prevention and management program in rural Gujarat, India from December 2007 to May 2008. This study was designed as a collaborative approach to equitably involve the community stakeholders in the planning, implementation, education and review process. Community-based participatory research was used to plan and tailor the intervention by engaging trained community health workers as change agents to provide lifestyle education, serve as community advocates, and collect data from 1,638 rural Indians (81.9% response rate). Ten culturally and linguistically appropriate health education messages were provided in face-to-face individual and group sessions (e.g., demonstrations of model meals and cooking techniques). Mean age was 41.9 ± 15.9 years. Overall point prevalence of diabetes, prediabetes, obesity, and hypertension were 7.2%, 19.3%, 16.7%, and 28%, respectively, with significant differences between the low socioeconomic status (SES) participants (agricultural workers) and the high SES participants (business community) due to differing diet and activity levels. The intervention significantly reduced blood glucose levels by 5.7 (0.32 mmol / L) and 14.9 mg/dL (0.83 mmol / L) for individuals with prediabetes and diabetes, respectively, and systolic and diastolic blood pressure by 8 mm Hg and 4 mm Hg, respectively, in the overall population. Knowledge of diabetes and cardiovascular disease improved by 50% in the high SES group and doubled in the low SES group; general and abdominal body fat percentage also decreased by ≤1%. Among individuals with diabetes, metabolic complications such as diabetic nephropathy and chronic kidney disease were noted. The study concluded that through collective engagement of the community, participatory programs can serve as a prototype for future prevention and management efforts, which are rare and underutilized in India.

3.4. Community-Based Physical Activity Intervention using Principles of Social Marketing: A Demonstration Project in Southern India[37]

The study aimed to develop and implement promotion of physical activity in a rural community by applying the principles of social marketing. The intervention targeted 485 people, 20–49 years of age, and residents of *Periakattupalayam* and *Rangareddipalayam* villages of Tamil Nadu. Health education by one-to-one counseling, written materials and community events were used to promote moderate intensity physical activity (brisk walking for 30 m on 4 days/week, primary through walking). Participants formed 30 walking groups under four coordinators, in a home-based setting with professional supervision and guidance, and village leaders, self-help groups and youth clubs were involved in promoting physical activity. Of the 485 subjects, 265 people (54.6%) engaged in brisk walking more than 4 days a week, while 156 subjects (32.2%) performed walking on 1–4 days per week during the intervention. The drop-out rate was 13.2% (64 subjects). Age, occupation and educational status were important determinants of participation and adherence to the physical activity program. It was found that the application of social marketing techniques in an intervention to promote physical activity was successful in a rural Indian community. Social marketing is being encouraged as a core public health strategy to control voluntary lifestyle behaviors such as smoking, drinking, drug use, physical activity and diet.[38]

4. LARGE-SCALE COMMUNITY EDUCATION PROGRAMS FOR PRIMARY PREVENTION OF DIABETES IN INDIA

Large-scale projects often utilize mass media, community screening, and existing infrastructure to reach large population groups (e.g., cities, states, or regions). Because of the scale of these projects, many are planned and implemented with several partner organizations, often including groups from different sections of health promotions [e.g., academic institutions, non-government organizations (NGOs), government groups]. Many of these programs may not include formal program assessments, focusing on measuring program reach only. It is important to note that reaching large numbers through awareness messages does not guarantee behavior change; however, these large-scale community programs still play an important role in improving diabetes knowledge and education.

4.1. PACE: Prevention Awareness Counseling Evaluation

The Chennai Urban Rural Epidemiology Study (CURES)[39] was a large epidemiological study on diabetes and its complications carried out in the year 2001–2002 in Chennai showing low diabetes knowledge. For example, among a representative sample of the Chennai population, only 22.2% knew that diabetes could be prevented and only 19% knew that diabetes could cause complications; among individuals with know diabetes knowledge was not much better, with only 41% reporting that diabetes could be prevented and only 40.6% understanding that diabetes could cause complications.[40] As a follow-up to CURES and in order to improve the awareness about diabetes, a large-scale community-based diabetes awareness and prevention program was taken up in Chennai called the Prevention Awareness Counseling and Evaluation (PACE) diabetes project.[41] PACE included the following components:

a. A free public awareness campaign with lectures and interactive programs. A total of 774 screening and education camps were conducted all over Chennai. Overall, 76,645 individuals were screened including 17% with known diabetes, 4% with newly diagnosed diabetes, and 7.5% with prediabetes.
b. One hundred and sixty four "PACE Education Counters" were opened at various bookshops, shopping complexes, food chain stores, and family physician clinics in Chennai, which provided free diabetes educational materials.
c. Mass media programs included a documentary film/radio program on diabetes and diabetes prevention and management messages provided though newspaper articles, cinema theater advertisements, and text messaging on mobile phones.
d. General Practitioners (GPs) were trained in diabetes management and prevention strategies. The aim of training was to increase awareness

about prevention and improve overall diabetes health care management practice. A total of 232 GPs were trained. There was a 20% increase in diabetes prevention and management awareness scores of participating GPs after the program.[42]

Assessment conducted after the PACE project (in 2007) showed improvements in diabetes awareness and knowledge compared with results of the CURES survey conducted in 2001–2002. Eighty-one percent of people surveyed after the PACE project had heard of a condition called diabetes compared to 75.5% in the CURES survey. Almost 74% of the city residents were also aware that the prevalence of diabetes was increasing as compared to 60.2% reported earlier during CURES. Significantly more people knew that diabetes could be prevented by a combination of diet and exercise. Respondents reporting that obesity, family history of diabetes, hypertension and mental stress could contribute towards diabetes also increased significantly after PACE ($p < 0.001$).[41]

4.2. MARG (The Path): Medical Education for Children/ Adolescents for Realistic Prevention of Obesity and Diabetes and for Healthy Ageing (August 2006–December 2008)[43]

This project was conducted by the Diabetes Foundation of India and focused on primary prevention with the aim of creating awareness about diabetes, obesity, lipid disorders and heart disease in children and adolescents in North India. The MARG program [funded by World Diabetes Foundation (WDF), Denmark] was the first large scale community intervention project in South Asia which focused on primary prevention not only of diabetes, but also of non-communicable diseases in general, through promotion of optimal dietary and lifestyle practices. Through various activities, like drama and healthy recipe demonstration, health educators and volunteers demonstrated how unhealthy eating and sedentary lifestyles can affect the health of school children. In addition, schools were encouraged to substitute unhealthy foods with healthier choices in the canteen (cafeteria). School volunteers and teachers have taken the initiative to continue the program by organizing healthy cooking demonstrations, poster making and extempore speaking competitions promoting healthy lifestyle choices.[44]

The MARG program reached 40,196 children (aged 8–18 years), 25,000 parents and 1500 teachers in three cities of North India (Delhi, Jaipur, and Agra) over a period of three years. Cross-sectional surveys reported low baseline knowledge and behaviour scores in 75–94% government and 48–78% private school children, across all age groups. Private school children, parents and teachers performed significantly better than government school subjects ($p < 0.05$). Following the intervention, scores improved in all children irrespective of the type of school ($p < 0.001$). A significantly greater improvement was observed in younger children (aged 8–11 years) as compared with those aged 12–18 years, in females compared with males and in government schools compared with private schools ($p < 0.05$ for all).[43]

The effectiveness (in terms of improving knowledge and changing anthropometric outcomes) of the MARG program was studied in a subset of urban adolescents in North India. Two schools matched for student strength and middle socioeconomic strata were randomly allocated to intervention or control group. Changes in nutrition-related knowledge, attitude, lifestyle practices, food frequency and body image of eleventh-grade students (15–17 years) in both schools were tested using a validated questionnaire. Anthropometric and biochemical measurements were made using standard methods. An 8-electrode multi-frequency bioelectrical impedance method of body fat estimation was used to carry out the segmental body composition analysis. At 6 months follow-up, significant improvement in several domains of knowledge was observed in intervention children ($n = 99$; males = 60; females = 39) compared with control school children ($n = 102$; males = 61; females = 41). In the intervention group, a significantly lower proportion of children consumed carbonated drinks (15.1%) and energy-dense unhealthy foods (8.9%), whereas significantly higher proportion brought tiffin (packed lunch) to school (14.9%) and brought a fruit in their tiffin (30.7%) compared with the control group ($p < 0.05$ for all comparisons). Significant decreases in mean waist circumference (95% CI = −2.43, −0.17), sagittal abdominal diameter (95% CI = −0.82, −0.09), waist-to-hip ratio (95% CI = −0.03, −0.004) and fasting blood glucose (95% CI = −0.09, 5.00) was seen in intervention compared with control school children. Thus, this multi-component model of nutrition and lifestyle education was effective in improving the nutrition-related knowledge, eating habits and lifestyle practices.[45]

4.3. Media Campaign for Prevention and Care of Diabetes, 'Jagran Pehel' New Delhi, North India (January 2008–January 2009)[46]

The joint initiative of WDF, Denmark and '*Jagran Pehel*'[19] was aimed at enhancing awareness about diabetes and its consequences among various stakeholders and to sensitize them to take appropriate action towards care and prevention by organizing a mass media campaign, road shows and screening camps. This project was executed in fourteen Indian states, targeting the general population, health care providers and policy makers. In the project, messages related to diabetes prevention and care were provided through several mass media initiatives, complementing each other and creating opportunities for interpersonal communication to reinforce the same messages. Rural areas received special attention. Initially a baseline knowledge, awareness and practice survey was conducted to assess the existing level of awareness, the use of media and available diabetes-related health services. The findings were used to design the campaign in order to make it more user-friendly. All the diabetes screening camps were preceded by a road show aimed at making people aware of the various aspects of diabetes by, for example, providing educational materials and having a contest on diabetes awareness. Those who had diabetes were referred to nearby health centres for counselling and care. Before the road shows and screening camps, local communities, key opinion leaders, doctors and health care professionals were mobilised to promote the road shows and screening camps and also to sensitise local stakeholders. In addition to these activities, print media and radio campaigns provided educational messages about diabetes and information about campaign events, and a diabetes helpline with SMS text messages was developed where members of the community could access information related to diabetes through their mobile phone.

The media campaign ran for 193 campaign days, covering 96 districts in fourteen states. At 410 screening camps, a total of 114,027 people were screened and 15,760 persons (or 13.8%) were detected for diabetes. More than 500 doctors participated in the campaign. The total population reached with awareness activities during the road shows exceeded 350,000 people. The newspaper-based media program had an estimated reach of

20 million readers in 14 states and included approximately 30 pages of broad sheet editoral newspaper coverage and 14.5 pages of advertisements. An estimated 431,870 s (approximately five full days) of radio air time was dedicated to the program. The total media and radio coverage of the campaign was estimated to have reached more than 60 million people. The toll free helpline number had a response rate of more than 59,850 messages.

4.4. Arogya World — New Diabetes Prevention mHealth Program in India with Nokia Life Tools[47]

In September 2011, Arogya World, in association with Nokia Life (previously known as Nokia Life Tools) and with the support of other organizations, committed to implementing a diabetes prevention mobile health (mHealth) program — subsequently called mDiabetes — among one million people in India over a period of two years. One of the first nationwide diabetes mHealth initiatives in a developing country, this effort is supported by a consortium of prominent organizations from multiple sectors in India and the US, including Nokia, Emory University, Biocon, LifeScan, Inc., Aetna and Synovate (now Ipsos). The commitment was formally announced at the 2011 Clinton Global Initiative meeting. Fifty-six diabetes awareness and prevention messages were developed with Emory University with a strong emphasis on science of behavior change. The messages were reviewed for cultural relevancy and technical accuracy by Arogya World's Behavior Change Task Force, which includes diabetes and communications experts from US and India, and were pre-tested by consumers. Messages were transmitted by Nokia to mobile phone consumers throughout India as text messages in twelve languages, free of cost, twice a week, for six months.

A comprehensive measurement and evaluation plan, with multiple phases of research, was also planned and implemented. The aim was to measure the program's effectiveness in increasing the adoption of healthy lifestyles known to prevent diabetes. This analysis is not yet published; however, the program has reported statistics on program reach. Since the program's inception in January 2012, about one million consumers have been recruited into the program and messages have reached Indian consumers 18 million times in 2012.[48]

4.5. CHETNA (Awareness): Childrens Health Education through Nutrition and Health Awareness, Diabetes Foundation (India)[49]

CHETNA and Rotary Club of Delhi South-East, through the Rotary South-East Charitable Foundation initiated this program to impart health education on the prevention of obesity, diabetes, and heart disease in school children from 10 schools in New Delhi. Lectures, posters, group discussions with children, parents and teachers, and health camps were devised to create awareness among the children about adopting healthy lifestyles so that onset of obesity related disorders can be prevented. This program covered almost 150,000 children, and was expanded to include nine more cities in India, to cover 500,000 children, making it the largest initiative against childhood obesity and prevention of diabetes in South Asia. However, no effectiveness studies have been reported.

4.6. Teacher: Trends in Childhood Nutrition and Lifestyle Factors in India[50]

The Teacher study was a multi-centre project that was undertaken in schools in 4 major cities of India: New Delhi, Agra, Bangalore, Pune. The aim was to obtain an in-depth understanding of nutrition and lifestyle behaviors that affect the health and well-being of urban Indians, particularly children. Data on knowledge and attitudes were collected and anthropometric measurements of children and their mothers were taken. The children and their mothers were given advice regarding healthy eating and physical activity and made aware of the various chronic diseases related to lifestyle behaviors (e.g., diabetes, obesity and heart diseases). The study results have not been reported.

4.7. DISHAA (Horizon): Diabetes and Obesity Awareness for Children/Adolescents and Adults[51]

This program was an initiative of National Diabetes, Obesity, and Cholesterol Diseases Foundation to enhance mass awareness about diabetes and obesity among children and adults through Lectures on "Diabetes: Causes, Consequences, Prevention and Care." This involved school health camps, public awareness campaigns, diabetes health camps, distribution of printed education material to children and adults, and message dissemination through media to act as change agents and using over 70 diabetologists, physicians and nutritionists as leaders for better lifestyles and prevention of diabetes in 50 cities of India. This is an ongoing program.

4.8. A Major Health Education Program Focusing on Women's Health and Nutrition[52]

A nutritional education program in India, which focused on middle aged and elderly women, was started with the help of a grant from the Department of Science and Technology. This project has been initiated in 8 cities and all women 30 years or older are targeted for proper nutrition and lifestyle advice and early detection of various diseases such as diabetes, obesity, heart problems and cancer. Mass awareness campaigns towards early detection and proper treatment of diabetes among the general public as well as among the medical and para-medical fraternity have also been initiated in Delhi, UP and Haryana. Medical counseling, medicines and insulin were also provided free of charge. This program is ongoing.

5. COMMUNITY-BASED DIABETES MANAGEMENT PROGRAMS IN INDIA

Although the projects described in this section focus primarily on prevention of diabetes-related complications, most promote diabetes prevention through screening and education. In addition, these programs show how private institutions and the Indian government are applying mass media, provider education, and technology to addressing the burden of diabetes in India.

5.1. Stop Diabetes — A Movement for Diabetes Free India — by Swasthya (Health) Diabetes Care and Supported by WDF in Gujarat, Western India (November 2010–February 2014) — WDF09-477[53]

This project aimed to implement a diabetes prevention program for the population of Gujarat and to train community doctors/nurses/other paramedical staff/interns in screening high-risk individuals and carrying out blood tests to diagnose diabetes and pre-diabetes. The awareness campaign was expected to reach more than 20 million people using various methods. The All India Institute of Diabetes and Research (AIIDR) implemented this project in Gujarat State in Western India in partnership with the Yash Diabetes Specialities Centre Private Limited, which provided technical support. The AIIDR also involved local NGOs, associations, private companies and educational institutions in the project, with the aim of broadening and securing a wider community ownership and involvement, thereby improving longer-term sustainability.

A comprehensive awareness campaign was initiated targeting the general public in the first phase of the project. The campaigns ran throughout the whole project period and were intense, highly visible and used various approaches to reach out to the audience, e.g., TV, radio, printed material, billboards, exhibitions etc., to reach out to as many people as possible, regardless of literacy level. Health care professionals (HCP) including GPs, medical officers, nurses, dieticians, diabetologists and diabetes educators already involved in the diabetes field, participated in seminars and workshops. After completion of training, the HCP shared their training experiences with their colleagues, trained their team members and disseminated the information learned at the sessions. One of the main responsibilities of the newly trained HCP was to organize awareness and screening camps at clinics, hospitals and at schools. Community volunteers were also trained in conducting yoga and other related lifestyle modification activities. Training HCP, teachers, school children and volunteers during the project period offered a sustainability plan to this translational effort. They were the ambassadors in the community who helped continue to raise awareness about diabetes even after project completion.

As a result of this project: 1,101 doctors were trained in early detection and proper management of diabetes, 4,065 other health care providers were trained in diabetes management, 139 awareness/screening camps were conducted, 33,557 people were screened for diabetes; 8,609 were diagnosed with previously unknown diabetes, 6,191 were screened for diabetes-related complications, and 50 television, 4 radio and 64 newspaper based campaigns were conducted; and a website was created.[54]

5.2. CRDPP: The Chunampet Rural Diabetes Prevention Project[55]

The majority of India's population (72%) resides in rural communities lacking trained medical staff, limited access to clinics, diabetes care centres, or public health centres, and often has low diabetes awareness and knowledge. Lack of access to sufficient care results in higher rates of undiagnosed diabetes,[56] delayed diagnosis, improper treatment, and higher rates of diabetes-related complications in these communities. CRDPP was developed with the aim of providing holistic diabetes care and promoting diabetes prevention in rural India through the use of telemedicine.[55] This project, which started in March 2007, was implemented by a diabetes care centre and research institute in Chennai India (Dr. Mohan's Diabetes Specialities Centre and the Madras Diabetes Research Foundation) funded by the WDF, Denmark, and undertaken in a cluster of 42 villages in and around Chunampet in Chithamur block of Kancheepuram district of Tamil Nadu in southern India.

One of the major problems faced by individuals with diabetes living in rural India is the lack of facilities for specialized screening and treatment of diabetes-related complications; patients often have to travel long distances to the nearest city for this purpose, which can result in insufficient care. Use of a mobile unit with a satellite provided by the Indian Space Research Organization (ISRO) with appropriate equipment and trained technicians has helped to bridge this gap and ensure increased accessibility to health services in rural areas. The van is equipped with a digital retinal camera, electrocardiography (ECG), doppler and biothesiometry and is used to screen for complications of diabetes. Village health workers (VHW) and research assistants (RA) are used to encourage and motivate all individuals with diabetes to undergo screening for complications. Retinal images are sent via satellite transmission to Chennai. Ophthalmologists at the tertiary care diabetes centre at Chennai review the photographs and provide consultations at an appointed time. Employing the VHW ensures long-term sustainability of the program as this allowed individuals with basic high school qualification, after undergoing rigorous training in basic health research techniques, to gain employment in their own village.[55,57]

With the help of the telemedicine van, 27,014 individuals (86.5% of the adult population) were screened in and around the 42 villages of

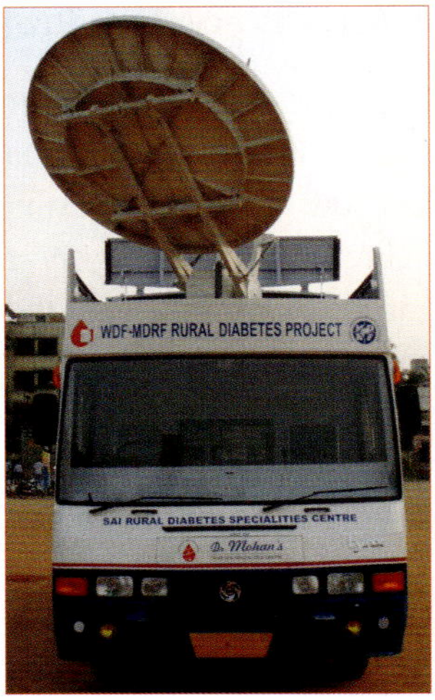

Infrastructure inside the Mobile Van	Personnel Needed
• Retinal Camera • Snellen visual activity chart • Doppler • Biothesiometry • ECG • V-Sat dish for telemedicine facility • Video conferencing equipment • Computer & printer	• Trained eye technician • Trained clinical technician • Information technology (IT) assistant • Dietitian

Fig. 3. Telemedicine van used in CRDPP (Mohan *et al.*, 2012).

Chunampet. There were 1,138 individuals (4.9%) with diabetes and 3,410 with prediabetes (14.6%). The mean glycated hemoglobin levels among the subjects with diabetes in the whole community decreased from 9.3 ± 2.6% to 8.5 ± 2.4% within a year of implementing this project. Less than 5% of patients needed referral for further management to the tertiary diabetes hospital in Chennai.[57] Thus, CRDPP can be used as a model for diabetes screening, prevention and health care delivery in rural areas of developing countries like India.[58] Other mobile diabetic retinopathy screening and treatment models exist in India[59,60] also serve as models for using telemedicine as a tool for screening for and preventing diabetes-related complications.

5.3. Innovative Low-Cost mHealth Toolkit[61]

A low-cost portable telemedicine kit called mHealth4U® was designed and developed for low- to middle-income countries as a sustainable telemedicine solution for the local delivery of primary healthcare within the household. The kit was developed at the School of Telemedicine and Biomedical Informatics, Sanjay Gandhi Postgraduate Institute of Medical Sciences, Lucknow as a part of research strategy on development of low-cost tele-health delivery tool,

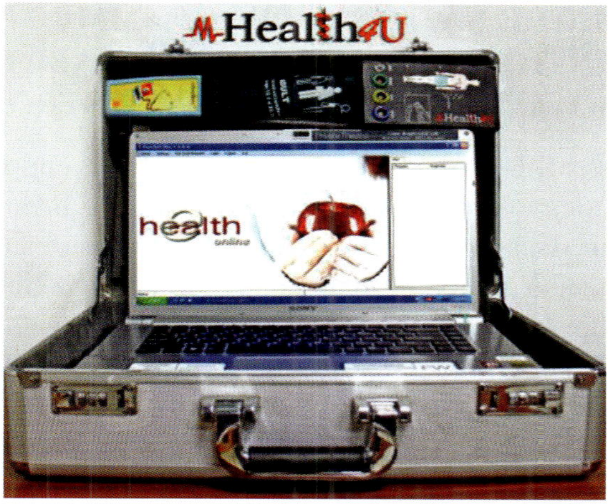

Fig. 4. mHealth4U® Tool Kit (Suitcase) — (Singh *et al.*, 2012).

under a research grant received from the Department of Information Technology, Ministry of Communication and IT, Government of India.

This telemedicine kit, available as a backpack or a suitcase (Fig. 4) each weighing 2–4 kg, includes a laptop with portable wireless broadband internet, a videoconferencing system, and Curesoft® Telemedicine software, which was specifically designed and developed for this kit as well as the ability to non-invasively perform blood pressure, spirometer, ECG, and blood oxygen saturation (SPO2) testing. The practitioner in a remote area can capture patient data in the form of audio, video, and images and forward them over the wireless broadband internet to a doctor for a diagnosis. A videoconference can then be established for real-time consultation with a specialist.

This mHealth toolkit has been tested in several proof of concept studies in multiple settings including rural hospitals, public festival celebrations, and in the field. These testing programs have shown that the toolkit could be successfully used to collect and transmit data, and conduct videoconference consultations in multiple settings. Furthermore, the toolkit ranked high in terms of use and acceptability for users in the field, including doctors and paramedical staff.

5.4. NPDCS: THE NATIONAL PROGRAMME FOR PREVENTION AND CONTROL OF DIABETES, CARDIOVASCULAR DISEASES AND STROKE[62]

The objectives of the NPDCS program are: (1) prevention of diabetes through identification of high-risk subjects and early intervention in the form of health education; (2) early diagnosis of disease and appropriate treatment; (3) reduction of morbidity and mortality with reference to the high-risk group; (4) prevention of acute and chronic metabolic, cardiovascular, renal and ocular complications of the disease; (5) provision of equal opportunities for physical attainment and scholastic achievement for the diabetic patients; and (6) rehabilitation of partially or totally handicapped individuals with diabetes. The Government of India started the NPDCS in some districts of Tamil Nadu, Jammu and Kashmir and Karnataka in 1987 to pilot test program components. Larger-scale piloting of the project started in 2008 with the objective of early diagnosis and appropriate management of diabetes, cardiovascular diseases (CVD) and stroke. The expected outcomes for the pilot phase were awareness generated on healthy lifestyles; health promotion at school, community and workplaces; and a decrease in the incidence of diabetes, CVD and stroke. NPCDCS was then expanded to include ten districts of ten states in 2010.

After completion of the initial pilot projects, the Union Cabinet gave its approval for the project and it is now being rolled out in 20,000 sub-centres and 700 community health centres in 21 states of the country. The National Rural Health Mission (NRHM) seeks to provide effective healthcare to rural population throughout the country with special focus on eighteen states, which have weak public health indicators and/or weak infrastructure. It aims at effective integration of health concerns with determinants of health like sanitation and hygiene, nutrition, and safe drinking water through a District Plan for Health. NPCDCS aims to utilise the existing framework provided by NRHM for optimising resources as well as ensuring seamless delivery of care to the patient. The cost of the program is shared between the centre and state in a ratio of 80:20.

6. GAPS IN T2DM TRANSLATIONAL RESEARCH IN INDIA

The initiatives outlined above are far from adequate to address the emerging epidemic of diabetes in India.[63] Some of the gaps in translational research in diabetes are as follows:

(1) *Lack of large-scale health surveillance* to make accurate prediction of prevalence, incidence, quality of care, complications, mortality, disability, costs is a major research gap for diabetes in India. Most of the aforementioned efforts in diabetes in India are regionalized or localized and cannot be easily generalized to the entire Indian population. Moreover, many pockets of India, especially the northeastern states, are highly neglected in many T2DM-related research efforts. Therefore, to measure the scale of the problem there is a need for reliable population-based epidemiological studies in diabetes and the role of lifestyle factors to implement socio-culturally relevant prevention programs. A framework for understanding the process of translating research to action as applicable to NCDs has been shown by The International Network of field sites with continuous Demographic Evaluation of Populations and Their Health (INDEPTH) which has 34 Health and Demographic Surveillance System (HDSS) in 17 different low-middle-income countries of which 10 are in Asia.[64] Such systems are urgently needed in many parts of India.

(2) *Inadequate* prevention efforts are apparent from the escalating numbers of people with diabetes and reported prevention efforts. There is a need to establish evidence-based services for effective prevention, diagnosis and care of T2DM. These services need to be rolled out as a government policy or programs to be implemented at all levels, along with appropriate evaluation methods built-in. Research is needed to determine cost-effective tools for diabetes prevention in India, and existing programs. Therefore, efforts initiated by the Government through the NPCDS should be evaluated to assess program cost, cost-effectiveness, impact, and reach. Moreover there are many prevention efforts ongoing but they are not backed by scientific evidence or reports. If the government encourages documentation of these reports either on a web-based

platform or through registration at specified government offices, it may help avoid duplication of work in the same areas and can also maximize individual efforts through networking and collaboration. It is, however, encouraging to note that joint ventures among developed countries such as the USA, UK and other European countries and centres of excellence in South Asia have been initiated to develop large-scale, community-oriented, and pragmatic intervention strategies.[65]

(3) *Audit and capacity building*: Evaluation of adherence to the national guidelines for T2DM prevention and management are required to ensure appropriate care is provided, and if not, how this may be improved. There is also an acute shortage of trained manpower in the field of diabetes care in India as doctors with a bachelor's degree in medicine are not equipped to deal with non-communicable diseases (NCDs) in general and diabetes in particular further impacting the quality of diabetes care in the country.[66] A case in point may be the treatment provided for people with pre-diabetes. In India, GPs are the first contact point for patients.[42] If GPs are unaware and do not follow the standard guidelines, prevention of diabetes may remain elusive. In addition, doctors alone cannot handle the diabetes burden in India; capacity building and community empowerment should be an integral component of every translational research activity to improve infrastructure for diabetes prevention and care through providers, paramedical staff, certified lifestyle coaches, community health workers, and community volunteers both in urban and rural areas. These individual can be trained in simple screening and prevention activities. The certificate course in Evidence Based Diabetes Management (CCEBDM), a joint program of the Public Health Foundation of India (PHFI) and Dr. Mohan's Diabetes Education Academy (DMDEA) has trained over 5,000 physicians in diabetes prevention, control and management from across 65 cities and 20 states of India.[67] Similarly, the National Diabetes Educator program (NDEP) was initiated with the primary aim to train diabetes educators in India and in its first cycle has trained 1,032 diabetes educators across India.[68] Programs such as these can help in capacity building in India.

(4) *Need of increased awareness of T2DM*: Awareness programs listed above may not be sufficient in the light of T2DM burden in India because of low coverage and predominance of these programs in the urban areas. A nationwide awareness program taking into account the

relevant social and economic settings and rolled out for the whole country in a phased manner, by a central body through a multi-sectoral approach can have the desired effect. A simple message such as increasing active travel (walking, bicycling, and public transport) can be a key modification in lifestyle that can reduce the growing burden of NCDs.[69]

(5) *Need for a well-integrated translational research*: There is an urgent need for supportive grants that test practical interventions in real world settings. In order for clinically relevant research to finally benefit the public at large, there is an urgent need for funding agencies on the lines of WDF and IDF (through their BRiDGES and D-START programs) to exclusively encourage translational research projects.

7. CONCLUSIONS

Progress in the control and prevention of T2DM in India is impeded by a health system that places a higher priority on communicable diseases and maternal and child health services and by a private health system driven by curative and therapeutic medicine.[70] Effective implementation of translational research for the prevention and management of diabetes, particularly in low- and middle-income countries, is thus a challenge but can be achieved through community empowerment. Prevention requires a multi-sectoral approach involving the Government, corporations, urban planners and the public. The Chunampet model (CRDPP) shows how this can be done even in a low resource, rural setting in India. For this to happen at a National level, the Government has to take on a more active role by involving major stakeholders while making policy decisions on health-related issues. A few recommendations specific to the area of diabetes translation could be to (a) screen and identify prediabetes (b) train lifestyle coaches and certify them (c) deliver lifestyle intervention through community, worksite and using technology such as mhealth and (d) evaluate the impact of such programs.

There is an obvious need to design strategies, which are both culturally and socioeconomically appropriate, for addressing lifestyle issues on a large scale. Approaches directed at people with pre-diabetes are likely to be the most cost-effective as up to 60% of cases of incident diabetes are attributable to IGT and/or IFG.[71] However, the provision of infrastructure and planning the logistics to support and sustain such an intervention on a large scale remains a challenge in any health care setting. Utilizing tools such as telemedicine, mhealth, trained lay health educators, community health workers, provider education and media could help to overcome some of the barriers to diabetes translation in the community.

ACKNOWLEDGMENTS

The authors would like to thank Ms. Nidhi Krishna, Research Assistant, Translational Research Dept., MDRF for her help in literature review, compiling the references and formatting the article.

REFERENCES

1. The Diabetes Atlas, e-Atlas. 5th ed. http://www.idf.org/diabetesatlas/. 2011 (Accessed May 2013, at http://www.eatlas.idf.org/Incidence/.)
2. Anjana RM, Pradeepa R, Deepa M *et al.* (2011) Prevalence of diabetes and prediabetes (impaired fasting glucose and/or impaired glucose tolerance) in urban and rural India: Phase I results of the Indian Council of Medical Research-INdia DIABetes (ICMR-INDIAB) study. *Diabetologia* **54**: 3022–3027.
3. The Diabetes Atlas, e-Atlas. 5th ed. 2012 update. 2012. (Accessed September 2013, at http://www.idf.org/sites/default/files/5E_IDFAtlasPoster_2012_EN.pdf.)
4. Mohan V, Sandeep S, Deepa R, Shah B, Varghese C. (2007) Epidemiology of type 2 diabetes: Indian scenario. *Indian J Med Res* **125**: 217–230.
5. Ramachandran A, Snehalatha C, Baskar AD *et al.* (2004) Temporal changes in prevalence of diabetes and impaired glucose tolerance associated with lifestyle transition occurring in the rural population in India. *Diabetologia* **47**: 860–865.
6. Amutha A, Datta M, Unnikrishnan IR *et al.* (2011) Clinical profile of diabetes in the young seen between 1992 and 2009 at a specialist diabetes centre in south India. *Prim Care Diabetes* **5**: 223–229.
7. Vikram NK, Tandon N, Misra A *et al.* (2006) Correlates of Type 2 diabetes mellitus in children, adolescents and young adults in north India: A multisite collaborative case-control study. *Diabet Med* **23**: 293–298.
8. Ramachandran A, Ramachandran S, Snehalatha C *et al.* (2007) Increasing expenditure on health care incurred by diabetic subjects in a developing country: A study from India. *Diabetes Care* **30**: 252–256.

9. Kapur A, Björk S, Nair J, Kelkar S, Ramachandran A (2004) Socio-economic determinants of the cost of diabetes in India. *Diabetes Voice* **49**:18–21.
10. Shobhana R, Rama Rao P, Lavanya A *et al.* (2002) Costs incurred by families having Type 1 diabetes in a developing country--a study from Southern India. *Diabetes Res Clin Pract* **55**: 45–48.
11. Park K (2005) Concept of health and disease. *Textbook of Preventive and Social Medicine*. Jabalpur, Madhya Pradesh, India: Banarsidas Bhanot, pp. 12–47.
12. Booth SL, Sallis JF, Ritenbaugh C *et al.* (2001) Environmental and societal factors affect food choice and physical activity: rationale, influences, and leverage points. *Nutr Rev* **59**: S21–S39; discussion S57–S65.
13. Narayan KM, Benjamin E, Gregg EW, Norris SL, Engelgau MM. (2004) Diabetes translation research: Where are we and where do we want to be? *Ann Intern Med* **140**: 958–963.
14. Marley J. (2000) Efficacy, effectiveness, efficiency. *Australian Prescriber* **23**: 114–115.
15. Garfield SA, Malozowski S, Chin MH *et al.* (2003) Considerations for diabetes translational research in real-world settings. *Diabetes Care* **26**: 2670–2674.
16. Woolf SH. (2008) The meaning of translational research and why it matters. *JAMA* **299**: 211–213.
17. Crossing the Abyss: From Research to Dissemination/Implementation to Better Health (2010). Available at http://research-practice.org/umbraco/Other%20Presenters/Szilagyi_From_Research_to_Dossemination_Implementation.pdf.
18. Narayan KMV, Echouffo-Tcheugui JB, Mohan V, Ali MK. (2012) Global prevention and control of type 2 diabetes will require paradigm shifts in policies within and among countries. *Health Affairs* **31**: 84–92.
19. Madhab A, Prasad VM, Kapur A. (2011) Gestational diabetes mellitus: Advocating for policy change in India. *Int J Gynaecol Obstet* **115**: S41–S44.
20. Nielsen KK, Courten MD, Kapur A. (2012) Health system and societal barriers for gestational diabetes mellitus (GDM) services — Lessons from World Diabetes Foundation supported GDM projects. *BMC Int Health Hum Rights* **12**: 33.
21. Ramachandran A, Snehalatha C, Mary S, Mukesh B, Bhaskar AD, Vijay V. (2006) The Indian Diabetes Prevention Programme shows that lifestyle modification and metformin prevent type 2 diabetes in Asian Indian subjects with impaired glucose tolerance (IDPP-1). *Diabetologia* **49**: 289–297.

22. Ramachandran A, Snehalatha C, Ram J *et al.* (2013) Effectiveness of mobile phone messaging in prevention of type 2 diabetes by lifestyle modification in men in India: A prospective, parallel group, randomized controlled trial. *Lancet Diabet Endocrinol,* online ahead of print.
23. Shetty AS, Chamukuttan S, Nanditha A, Raj RK, Ramachandran A. (2011) Reinforcement of adherence to prescription recommendations in Asian Indian diabetes patients using short message service (SMS) — A pilot study. *J Assoc Physicians India* **59**: 711–714.
24. A Pragmatic and Scalable Strategy Using Mobile Technology to Promote Sustained Lifestyle Changes to Prevent Type 2 Diabetes in India and the UK (2013). (Accessed July 2013, at http://ichgcp.net/clinical-trials-registry/NCT01570946.)
25. Weber MB, Ranjani H, Meyers GC, Mohan V, Narayan KM. (2012) A model of translational research for diabetes prevention in low and middle-income countries: The Diabetes Community Lifestyle Improvement Program (D-CLIP) trial. *Prim Care Diabetes* **6**: 3–9.
26. Weber MB, Ranjani H, Ali MK *et al.* (2013) Changes in anthropometric measurements in asian indians enrolled in a lifestyle intervention program: one year results of the D-CLIP Trial. *World Diabetes Congress*. Melbourne, Australia.
27. ASCEND Research Network: Controlled Trial of the Kerela Diabetes Prevention Program (K-DPP). (Accessed August 2013, at http://www.med.monash.edu.au/ascend/docs/as39-kdpp.pdf.).
28. Daivadanam M, Absetz P, Sathish T *et al.* (2013) Lifestyle change in Kerala, India: Needs assessment and planning for a community-based diabetes prevention trial. *BMC Public Health* **13**: 95.
29. Mohan V, Shanthirani CS, Deepa M, Datta M, Williams OD, Deepa R. (2006) Community empowerment — a successful model for prevention of non-communicable diseases in India — the Chennai Urban Population Study (CUPS-17). *J Assoc Physicians India* **54**: 858–862.
30. Deepa M, Anjana RM, Manjula D, Narayan KM, Mohan V. (2011) Convergence of prevalence rates of diabetes and cardiometabolic risk factors in middle and low income groups in urban India: 10-year follow-up of the Chennai Urban Population Study. *J Diabetes Sci Technol* **5**: 918–927.
31. Shanthi Rani CS, Rema M, Deepa R *et al.* (1999) The Chennai Urban Population Study (CUPS) — Methodological details — (CUPS Paper No.1). *Int J Diabet Develop Countries* **19**: 149–157.
32. Mohan V, Shanthirani S, Deepa R, Premalatha G, Sastry NG, Saroja R. (2001) Intra-urban differences in the prevalence of the metabolic syndrome

in southern India — the Chennai Urban Population Study (CUPS No. 4). *Diabet Med* **18**: 280–287.

33. Stevens J, Truesdale KP, Wang CH, Cai J. (2009) Prevention of excess gain. *Int J Obes (Lond)* **33**: 1207–1210.
34. World Health Organization (2005) Improving the built environment in India. Preventing chronic disease — A vital investment. Geneva.
35. Balagopal P, Kamalamma N, Patel TG, Misra R. (2008) A community-based diabetes prevention and management education program in a rural village in India. *Diabetes Care* **31**: 1097–1104.
36. Balagopal P, Kamalamma N, Patel TG, Misra R. (2012) A community-based participatory diabetes prevention and management intervention in rural India using community health workers. *Diabetes Educ* **38**: 822–834.
37. Subitha L, Soudarssanane MB, Murugesan R. (2013) Community-based physical activity intervention using principles of social marketing: A demonstration project in southern India. *Natl Med J India* **26**: 12–17.
38. Gordon R, McDermott L, Stead M, Angus K. (2006) The effectiveness of social marketing interventions for health improvement: What's the evidence? *Public Health* **120**: 1133–1139.
39. Deepa M, Pradeepa R, Rema M *et al.* (2003) The Chennai Urban Rural Epidemiology Study (CURES) — study design and methodology (urban component) (CURES-I). *J Assoc Physicians India* **51**: 863–870.
40. Mohan D, Raj D, Shanthirani CS *et al.* (2005) Awareness and knowledge of diabetes in Chennai — the Chennai Urban Rural Epidemiology Study [CURES-9]. *J Assoc Physicians India* **53**: 283–287.
41. Somannavar S, Lanthorn H, Pradeepa R, Narayanan V, Rema M, Mohan V. (2008) Prevention awareness counselling and evaluation (PACE) diabetes project: A mega multi-pronged program for diabetes awareness and prevention in South India (PACE- 5). *J Assoc Physicians India* **56**: 429–435.
42. Harish R, Padmaia U, Mehta AV, Anbalagan VP, Somannavar S, Mohan V. (2012) Improvement in knowledge of Diabetes among general practitioners after a structured diabetes training program (PACE-7) *TAPI J* **4**.
43. Shah P, Misra A, Gupta N *et al.* (2010) Improvement in nutrition-related knowledge and behaviour of urban Asian Indian school children: Findings from the 'Medical education for children/Adolescents for Realistic prevention of obesity and diabetes and for healthy aGeing' (MARG) intervention study. *Br J Nutr* **104**: 427–436.
44. Singhal N, Misra A, Shah P, Gulati S. (2010) Effects of controlled school-based multi-component model of nutrition and lifestyle interventions on

behavior modification, anthropometry and metabolic risk profile of urban Asian Indian adolescents in North India. *Eur J Clin Nutr* **64**: 364–373.
45. Singhal N, Misra A, Shah P, Rastogi K, Vikram NK. (2010) Secular trends in obesity, regional adiposity and metabolic parameters among Asian Indian adolescents in north India: A comparative data analysis of two selective samples 5 years apart (2003, 2008). *Ann Nutr Metab* **56**: 176–181.
46. Media campaign for prevention and care of diabetes WDF07-295. (Accessed August 2013, at http://www.worlddiabetesfoundation.org/projects/delhi-india-wdf07-295.)
47. Arogya World Launches New Diabetes Prevention mHealth Program in India with Nokia Life Tools (2011) (Accessed August 2013, at http://www.arogya-world.org/arogya-world-launches-new-diabetes-prevention-mhealth-program-in-india-with-nokia-life-tools/.)
48. Saligram N. (2012) Non-communicable diseases: Smart policy is needed to address this public health crisis. *Community Health Partnerships* 28–31.
49. Bhardwaj S, Misra A, Khurana L, Gulati S, Shah P, Vikram NK. (2008) Childhood obesity in Asian Indians: A burgeoning cause of insulin resistance, diabetes and sub-clinical inflammation. *Asia Pac J Clin Nutr* **17**: 172–175.
50. 'TEACHER'. (Accessed July 2013, at http://www.diabetesfoundationindia.org/programs.htm.).
51. Diabetes and Obesity in India: Focus on Lifestyle of Young Individuals (Accessed August 2013, at http://www.cseindia.org/userfiles/nutrition.PDF).
52. A Major Health Education Program Focusing on Women's Health and Nutrition (Accessed August 2013, at http://www.diabetesfoundationindia.org/programs.htm).
53. STOP DIABETES — A Movement for a Diabetes Free India (Accessed August 2013, at http://www.stopdiabetesindia.org/index.php).
54. Diabetes prevention programme WDF09-477 (Accessed August 2013, at http://www.worlddiabetesfoundation.org/projects/gujarat-india-wdf09-477).
55. Prathiba V, Rema M. (2011) Teleophthalmology: A model for eye care delivery in rural and underserved areas of India. *Int J Family Med* **2011**: 683267.
56. Suresh S, Deepa R, Pradeepa R, Rema M, Mohan V. (2005) Large-scale diabetes awareness and prevention in South India. *Diabet Voice* **50**: 11–14.
57. Mohan V, Deepa M, Pradeepa R *et al.* (2012) Prevention of diabetes in rural India with a telemedicine intervention. *J Diabet Sci Technol* **6**: 1355–1364.
58. Patel V, Chatterji S, Chisholm D *et al.* (2011) Chronic diseases and injuries in India. *Lancet* **377**: 413–428.

59. Murthy KR, Murthy PR, Kapur A, Owens DR. (2012) Mobile diabetes eye care: Experience in developing countries. *Diabetes Res Clin Pract* **97**: 343–349.
60. Rani PK, Raman R, Agarwal S *et al*. (2005) Diabetic retinopathy screening model for rural population: Awareness and screening methodology. *Rural Remote Health* **5**: 350.
61. R. SIMSD (2012) Innovative Low Cost mHealth tool kit. Proceedings of the First International Conference on Intelligent Infrastructure at the 47th Annual National Convention Computer Society Of India, December 1–2, 2012. Science City, Kolkata, India.
62. Nationalal Programme for the Prevention and Control of Cancer, Diabetes, Cardiovascular Disease and Stroke (NPCDCS): Operational Guidelines (Accessed March 2013, at http://health.bih.nic.in/Docs/Guidelines/Guidelines-NPCDCS.pdf).
63. Walgate R. (2008) Diabetes research for developing countries. *N Biotechnol* **25**: 111–116.
64. Krishnan A, Nongkynrih B, Kapoor SK, Pandav C. (2009) A role for INDEPTH Asian sites in translating research to action for non-communicable disease prevention and control: A case study from Ballabgarh, India. *Global Health Action* **2**: 76–83.
65. Ramachandran A, Snehalatha C, Samith Shetty A, Nanditha A. (2013) Primary prevention of Type 2 diabetes in South Asians — challenges and the way forward. *Diabet Med* **30**: 26–34.
66. Venkataraman K, Kannan AT, Mohan V. (2009) Challenges in diabetes management with particular reference to India. *Int J Diabetes Dev Ctries* **29**: 103–109.
67. Hasan H, Zodpey S, Saraf A. (2011) Diabetes care in India: Assessing the need for Evidence-Based education. *South–East Asian J Med Educ* **5**: 15.
68. Joshi S, Joshi SR, Mohan V. (2013) Methodology and feasibility of a structured education program for diabetes education in India: The National Diabetes Educator Program. *Indian J Endocrinol Metab* **17**: 396–401.
69. Millett C, Agrawal S, Sullivan R *et al*. (2013) Associations between active travel to work and overweight, hypertension, and diabetes in India: A cross-sectional study. *PLoS Med* **10**: e1001459.
70. Siegel K, Narayan KM, Kinra S. (2008) Finding a policy solution to India's diabetes epidemic. *Health Aff (Millwood)* **27**: 1077–1090.
71. Simpson RW, Shaw JE, Zimmet PZ. (2003) The prevention of type 2 diabetes — lifestyle change or pharmacotherapy? A challenge for the 21st century. *Diabetes Res Clin Pract* **59**: 165–180.

Chapter 14: Diabetes Prevention in the Middle East and North Africa Region

*Adel A El-Sayed**, *Eman Sabet and Amal Khalifa*

1. INTRODUCTION

Diabetes is a major 21st century health and development challenge to which no region or country in the whole world is immune. The epidemiologic evidence[1] suggests that unless effective preventive measures are implemented, the prevalence of this disease will continue to rise globally. Diabetes prevention is of particular importance in the case of the Middle East and North Africa (MENA) Region due to the high burden of diabetes in this region. The burden of diabetes in MENA Region has two arms: epidemiologic and economic.

1.1. The Epidemiologic Burden of Diabetes in the MENA Region

The greatest burden of diabetes is increasingly falling on low- and middle-income countries. It is estimated that developing countries in Asia and in the Middle East in particular, will have the largest increases in the prevalence of diabetes by 2030.[2]

IDF MENA Region represents 20 diabetes organizations in 21 countries and has one of the highest rates of diabetes in the world.[3] The prevalence of type 2 diabetes has increased dramatically in the countries of the MENA Region over the last few decades, a trend that parallels increased industrial development. The wealth generated by oil-rich resources in countries of the Arabian Gulf is a prominent example of these changes which have led to improved living standards. The resultant rapid

*Corresponding author. Email: el_sayedadel@hotmail.com
Internal Medicine, Sohag Faculty of Medicine, Sohag University, Sohag–Egypt.

economic development and urbanization have changed the lifestyle of the people and have led to reduced levels of physical activity, increased intake of refined carbohydrates, rise in obesity[4]; and aging of these populations.[5] These factors have led to an increase in risk factors for type 2 diabetes and a rapid increase in its prevalence. Consequently, diabetes has become a major public health problem in the region and imposes a considerable strain on individuals, family members and carers; as well as on health systems in the region.

The highest prevalence of diabetes is seen in the countries of the Arab Gulf Region, with four of these countries (Saudi Arabia, Kuwait, Qatar and Bahrain) all reporting prevalences of greater than 20%; and a fifth country in the same locality (United Arab Emirates) reporting a prevalence of nearly 19%.[5] Other countries in the Region — which are not as rich as the Gulf States — such as Egypt and Lebanon have also very high prevalence of diabetes by international standards. The largest number of cases in the MENA Region is in Egypt, Pakistan and Iran reflecting their status as the countries with the largest populations in the region.

The most important risk factors for development of diabetes in the region are:

Obesity is directly related to the risk of developing type 2 diabetes.[6–8] It predicts diabetes in both genders and in different ethnic groups.[9,10] A meta-analysis of ten studies revealed an odds ratio of 2.14 for obese subjects developing type 2 diabetes.[11] In the MENA Region the prevalence of obesity in adults, adolescents, and children is extremely high ranging between 2–55% in adult females and 1–30% in adult males while the prevalence in adolescents and children range from 5–14%.[12–17] One important problem with childhood obesity is that it generally persists into adulthood.[18]

Modernization of large cities and towns in MENA Region increased urbanization and exposure of the population to a more Western lifestyle.[19]

Dietary habits have radically changed in the Region during the last few decades secondary to the economic improvement and Westernization. Instead of consuming dates, milk, fresh vegetables and fruit, whole wheat bread and fish, local people have now shifted to consuming foods rich in high saturated fats and refined carbohydrate diets with low fiber intake.[20]

Physical inactivity dramatically increased in the MENA Region countries due to rapid economic development and significant changes in socioeconomic status and lifestyle. The economic growth has led to increased availability of cars, greater use of machines at home and work, access to cheap migrant labor, widespread use of computers, televisions and electronic gaming devices which have created an environment that encourages sedentary lifestyles. Studies showed that not only the rich Gulf states populations lead a sedentary life, but also much less affluent countries as only 2% of Egyptian adults exercise daily.[21]

1.2. The Economic Burden of Diabetes in the MENA Region

The countries of the MENA Region are divided according to their economic status into: Low-Middle-Income Countries (LMIC), Upper Middle-Income Countries (UMIC), and High-Income Countries (HIC):

Data region	Countries
MENA-LMIC-Central	Iraq, Jordan, State of Palestine, Syrian Arab Republic, Yemen
MENA-LMIC-East	Afghanistan, Pakistan
MENA-LMIC-West	Egypt, Morocco, South Sudan, Sudan, Tunisia
MENA-UMIC	Algeria, Islamic Republic of Iran, Lebanon, Libya
MENA-HIC-Central	Bahrain, Kuwait, Oman, Qatar, Saudi Arabia, United Arab Emirates

Although the MENA Region reports extremely high numbers of type 2 diabetes patients, it is estimated — in the last published 5th Edition IDF Atlas[22] — that only USD 10.9 billion is spent on diabetes-related costs in the MENA Region compared to the USA and Europe, which spend proportionately more on diabetes-related expenses (USD 223 billion and 131 billion USD respectively).[23] The marked discrepancy between the economic level and expenditure of different MENA Region countries makes the situation even worse in the larger and lower economic countries. Future predictions of health expenditure on diabetes are difficult to make but it is likely to increase dramatically, driven both by the increased number of people who are predicted to have diabetes, and the progressive aging of the population, which will lead to an increase in the number of individuals with diabetes complications and therefore requiring more expensive medical care. Costs to health systems will therefore increase through an increase in the resources needed to manage diabetes (such as prescription of drugs), the intensive management of associated comorbidities (such as hypertension and dyslipidaemia), and the management of complications (such as renal and cardiovascular diseases). This increase is apparent in the figures of 2013 when health expenditure on diabetes is estimated at $13 billion according to the 6th Edition IDF Diabetes Atlas.[5]

2. PREVENTION OF DIABETES IN THE MENA REGION

A group of excellent studies published during the early years of this century had demonstrated unequivocally that type 2 diabetes is a preventable disease and life style modification (and to a lesser extent several pharmacological agents) can decrease the rate of progression of individuals with prediabetes to frank diabetes.[24] Later studies focused on defining those who are particularly at high-risk of future development of type 2 diabetes. It is widely accepted now that using a simple questionnaire that assesses easily available information such as family history, cardiovascular risk factors, age, and waist-to-hip circumference ratios is an easily implementable first step for identifying those at risk. The use of other diagnostic tests such as HbA1c in this process proved to be less effective and was associated with a high proportion of false-negative test results.[25] Once identified, high risk individuals should undergo routine and inexpensive screening tests for diabetes such as measuring levels of plasma and urine glucose, and possibly undergo an oral glucose tolerance test (OGTT), especially when the presence of type 2 diabetes is strongly suspected.[3] Type 2 diabetes can then be prevented or its progression impeded by implementing lifestyle changes. Modification of lifestyle has no costs associated with it, is usually free of side effects, and can be as, or more, beneficial than some pharmacological approaches.[2] These lifestyle changes are often designed to reduce obesity, which is increased by excessive energy intake and low levels of physical activity.[26,27] Importantly, current guidelines suggest that only modest but regular exercise as being a beneficial strategy in the prevention of type 2 diabetes.[28]

Since these data were made available, projects for diabetes prevention have been developed, and are still progressing in different parts of the world. In the MENA Region with all its diabetes-related problems, the situation is not proportionately ideal. Although there are many studies and projects in the region which are related to diabetes prevention, like those which address diabetes education, healthy food and physical exercise, the studies which are specifically designed for prevention of diabetes or include that objective in their targets are inadequate. The latter initiatives are the only ones considered in this chapter. We used internet search, personal data and personal communications with individual authors and member associations of the MENA Region to collect the required data about diabetes prevention in the Region. Many of the projects obtained have only recently been started and their results not yet published, reflecting the recent interest in diabetes prevention in the MENA Region.

The efforts of diabetes prevention in the MENA Region can conveniently be divided into three levels:

1. Regional
2. Sub-Regional
3. Individual Country

2.1. Regional Efforts

The regional efforts for diabetes prevention started as early as 1993 by "a call for action" from the Eastern Mediterranean Regional Office EMRO of the World Health Organization (WHO) for the prevention and control of diabetes mellitus.[29] However, because of the lack of valid screening tests and well-developed health care systems in the countries of the Region, this call had not been translated into significant results and only a few countries responded to it.

Very recently, the MENA regional efforts had been revived when the International Diabetes Federation (IDF) Middle East and North Africa MENA Region and the WHO East Mediterranean Regional Office (EMRO) developed a Collaboration Agreement to work together for the cause of diabetes. The draft agreement is being revised and will be signed in 2014.

In this agreement, diabetes prevention is specifically mentioned and targeted. A specific Task Force on Childhood Obesity will focus on long-term prevention of diabetes in different countries of the region taking into consideration the huge problem of childhood obesity as one of the most important preventable risk factors for the high incidence of diabetes in the MENA Region. The plan outlines have been determined and the initiative is expected to start at the time of the joint WHO/IDF Symposium which will be held in Luxor-Egypt in December 2014.[30]

2.2. Sub-Regional Efforts: The Arab Gulf State Model

The Arab Gulf States have a peculiar problem with diabetes. Five of the top ten countries with the highest diabetes prevalence belong to the Gulf Area. The Gulf States are characterized by their small populations and substantially high income status due to oil production. As a result of these common characteristics, it is natural that they cooperate and have developed the Gulf Cooperation Council (GCC) which is responsible for organizing common plans in different areas, health being one important aspect.

The Health Ministers in the Gulf States held a number of conferences about the problem of diabetes in their area and developed the Gulf Program for Diabetes Control.[31]

The 61st conference of the Health Ministers (held in Geneva on 24/5/2006) assigned the specialized Gulf committee to undertake the process of development and update of the program through the following:

(1) Review of the Gulf Program for Diabetes Control in the light of recent scientific updates, and after evaluation of the achievements in various stages, reasons for delay and how to overcome them, setting an executive work plan including preventive and promotional aspects.
(2) Study the current diabetes epidemic in the Council States, the objectives realized in the Gulf Program for Diabetes Control, and the reduction of diabetes incidence and its complications for a 10-year period (based on recommendations for the 53rd meeting of the Executive Body).

The Health Ministers in their 62nd conference held in Kuwait (23–24/1/2007) expressed their great concern about the steady increase of the diabetes problem in the Gulf community and the associated-large economic and community burdens. In addition, they emphasized the importance that the specialized technical committee should have an expanded meeting with participation of concerned deputy ministers with the objectives of:

(1) Developing an integrated, updated executive plan to be raised to their Ministers of Health and hence to the leaders of the Cooperation Council States to gain the required commitment to control this disease.
(2) Designing a Gulf Study with unified methodology that deals with epidemiology, burden of disease and economics of diabetes. This study shall be community-based.

The expanded meeting of the Gulf Committee for Diabetes Control was held in Kuwait (16–17/4/2008) with participation of the concerned deputy ministers and resulted in the following noteworthy outcomes:

- Setting the Joint statement for the Health Ministers' Council for the Cooperation Council States about Diabetes.
- Considering the working paper submitted by the Director General of the Executive Board for updating and developing the Gulf plan, a scientific and practical integrated approach for that purpose.
- Setting the Gulf Executive plan for diabetes control (2008/2018).
- Setting the method of preparing and designing the unified Gulf research for epidemiology burden and economics of diabetes.

2.2.1. *The proposed Interim Operational Plan (2008–2009)*

Based on the request of the Director General of the Executive Board, the meeting for the Specialized Technical Committee was held alongside the Diabetes Economics Conference "Diabetes Economics — Vital Investment"). The principal focus was on the next steps to combat diabetes. It was agreed to divide the Gulf plan into five stages, where each stage is evaluated, reviewed and the progress assessed as well as shortcomings. Thereafter, a plan for the next stage is set. This plan included a section for diabetes prevention.

2.2.2. *Prevention*

(a) Primary Prevention Program

A section about risk factors and prevention of diabetes; dissemination of educational information in newspapers, symposia, TV, and essays in newspapers.

This extensive effort and expensive funding for diabetes control in the Gulf States resulted in increasing the establishment of public-private partnerships to jointly deliver prevention messages and increase the availability of specialized centres and clinics. However, efforts aimed at controlling the growing threat of diabetes have not effectively outpaced the increasing number of new cases and associated comorbidities. The current approach for diabetes control focuses primarily on awareness creation, diagnosis and treatment of the disease and this has not yielded the best results in containment.[32] No specific results for these efforts in terms of diabetes prevention have been published so far.

2.3. Individual Country Level

There are a number of countries in the MENA Region with projects for diabetes prevention at different stages of implementation. Many of these projects are not published yet.

2.3.1. *Diabetes prevention in Pakistan*

The diabetic population in Pakistan is very high, ranking seventh among countries with the largest number of reported diabetic cases. In 2007, there were 6.9 million individuals with diabetes in Pakistan, which is expected to increase to 11.5 million by 2025 according to the IDF.[33]

Riaz *et al.* tried to develop and evaluate a risk score to predict people at high-risk of developing type 2 diabetes in Pakistan. The diabetes risk score was developed by using simple parameters namely age, waist circumference, and family history of diabetes. Odds ratios of the model were used to assign a score value for each variable and the diabetes risk score was calculated as the sum of those scores. They concluded that a simple diabetes risk score, based on a set of variables, can be used for the identification of high-risk individuals for early intervention to delay or prevent type 2 diabetes in the Pakistani population.[34]

Akhter *et al.*[35] are currently conducting a study entitled "A translational randomized trial of culturally specific and cost-effective life style intervention for the prevention of type 2 diabetes in Pakistan" (Pakistan Diabetes Prevention Program or PDPP). The study is being performed at Aga Khan University Hospital (Karachi, Pakistan) and is supported by the IDF aiming to address the key issues in the prevention of type 2 diabetes. The study is planned for a 3-year period (September 1, 2011–September 1, 2014). The main objectives are:

1. To implement culturally tailored diabetes prevention program through lifestyle intervention into real life settings in communities of Ninhbinh province.
2. To evaluate the effectiveness, cost-effectiveness, feasibility, acceptability and sustainability of lifestyle intervention programs by assessing changes among various groups.
3. To determine the impact of dietary culture and city planning on incidence of obesity and diabetes.
4. To set up a community- based model of diabetes prevention by raising public awareness of diabetes and diabetic risk factors and to promote healthy eating along with physical activity in the target population.

Approximately 20,000 people are to be screened for diabetes risk factors using a non-invasive diabetes risk score system. Adults from both sexes aged 30–64 years are eligible for inclusion in the study, while those diagnosed to have diabetes mellitus, pregnant women or those with chronic psychological or physical disabilities are excluded. Those found to be at increased risk will be given an oral glucose tolerance test (OGTT). Those identified after as having metabolic syndrome, or pre-diabetes will have the opportunity to take part in the Pakistan Diabetes Prevention Study lifestyle intervention. This consists of culturally adjusted preventive strategies focusing on diet and physical activity in real-life settings. Diabetes awareness events and preventive programmes will be organized as part of this study. It is expected that these events will have a substantial effect in terms of diabetes education and health awareness throughout the wider population.

Results to September 2012: 8,640 people from four communities have been screened based on simple parameters, including family history of diabetes, abdominal adiposity, age and level of physical activity. Scores for different parameters with the age cut off of 64 is taken as eligibility criteria for performing the 75 g OGTT. Of the 8,640 participants, 48% (4,139) had a score of 60. 1,180 OGTTs have been performed so far with 32% found to have pre-diabetes and 13.4% diabetes (using ADA diagnostic criteria). The lifestyle intervention started in October 2012 in those found to be at high-risk. The main goals of intervention will focus on: weight reduction ≥5%, moderate intensity physical activity ≥30 min daily, dietary fat <30 proportion of total energy, saturated fat <10%, and fiber ≥ 15 g/1,000 kcal. There will be 9 sessions during the two year follow-up period.

Study outcomes: All study outcomes will be evaluated after 2 years of intervention and include incidence of type 2 diabetes, assessment of components of the metabolic syndrome and cost-effectiveness by assessing the incremental costs and benefits per case of diabetes prevented and per quality adjusted life year (QALY). The impact of city planning on prevalence of obesity and type 2 diabetes will also be assessed; communities will be divided according to the number and accessibility of parks. Communities with a large number of parks will be compared with those having no parks. Change in the incidence of diabetes and obesity after 2 years of lifestyle intervention will be compared between these two communities. In this way, it would be feasible to convince local authorities to incorporate findings into their agenda for future urban design.

2.3.2. *Diabetes prevention in the Islamic Republic of Iran*

The Islamic Republic of Iran is one of the first countries to have responded to "a call for action" from the Eastern Mediterranean Regional Office of the WHO for the prevention and control of diabetes mellitus.[29]

The Islamic Republic of Iran activities for the prevention and control of diabetes have been initiated as a pilot study in 3 rural areas since 1991, but because of the lack of valid screening tests and well-equipped health centers they were discontinued in 1993. Nonetheless, in 1996, a report covering the diabetes situation was presented to WHO and a vital step was taken towards diabetes prevention.[36] The same year, the Iranian National Advisory Committee resumed its work, and a new comprehensive national strategy was designed, with the support of the health authorities concerned, for the prevention and control of type 2 diabetes.

(a) The Health Care System in the Islamic Republic of Iran includes

1. *The District Level*
   The district has been the smallest autonomous unit in the primary health care network. Apart from the sections involved in overall planning, evaluation and supervision, which are located within higher-level facilities, all components of the health care system function at the district level.[37] The district is therefore the most appropriate location for problem recognition and identification of objectives specific to the area.
2. *The Health House*
   Health houses are located in villages and are the most outlying rural facility in the network. Each health house is capable of serving about 1,500 people, and often covers up to four satellite villages in addition to the main village. The main function of a health house is to offer primary health care services to the community it serves. Some of the most important tasks (among others) of the community health worker are:
   - Public health education and encouragement of community participation.
   - Family health care services (family planning services, immunization for children <5, health care for school age children).
   - Disease control services (communicable and noncommunicable diseases).
   - Patient care and referral to the rural health centers when necessary.
   - Environmental health activities.
   - Data collection, documentation, and regular reporting.

3. *The Rural Health Center*

   The rural health center is a village-based facility which supervises the health house in its own village and usually four other health houses in neighboring villages. Each rural health center covers an average of 90,000 people.

   The rural health center's main responsibilities related to prevention of non-communicable disease prevention are:

   - Monitoring, supervising, and supporting 3–5 health houses.
   - Providing out-patient care and screening of individuals referred to the health house.
   - Performing basic laboratory tests.
   - Providing maternity facilities.
   - Environmental health services.
   - Data collection and regular reporting.

The national program for the prevention and control of type 2 diabetes was designed in 1996.

The aim of this program is primary, secondary, and tertiary prevention through community and high-risk screening and the integration of diabetes care into the primary healthcare network. The Ministry of Health and Medical Education, with the coordination of the National Diabetes Advisory Committee, launched 6 comprehensive workshops about diabetes for physicians, nurses and nutritionists in 1997 and 1998, in which about 60 physicians, 60 nurses and 60 nutritionists participated each year.

(b) Program objectives

1. *General objectives*

Prevention and control of type 2 diabetes and its complications in the Islamic Republic of Iran.

2. *Specific objectives*

Primary prevention is a specific objective and aims to reduce the prevalence and incidence of type 2 diabetes and also to reduce the prevalence and incidence of modifiable predisposing factors to the condition (obesity, physical inactivity, unhealthy diet, etc).

Strategies for achieving these objectives are to:

- Modify life-styles in high-risk Iranian populations.
- Control and reduce the predisposing factors of diabetes.
- Screen those at risk of type 2 diabetes.
- Control and follow up high risk populations.
- Enhance the perception and knowledge of the community and health care personnel on diabetes, its predisposing factors and its complications.

Secondary prevention aims to prevent and reduce short-term and long-term complications and to postpone their development, to alter the natural course of the disease and stop its progression.

Tertiary prevention aims to reduce (and postpone) the number of disabilities and deaths caused by diabetes and its complications.

3. *Outcome*

- Reduce economic costs imposed by diabetes and it complications.
- Reduce disabilities caused by diabetes and its complications.
- Reduce the mortality rate of diabetes and its complications.
- Increase years of effective life.

A cluster-controlled trial was also conducted in 2002–2005 in the Islamic Republic of Iran.[38] The study aim was to assess the effect of lifestyle modification on risk factors for non-communicable diseases (NCDs) and the development of type 2 diabetes at the community level.

- Materials and methods

1. *Study population*

A total of 10,368 individuals aged ≥20 years were enrolled in the study and 3,931 participants were selected as the lifestyle intervention group.

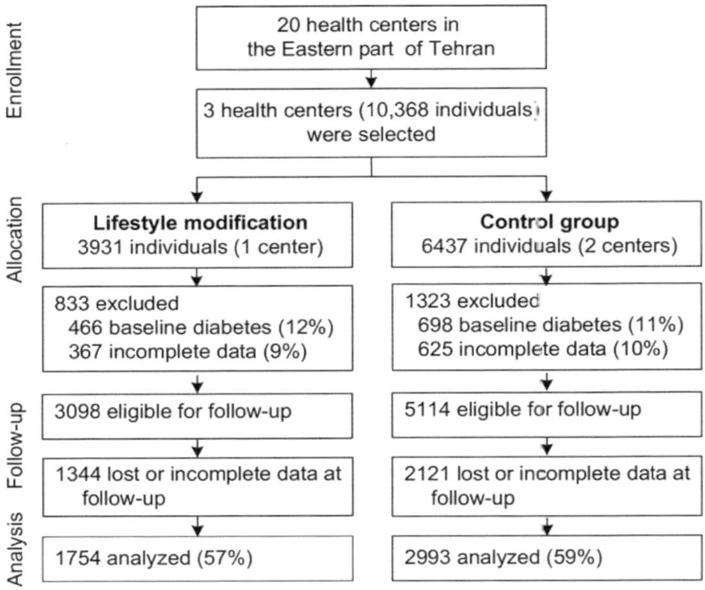

2. *Lifestyle interventions*

Interventions were aimed at lifestyle modification through primary prevention for noncommunicable diseases (NCDs) by improving nutrition and dietary pattern, increasing physical activity levels, and reducing cigarette smoking.

Nutrition educational classes were held four days of the week. Methods of education included face-to-face consultation, educational videos and slides, and nutritional education and consultation, which involved demonstrations of healthy food preparation. Public conferences on occasions such as the World Diabetes Day or World No-Tobacco Day were held to promote the importance of healthy lifestyle behaviors.

3. *Clinical and laboratory measurements*

Examinations were performed at baseline and follow-up in both intervention and control groups. A brief physical examination was performed including blood pressure and anthropometric measurements. A blood sample was taken 12–14 hr after an overnight fast.

For the OGTT, 75 g of anhydrous glucose was administered orally and a blood sample was taken 2 hours later. Cholesterol, triglyceride and high-density lipoprotein cholesterol (HDL-C) were measured. All measurements were conducted by the same method at baseline and follow-up examinations.

• *Results*

After a mean follow-up period of 3.6 years, 188 new cases of type 2 diabetes were diagnosed. The incidence rate of type 2 diabetes after follow-up was 12.2/1,000 person-years and 8.2/1,000 person-years in the control and intervention groups, respectively. The lifestyle intervention was highly effective in both genders, those aged >65 years, individuals with BMI >30 kg/m^2, and those with normal or prediabetic FPG and 2 hr-post-load glucose levels.

Women in the intervention group, but not in the control group, had a greater decrease in their total cholesterol [0.07 mmol/L (2.8 mg/dL), $p>0.001$)] and less of a decrease in their HDL-C [0.03 mmol/L (1.1 mg/dL), $p>0.05$] compared to the control group.

The rate of smoking cessation (current smokers who quit smoking at follow up) was 70% higher in the intervention than in the control group.

Overweight individuals (BMI >25 kg/m^2) in the intervention group were twice as likely as those in the control group to lose at least 5% of their baseline weight during the follow-up.

2.3.3. *Diabetes prevention in Kuwait*

Kuwaiti national activities for prevention of diabetes include:

1. National Program for the Prevention of Overweight and Obesity (NPPOO).

   Obesity constitutes a major health problem in Kuwait.[39,40] The first NPPOO was launched in Kuwait in 2004 by establishing obesity clinics in the Primary health care units (PHC). Training courses on implementation of clinical guidelines on prevention and management of obesity for the working team were completed in December 2006. Twelve obesity clinics in 3 districts are now working in full capacity. The team participates in health education activities and annual world health events as well as production of awareness publications (booklets, leaflets, posters, etc).

2. Healthy breakfast/snack project in primary schools for children 6–11 year olds was started in 2009. The project was performed in collaboration between Ministry of Education (MOE) and Ministry of Health (MOH); healthy snacks were prepared and supervised by MOH regarding their composition and caloric content. The program includes training of schools staff/administration team to support plans and objectives and recommending physical education as core subject in the schools. It was evaluated after one year for acceptance by children and then applied to the higher schools.
3. Increase health/nutrition awareness: A book entitled "Facts of Life" was first reviewed and edited by MOE/MOH. The contents were adapted from UNICEF and included facts about healthy lifestyle and good nutrition to raise health/nutrition awareness among school students. It was edited to suit the target age group of 14 year-old youngsters. The trial implemented in 2009–2010 was greatly successful with more than 80 schools participating. Repeated again in 2010–2011, with modifications, resulted in greater school and student participation. There was preliminary agreement that it will become a part of the school curriculum in 2014.[41]
4. Program for the prevention of NCD including diabetes was launched in March 2013.[41]
5. Dasman Diabetes Institute: A tertiary care organization dedicated to fight diabetes and related risk factors through a holistic approach bringing together under one roof treatment, education, prevention, healthy living and research.[41]

(a) *Research projects*[41]

- Kuwait Diabetes Epidemiology Program:
  A population-based study of diabetes and obesity in Kuwait was started in April 2011. They plan to study 14,000 residents (Kwts/non-Kwts), randomly selected through the Civil Service Authority, interviewed and screened for risk factors.
- Obesity, Metabolic syndrome and type 2 diabetes risk in Children and Adolescents from Multiethnic Origins in Kuwait: A prospective cohort

study started in May–June 2011, they planned to screen 17,280 school children, aged 6–18 years, randomly selected from government and private schools, Kuwaitis and non-Kuwaitis. The project consists of an extensive questionnaire and screen for all risk factors. The identified group will join a preventive program of lifestyle modification and will be followed for 10 years.

- The initiation of the Childhood Onset Diabetes electronic Registry (CODeR).

(b) *Education programs*[41]

- Patient Education
  In addition to education programs for diabetic patients, regular healthy cooking sessions are also given.
- Professional Education
  Includes postgraduate Certificate/Diploma/MSc in Diabetes Care, postgraduate fellowship in diabetes from Kuwait University, courses of nutrition education for dietitians of the Ministry of Health, courses of nutrition education for school teachers aiming to increase awareness about basic nutrition, identification and management of hypo- and hyperglycemia among students with diabetes, healthy foods and better choices during school hours.
- Community Awareness Program
  Aiming to increase public awareness toward the relationship between diet, food choices and the prevention of disease.
- Educational Kitchen and Healthy Cooking
  Regular session on healthy cooking for groups of individuals with diabetes and their families, public and schools; the sessions are run by specialized chefs.
- Education for school children.
- Regularly host schools teach children about importance of breakfast, dietary fiber and other nutrition-related topics.
- Education programs via a diversity of stimulating, informative, interactive and internationally accepted programs covering healthy eating, healthy shopping tours at supermarkets, weight management and physical exercise.

(c) *Kuwait Diabetes Society program* includes regular community screening in malls, schools and collaborating with other non-governmental organizations (NGO) and annual celebration of the WDD.

2.3.4. *Diabetes prevention in Tunisia*

Tunisia is facing an epidemiological transition and the prevalence of diabetes is dramatically increasing. This epidemic is developing in association with obesity, which represents an important risk factor of type 2 diabetes. Childhood obesity constitutes a major public health challenge in Tunisia and worldwide.

Therefore, Hassan Ghannem and colleagues[42] propose to implement and evaluate a school-based intervention to manage overweight and obesity among school adolescents aged 14–16 years in the region of Sousse, Tunisia. This will be a one-year behavioral intervention that will include nutritional, physical activity and psychological components. Parental involvement is mandatory.

Objectives

1. To demonstrate the feasibility of a school-based management program for obese and overweight adolescents in Sousse, Tunisia.
2. To demonstrate the effectiveness of a one year intervention program to manage obesity and overweight among school children in Sousse, Tunisia by:
   - Increasing by 10% the proportion of school children who follow a balanced diet.
   - Increasing by 10% the proportion of school children who follow a regular physical activity.
   - Decreasing body mass index mean by 1.5 kg/m^2 after a one year intervention.

Methodology, study design and intervention

- Evaluation of lifestyle habits and body mass index among obese and overweight school children in Sousse, Tunisia with pre- and post intervention evaluation.

– Managing overweight and obese school children considered at high risk for diabetes in the intervention group. Overweight and obese school children in the control group do not have any specific intervention other than what the school medical team would advise.

Intervention program

During a one year intervention from December 2012 to the end of November 2013, recruited school children will be managed for overweight. There will be two intervention strategies: collective intervention for all recruited children (overweight and obese) and an individual intervention only for obese children who require intensive management.

(1) Collective intervention

The intervention group is including collective sessions with groups of almost 15 school children. They are organizing three types of interventions in each college.

– Collective sessions for overweight and obese children in schools about healthy eating.
– The second session is undertaken by physical activity teachers of each school to motivate children to exercise in schools and with their families outside of schools. Teachers are also proposing a program of twice-a-week physical activity sessions in schools for overweight and obese school children (independent of physical activity in school sessions).
– The third intervention is a workshop with children and their parents conducted by a dietician about healthy cooking.

(2) Individual intervention

Consenting participants will complete a 24-hr food and physical activity recall questionnaire and participate in metabolic control and biomedical measures: blood pressure, bodyweight, height, waist circumference, lipid, insulin and glycemic levels measured at baseline, at the end of the one year intervention and six months after the end of the intervention.

The first meeting considered all overweight and obese children recruited in the study. Then, only obese children will be invited to a consultation every three months.

2.3.5. *Diabetes prevention in Oman*

In Oman, a simple diabetes risk score was developed to identify individuals with high-risk of developing type 2 diabetes. The score had high sensitivity and specificity in two cohort studies and was able to identify most individuals at high-risk of developing type 2 diabetes in community based settings. Of interest, the Thai, Dutch, Finnish, and Danish diabetes risk scores performed poorly in Omani Arabs.[43]

Insulin secretion and sensitivity after an OGTT differ in various ethnic groups. A study comparing normal glucose tolerance (NGT) and impaired glucose tolerance (IGT) in which subjects from different ethnic backgrounds (718 subjects of Arabic, Japanese, and Mexican-American descent) received an OGTT and had plasma glucose and insulin levels recorded every 30 m using the Matsuda index of insulin sensitivity. Regardless of their ethnic backgrounds, individuals with IGT had both impaired insulin secretion and sensitivity compared to NGT subjects. However, reduced insulin secretion was highest in Arabs (80%), while lower in Japanese (55%) and Mexican-Americans (41%). Conversely, decreased insulin sensitivity was greatest in Mexican-American (30%), lowest in Arabs (11.5%), and intermediate in Japanese (23%).[44] These data suggest that Arab individuals with diabetes experience impaired insulin secretion to a greater extent than decreased insulin sensitivity. It would be useful if such studies considered different ethnic Arabic groups (Arabs from African descent versus those from Caucasian descent).

2.3.6. *Diabetes prevention in Saudi Arabia*

A Chronic Metabolic Disorders Primary Prevention Program was initiated in 1999. The program started in Riyadh at King Saud Housing, Dirab, one of the Primary Healthcare portals of the Saudi National Guard Health Affairs providing care to more than thirty thousand National Guard Employees and their families.[45]

The Program was aimed at assessing the prevalence of the various risk factors for diabetes and coronary heart disease in the catchment population and initiate preventive measures to reduce such risk. The interventions consisted of encouraging the participation of individuals and families in lifestyle change initiatives and then following up. Initial screening started on August 1, 1999 and continued untill June 8, 2000. Individuals aged 15 years or older were invited to participate excluding known diabetic patients and pregnant women. Examination included height, weight and blood pressure measurements. Fasting blood samples were taken for blood glucose and total cholesterol measurements, followed by a 2 hour post-prandial serum glucose measurement after oral administration of a 75 gram glucose load.

Follow-up started in May 2001, with the development of a call-recall assessment of all registered individuals. Five thousand persons were screened during the initial campaign. Additional individuals were included during the follow-up period and a total of 6,235 persons had been screened and registered by the end of 2005.

Results of Initial Screening

Sixty-eight percent of those screened and registered were males. The average age of the participants was 28 ± 11 years with 49% being less than 45 years. Only 6% were newly diagnosed as having diabetes. The prevalence of other risk factors was as follows: hypertension 9%, hyperlipidemia 26%, impaired glucose tolerance 7%, impaired fasting glucose 6%, with a cutoff of 6.1 mmol/L (110 mg/dL) and 24% with a cutoff of 5.6 mmol/L (100 mg/dL), overweight 28%, obesity 23%, and morbid obesity 2%. The prevalence of smoking was 18% and 73% of the population had at least one risk factor.

Follow-up and Interventional Program Results

Results of investigation were provided to all participants and educational sessions and follow-up visits were conducted according to their health status. Lifestyle change consultations were provided and weight reduction was encouraged. In addition to community-based programs comprising healthy activities, physiotherapists recruited and trained women inside the healthcare facilities.

Results of Lifestyle Interventional Program for Primary Prevention of Diabetes and Coronary Heart Disease at King Saud City Family and Community Medicine, Dirab, National Guard Health Affairs, Riyadh

Year	Converted from Impaired Glucose Tolerance to Normal	Converted from Impaired Fasting Glucose to Normal	Converted from Hyperlipidemia (Total Cholesterol) to Normal	Reduced weight by at least 2 KG
May 2001–May 2002	3	0	2	2
May 2002–May 2003	8	8	23	152
May 2003–May 2004	16	12	21	13
May 2004–May 2005	18	7	45	33
May 2005–February 2006	5	5	22	25
Total	50	32	113	225

2.3.7. *Diabetes prevention in Egypt*

Currently, Egypt stands among the top countries worldwide with the highest diabetic population in those aged 20–74.[23] This forms a severe burden not only on the health status of the community but also on the already compromised health care budget of the country. Diabetes prevention by weight control and physical excercise proved to be the most suitable solution for this problem.[45–47]

The European IMAGE project includes a European guideline for diabetes prevention together with a practical toolkit for the implementation of prevention programs. In this context, IMAGE developed an adequate education program for health care professionals to prevent diabetes as well as the establishment of quality standards.[48–50]

Diabetes prevention programs have not yet been established in Egypt until recently. El-Sayed and Schwarz designed a project for prevention of diabetes in Upper Egypt called IMAGE EGYPT. Before the clinical trial could be initiated, prevention managers (PM) were trained. PM are a group of health care professionals whose training was based on a curriculum adapted to suit local needs. After training, the Egyptian PM were able to deliver preventive intervention. The study is designed to be carried out in Sohag and El-Menia Governates in Upper Egypt and should be completed by the end of 2014.

(a) *Purpose*

The purposes of this study are to implement a diabetes prevention program in Upper Egypt, to assess the ability of adapted behavioral change methods transferred by specifically trained PM and to improve specifically determined markers.

The primary objective is to determine if a successful implementation of a diabetes prevention program will be associated with improved metabolic control determined by waist circumference (WC), blood pressure and HbA1c as primary endpoints.

Secondary Objectives:

Change in blood lipids
Change in motivation to improve healthy lifestyle
Change in quality of life

(b) *Study Design*

The study population consists of non-diabetic males and females 40–70 years who are at high-risk to develop type 2 diabetes. The study aims to screen 2000 non-diabetic individuals in both governates.

The FINDRISC and the Heart Score scales questionnaire will be used to identify those with type 2 diabetes and cardiovascular disease. This simple questionnaire was first validated as a tool for diabetes risk determination[45,46] and then adapted to the Arabic (especially Omani) population.[43] Questionnaires will be translated into Arabic by two independent certified translators. Furthermore, questionnaires will be administered to 10 non-medical individuals for evaluation of the clarity and simplicity of the questions. After reaching consensus, the questionnaires will be used for field-work. The answers to the FINDRISC questionnaire add up to a score of 26 points. High-Risk of Type 2 diabetes (T2D-HR) will be defined as a score >14 points on the FINDRISC questionnaire and those with a lower score will receive written information about the benefit of a healthy diet and exercise. Subjects with a high FINDRISC score will be offered an opportunity to participate in the intervention program which will be performed in group sessions. Persons with a very high score (20 and above) have a siginificant risk of having undiagnosed diabetes and will be advised to visit their physicians for further diagnostic evaluation. If diabetes is excluded, those individuals will be invited to participate in the intervention program. All T2D-HR identified individuals, will be invited to a clinic visit before and after intervention as well as after 6 and 12 months. During these clinic visits, height, weight, WC, blood pressure, total cholesterol, triglycerides and HDL cholesterol will be measured. A standard OGTT with 75 g of glucose and a 2-hr post-load blood glucose determination will be performed as well.

Inclusion Criteria

- High risk of type 2 diabetes with a FINDRISC score > 14 points.
- Minimum age of 40 years and maximum age of 70 years.
- Willingness to participate in the study and agree to the study proposal.
- Willingness to complete all study visits and study procedures
- HbA_{1c} ≤6.5%.

Exclusion Criteria

- Persons with a FINDRISC score higher than 20 points and subsequent newly diagnosed type 2 diabetes.
- Persons with previously diagnosed type 2 diabetes.
- Persons utilizing a lifestyle intervention program regularly during the previous 12 months.
- Patients treated with oral anti-diabetic drugs or with insulin.
- Persons with a BMI >35kg/m^2.
- Persons with the following impairments which, in the opinion of the investigator, would seriously compromise the integrity of the study:
  - Significant visual impairment
  - Significant hearing impairment

- Cognitive disorders
- Significant unstable comorbidities (notable changes within the past three months)
- Any other condition per the investigator's discretion

Trial Groups

This prospective, randomized, open clinical outcome study will be conducted at two clinical sites (Sohag and El-Menia) with a total of 200 prediabetic patients.

The observation period per patient is designed for 1 year.

Once a year, all patients enrolled in the intervention program will be invited to visit the health centre for clinical assessment (including an OGTT).

Intervention Group

In those with T2D-HR, intervention programs on lifestyle modification consisting of four sessions, will be conducted by PMs (e.g., physician and nurses) at each participating health care center. The length of each session will be 90 m. The intensive program duration is four weeks (one session per week). These sessions will be practical and interactive. Group sessions will demonstrate several ways to reduce the risk of getting diabetes through life style changes (food intake and daily exercise). Training will be done in smaller groups (10–15 participants), allowing for individualized interaction between the subjects and trainers, answering questions and deciding on individualized intervention goals.

The first session will include general information on diabetes, obesity, and their risk factors. The second session will review the principles of healthy nutrition and the third, the basis and benefits of increasing physical activity and losing weight. The fourth session will review the previous lessons with additional focus on maintenance. Intensive assistance and support will include various educational and training materials such as handbooks, brochures, posters and calendars.

The continuous intensive intervention program will include mailing of letters every two months and questionnaires every 6 months, or SMS every week to reinforce the key messages of type 2 diabetes prevention with reminders for weight control, physical activity and healthy diet, and clinic visits recalls.

(c) *Control Group*

The control group will only receive standard information about healthy lifestyles in written form such as brochures without a structured intervention program. There will be no continuous support by telephone calls, SMS or newsletter as in the intervention group.

(d) *Study Procedure*

The target subjects will receive an invitation letter to participate in the program signed by their physicians. All those who agree to participate will be informed about the program details.

– Screen persons with FINDRISC to identify people at risk.
– Assign to intervention or control groups for the two regions.

The PM will manage diabetes risk in subjects in the control group, as is currently done. Care will be provided as usual and will be performed in control subjects at baseline, 6 and 12 months. Subjects will also have access to written lifestyle education and all other usual care practices.

For subjects in the intervention group, the prevention manager will manage lifestyle intervention with the IMAGE Toolkit and the trainer manual based on the IMAGE PM curriculum.

REFERENCES

1. Alberti KG, Zimmet P, Shaw J. (2007) International Diabetes Federation: A consensus on type 2 diabetes prevention. *Diabet Med* **24**: 451–463.
2. Wild S, Roglic G, Green A, Sicree R, King H. (2004), Global prevalence of diabetes: Estimates for the year 2000 and projections for 2030. *Diabetes Care* **27**: 1047–1053.
3. Alhyas L, McKay A, Balasanthiran A, Majeed A. (2004) Prevalences of overweight, obesity, hyperglycaemia, hypertension and dyslipidaemia in the Gulf: systematic review. *J R Soc Med* **2**: 55. Wild S, Roglic G, Green A,

Sicree R, King H. (2004) Global prevalence of diabetes: estimates for the year 2000 and projections for 2030. *Diabetes Care* **27**: 1047–1053.

4. Badran M, Laher I. (2011) Obesity in arabic-speaking countries. *J Obesity* **2011:** 686430.
5. International Diabetes Federation (2013) *IDF Diabetes Atlas*, International Diabetes Federation, Brussels, Belgium, 6th ed. In press.
6. Bray GA. (1978) Definition, measurement, and classification of the syndromes of obesity. *Int J Obesity* **2**: 99–112.
7. Nguyen N, Magno C, Lane K, Hinojosa M, Lane S. (2008) Association of hypertension, diabetes, dyslipidemia, and metabolic syndrome with obesity. Findings from the National Health and Nutrition Examination Survey, 1999 to 2004. *J Am College Surgeons* **207**: 928–934.
8. Sjöström L, Lindroos A, Peltonen M. (2004) Lifestyle, diabetes, and cardiovascular risk factors 10 years after bariatric surgery. *New England J Med* **351**: 2683–2693.
9. Chan M, Rimm E, Colditz G, Stampfer M, Willett W. (1994) Obesity, fat distribution, and weight gain as risk factors for clinical diabetes in men. *Diabetes Care* **17**: 961–969.
10. Colditz G, Willett C, Rotnitzky A, Manson E. (1995) Weight gain as a risk factor for clinical diabetes mellitus in women. *Ann Inter Med* **122**: 481–486.
11. Freemantle N, Holmes J, Hockey A, Kumar S. (2008) How strong is the association between abdominal obesity and the incidence of type 2 diabetes? *Int J Clin Practice* **62**: 1391–1396.
12. Al-Sendi A, Shetty P, Musaiger A. (2003) Prevalence of overweight and obesity among Bahraini adolescents: A comparison between three different sets of criteria. *Eur J Clin Nutr* **57**: 471–474.
13. Bener A. (2006) Prevalence of obesity, overweight, and underweight in Qatari adolescents. *Food Nutr Bull* **27**: 39–45.
14. Malik M, Bakir A. (2007) Prevalence of overweight and obesity among children in the United Arab Emirates. *Obesity Rev* **8**: 15–20.
15. Nasreddine L, Mehio-Sibai A, Mrayati M, Adra N, Hwalla N. (2010) Adolescent obesity in Syria: Prevalence and associated factors. *Child Care Health Dev* **36**: 404–413.
16. Sibai A, Hwalla N, Adra N, Rahal B. (2003) Prevalence and covariates of obesity in Lebanon: Findings from the first epidemiological study. *Obesity Res* **11**: 1353–1361.
17. Sorkhou I, Al-Qallaf K, Al-Shamali N, Hajia A, Al-Qallaf B. (2003) Childhood obesity in Kuwait — prevalence and trends. *Family Med* **35**: 463–464.

18. Serdula M, Ivery D, Coates R, Freedman D, Williamson D, Byers T. (1993) Do obese children become obese adults? A review of the literature. *Preventive Med* **22**: 167–177.
19. Madanat H, Troutman K, Al-Madi B. (2008) The nutrition transition in Jordan: The political, economic and food consumption contexts. *Promot Educ* **15**: 6–10.
20. Musaiger A. (2002) Diet and prevention of coronary heart disease in the ArabMiddle East countries. *Med Principles Practice* **11**: 9–16.
21. Musaiger A. (2004) Overweight and obesity in the Eastern Mediterranean Region: can we control it? *Eastern Mediterranean Health J* **10**: 789–793.
22. International Diabetes Federation (2011) *IDF Diabetes Atlas*, International Diabetes Federation, Brussels, Belgium, 5th ed. (Available at http://www.idf.org/diabetesatlas)
23. Mohammad B, Ismail L. (2012) Type II Diabetes Mellitus in Arabic-Speaking Countries. *Int J Endocrinol* **2012**: 902873.
24. Salpeter S, Buckley N, Kahn J, Salpeter E. (2008) Meta-analysis: Metformin treatment in persons at risk for diabetes mellitus. *Am J Med* **121**: 149–157.
25. Pinelli N, Jantz A, Martin E, Jaber L. (2011) Sensitivity and specificity of glycated hemoglobin as a diagnostic test for diabetes and prediabetes in Arabs. *J Clin Endocrinol Metab* **96**: E1680–E1683.
26. Astrup A, Dyerberg J, Selleck M, Stender S. Nutrition transition and its relationship to the development of obesity and related chronic diseases. *Obesity Rev* **9**: 48–52.
27. Bassuk S, Manson J. (2005) Epidemiological evidence for the role of physical activity in reducing risk of type 2 diabetes and cardiovascular disease. *J Appl Physiol* **99**: 1193–1204.
28. Fritz T, Wändell P, Åberg H, Engfeldt P. (2006) Walking for exercise — does three times per week influence risk factors in type 2 diabetes? *Diabetes Res Clin Practice* **71**: 21–27.
29. Diabetes Prevention and Control (1993) A call for action. Alexandria, Egypt, World Health Organization, Regional Office for the Eastern Mediterranean.
30. Personal information.
31. sgh.org.sa/en-us/technicalprograms/noncommunicablediseases/diabetesmellitusprevention/overview.aspx
32. Staff Writer (2013) Is Enough Being Done To Manage The GCC Diabetes Time Bomb?, *Gulf Business*.

33. International Diabetic Federation Atlas. 2006 showing prevalence of diabetes in 2007 and future projection for 2025 [Internet]. [updated 2009] (Available at http://www.eatlas.idf.org/index1397.html)
34. Riaz M, Basit A, Hydrie MZ, Shaheen F, Hussain A, Hakeem R, Shera AS. (2012) Risk assessment of Pakistani individuals for diabetes (RAPID). *Prim Care Diabetes* **6**: 297–302.
35. Akhter J, Ahmed A, Iqbal R, Abdul Jabbar, Zaidi S. A translational randomized trial of culturally specific and cost-effective life style intervention for the prevention of type 2 diabetes in Pakistan (Pakistan diabetes prevention program PDPP) (ongoing study in Aga-Khan University Hospital (Karachi, Pakistan) supported by International Diabetes Federation) by personal communication.

35a. http://clinicaltrials.gov/ct2/show/NCT01530165.

36. Azizi F, Gouya MM, Vazirian P, Dolatshahi P, Habibian S. (2003) Screening for type 2 diabetes in the Iranian national programme: a preliminary report. *Eastern Mediterranean Health J* **9**: 1122–1127.
37. Shadpour K. (1994) *The PHC Experience in Iran*. Tehran, United Nations Children's Fund.
38. Harati H, Hadaegh F, Momenan AA, Ghanei L, Bozorgmanesh MR, Ghanbarian A, Mirmiran P, Azizi F. (2010) Reduction in incidence of type 2 diabetes by lifestyle intervention in a Middle Eastern Community. *Am J Prev Med* **38**: 628–636.
39. Ng SW, Zaghloul S, Ali HI, Harrison G, Popkin BM. (2011) The prevalence and trends of overweight, obesity and nutrition-related non-communicable diseases in the Arabian Gulf States. *Obes Rev* **12**: 1–13.
40. Al Rashdan I, Al Nesef Y. (2010) Prevalence of overweight, obesity, and metabolic syndrome among adult Kuwaitis: results from community-based national survey. *Angiology* **61**: 42–48.
41. Personal Communication.
42. Personal Communication.
43. Al-Lawati J, Tuomilehto J. (2007) Diabetes risk score in Oman: A tool to identify prevalent type 2 diabetes among Arabs of the Middle East. *Diabetes Res Clin Practice* **77**: 438–444.
44. Abdul-Ghani M, Matsuda M, Sabbah M. (2007) The relative contributions of insulin resistance and beta cell failure to the transition from normal to impaired glucose tolerance varies in different ethnic groups. *Diabetes Metab Syndr* **1**: 105–112.
45. Personal Communication.

46. Tuomilehto J, Schwarz P, Lindstrom J. (2011) Long-term benefits from lifestyle interventions for type 2 diabetes prevention: time to expand the efforts. *Diabetes Care* **34**: S210–S214.
47. Gilliies Cl, Abrams KR, Lambert PC, Cooper NJ, Sutton AJ, Hsu RT. (2007) Pharmacological or lifestyle interventions to prevent or delay type 2 diabetes in people with impaired glucose tolerance: Systematic review and meta-analysis. *BMJ* **334**: 299.
48. Lindstrom J, Ilanne-Parikka P, Peltonen M, Aunola S, Eriksson JG, Hemia K. (2006) Sustaine reduction in the incidence of type 2 diabetes by lifestyle intervention: Follow-up of the Finnish Diabetes prevention study. *Lancet* **368**: 1673–1679.
49. Lindstrom J, Neumann A, Shappard KE, Gilis-Januszewska A, Greaves CJ, Handke U. (2010) Take action to prevent diabetes- The IMAGE toolkit for the prevention of type 2 diabetes in Europe. *Horm Metab Res* **42**: S37–S55.
50. Pajunen P, Landgraf R, Muylle F, Neumann A, Lindstrom J, Shwartz PE. (2010) Quality indicators for the prevention of type 2 diabetes in Europe-IMAGE. *Horm Metab Res* **42**: S56–S63.
51. Paulweber B, Valensi P, Lindstom J, Lalic NM. (2010) Greaves CJ on behalf of the IMAGE study group A. European evidence-based guidelines for the prevention of type 2 diabetes. *Horm Metab Res* **42**: S3–S36.

Chapter 15: Prediabetes and Diabetes Prevention in South Africa

Naomi Levitt, Krisela Steyn† and Kirsty Bobrow‡*

1. INTRODUCTION

South Africa is a middle-income country of great diversity culturally, linguistically and socioeconomically. Although the country is amongst the most affluent in sub-Saharan Africa, it has one of the highest GINI coefficients globally, ie income inequality globally, and is in the grip of a complex and rapid epidemiological transition.[1] This has seen the emergence of a multiple disease burden namely infectious diseases such as tuberculosis and HIV/AIDS, non-communicable diseases (NCDs), persisting childhood malnutrition and diarrhoea, as well as interpersonal violence and accidents.[2] The term colliding epidemics is frequently used to characterise the current situation between chronic infectious diseases and NCDs.[3,4] The extent of the HIV/AIDS epidemic and the early years of lack of access to antiretroviral therapy (ART) saw a dramatic fall in life expectancy from 62 years in 1992 to 53 years in 2010. This has reversed in 2012 as life expectancy had recovered to 60 years, testament to the rapid expansion of the ART programs. On the other hand, there has been little change in overall mortality from NCDs over the past ten years.[5]

*Corresponding author. Email: naomi.levitt@uct.ac.za
Chronic Disease Initiative for Africa and Division of Diabetic Medicine and Endocrinology, Department of Medicine at Groote Schuur Hospital and University of Cape Town.
†Chronic Disease Initiative for Africa. C/o Department of Medicine, Faculty of Health Sciences, University of Cape Town, P/bag X3, Observatory 7935, South Africa.
‡Nuffied Department of Primary Care Health Sciences, University of Oxford; Chronic Disease Initiative for Africa.

The first South African Burden of Disease study provided evidence that diabetes is a major contributor to the burden of disease in South Africa.[5] The study estimated that the diabetes prevalence in people over the age of 30 was already 5.5% in the year 2000. Further that diabetes accounted for 4.3% of deaths and a total of 258,000 disability-adjusted life year (DALYs) in this age group. By 2009, the estimated prevalence had risen to 9.0% in the same age range, representing approximately 2 million cases of known diabetes. The estimated mortality rates had risen and the non-fatal disease burden, examined for the first time, was considerable. In 2009, an estimated 8,000 new cases of blindness and 2,000 new amputations were reported to be caused by diabetes in addition to which 78,900 years lived with disability (YLD) was attributed to diabetes related to retinopathy, amputations, attributable stroke and ischemic heart disease.[6]

National prediabetes prevalence rates are not known in this highly diverse country in which black Africans are in the majority (79.2% of the population). The most recent estimates of the prevalence of prediabetes are drawn from two studies conducted in Cape Town. In the adult 'colored' or mixed ancestral population the crude prevalence of prediabetes, impaired glucose tolerance (IGT) and impaired fasting glucose (IFG), was 19.7% and crude prevalence of type 2 diabetes was 28.2% [age-adjusted 26.3% (95% confidence interval (CI) 22.0–30.3)].[7] These figures are considerably higher than those reported in the adult urban Black population (crude prediabetes prevalence 11.7% and that of diabetes 12% in people 24 to 74 years of age).[8]

The major drivers of the diabetes epidemic are largely similar to those found elsewhere namely, the adoption of unhealthy lifestyles with a change in dietary patterns, and a decrease in physical activity with a resulting rise in obesity rates, as well as urbanisation and demographic changes such as an ageing population.[9] Of these, the greatest risk factor is undoubtedly the frighteningly high rate of overweight/obesity, particularly amongst women. Indeed, South Africa has among the highest prevalences of overweight/obesity globally. In the recently released SANHANES, the prevalence of overweight and obesity in adult women was 24.8% and 39.2% and in adult men 20.1% and 10.6%, respectively. The reasons underpinning this unwelcome distinction are complex (Fig. 1).[10]

Multiple data sources suggest that the nutrition transition, from a traditional diet high in carbohydrate and fibre and low in fat, to a diet higher in

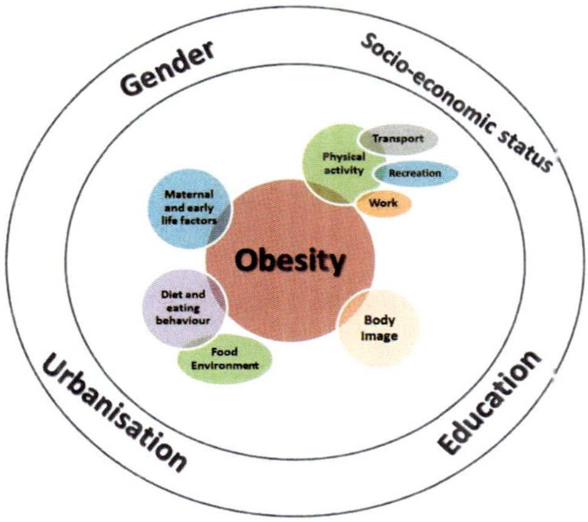

Fig. 1. Social determinants of obesity in African women (adapted from Ref. [10]).

fat and salt, is evident and associated with urbanisation trends. The dietary transition is strongly influenced by large commercial entities, referred to as 'Big Food,' that dominate the food and beverage environment. Indeed, in 2007 the 10 largest packaged food companies in South Africa account for almost twice the global average of the processed foods market in 2007.[11] Chain retailers now control over half of food sales in South Africa and South Africa has become a major importer of processed food products. These developments contribute to a significant diabetogenic food environment.[12]

Important cultural and socioeconomic factors also need to be taken into consideration in understanding the obesity epidemic. These include food insecurity. For example the recollection of childhood hunger has been associated with obesity in women.[13] While education as a marker of socio-economic status, is still positively associated with obesity, unlike the situation in high-income countries.[2] Another is the perception of ideal body size. Among the African population, many studies have reported that overweight is the desired state, because it is perceived to be associated with dignity, respect, wealth, strength, attractiveness, happiness, health and not having HIV/AIDS. In addition, even in overweight young girls there has been a consistent false perception that their weight was normal.[14] Yet evidence is beginning to accumulate that these attitudes are changing. For example young girls are beginning to report positive attitudes about being thin, such as feeling more like a girl, but at the same time, expressing positive feelings about being fat. Puoane *et al.* have proposed that is due to the opposing influences of the traditional positive attitude toward overweight in black African women and the visual images of western women on TV and movies where the preferred female shape is clearly slim.[14]

1.1. Current Non-Communicable Disease (NCD) Policy Initiatives

To date, policies for the prevention of prediabetes and diabetes have been imbedded in national policy initiatives for NCDs. In the period prior to the United Nations Summit on NCD in September 2011,[15] the South African National Department of Health was actively engaged in national, regional (the Brazzaville Declaration on NCD Prevention and control for the WHO African region)[16] and international (First Global Ministerial Conference on Healthy Lifestyles and Non-communicable Disease Control in Moscow, 28–29 April 2011.[15]

The Minister of Health called a National Summit on the Prevention and Control of NCD in early 2011. This culminated in the adoption of a NCD declaration with a strategy comprising three major components (see Fig. 2) together with 10 targets (see panel 1) to be reached by 2020 in order to reduce the impact of NCD in South Africa. It is notable that diabetes is only specifically mentioned in one of the targets, i.e., increasing diabetes control by 30%. Nevertheless, successfully addressing risk factors for diabetes such as obesity, physical inactivity and smoking is likely to impact the burden of diabetes in the long-term. The National Department of Health's Strategic Plan for the Prevention and Control of NCD 2013–2017 (SA strategic plan) was finally formally launched in August 2013.[17] This provides details of population-based interventions required to reduce lifestyle risk factors for NCD. Further, it speaks to the extensive restructuring needed for transformation of the public sector primary care health services to adequately provide for patients with NCDs and their risk factors.

1.2. Population Health Initiatives

Population health initiatives have predominantly consisted of regulatory-based policies and associated community education programs. A recent

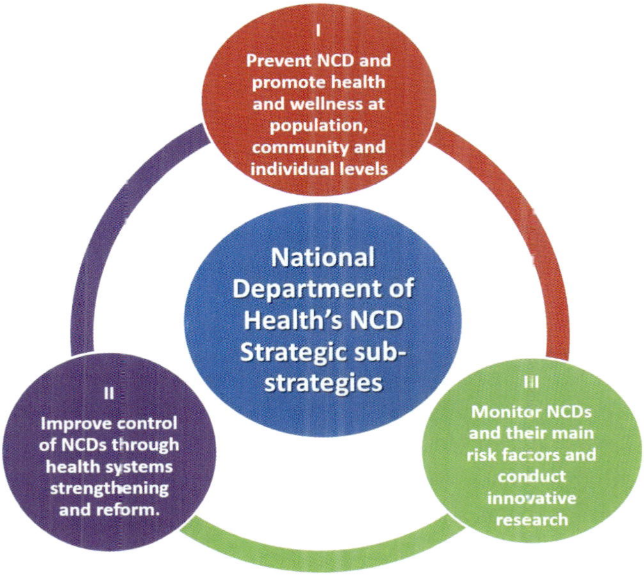

Fig. 2. The major components of the National Department of Health Strategic plan on NCD.[17]

Panel 1: THE 10 NCD GOALS AND TARGETS FOR 2020.

REDUCE

- premature mortality from NCDs by 25%
- tobacco use by 20%
- alcohol intake by 20%
- mean population salt intake to less than 5 g per day
- prevalence of overweight and obesity by 10%
- prevalence of high blood pressure by 20%.

INCREASE

- prevalence of physical activity by 10%
- percentage of people controlled for hypertension, diabetes and asthma by 30%
- the number of people screened and treated for mental disorders by 30%
- the coverage and uptake of cervical cancer screening among women (especially those with previous STI).

description of the 10 'Best Buys' for the prevention and control of heart disease, diabetes and stroke in the African region included food control legislation and public education, promotion of physical activity and the maintenance and extension of tobacco control activities.[18]

A 'Healthy Lifestyle Campaign' was central to the National Department of Health's strategic priorities for 2004–2009. This campaign had five main pillars which included: healthy nutrition, tobacco control, promotion of physical activity and combating the abuse of alcohol.[19]

1.2.1. *Nutrition policies and initiatives in South Africa*

Promoting healthy nutrition has been one of the focus areas of the National Department of Health for more than two decades. The following section highlights the developments and changing approaches in nutrition policy and programs as they relate to the prevention of pre-diabetes and diabetes.

1.2.2. *Initiatives led by the National Department of Health*

In general, until relatively recently, the attention of the country's nutrition researchers and policy makers has focused almost exclusively on under-nutrition. In fact, the term malnutrition was and is still widely assumed to mean under-nutrition.

Traditionally, routinely published data on the nutritional status of children in particular, reported on under-nutrition without any reference to overweight or obesity. When the African National Congress government came to power in 1994, after decades of enforced racial segregation and inequality during apartheid, addressing under-nutrition and micronutrient deficiencies was one of the first aspects of health to receive attention. The resulting Integrated Nutrition program (INP), planned to be part of the Primary Health Care package for the country,[20] had the overall aim of reducing the prevalence of 'malnutrition' (meaning under-nutrition). The INP emphasized exclusive breastfeeding until six months of age thereafter introducing appropriate complementary foods with on-going breastfeeding until 24 months of age and beyond, ensuring optimal growth of infants and young children, promoting health of women and in particular pregnant and lactating women and to prevent an increase in mortality due to diseases of lifestyle. Indeed, it continues to be essential to address under-nutrition and hunger in large segments of the population. However, the complex interaction between over- and under-nutrition amongst poorer South Africans is predisposing them to ever increasing risk of overweight and obesity, and in turn prediabetes and diabetes.[3]

There is still a focus on under-nutrition in the Department of Health's most recent revision of the INP, encapsulated in the 'Roadmap for Nutrition in South Africa. 2013–2017', although less so than in the 1995 program.[21] The roadmap describes the key focus areas, policies, targets groups and support systems available for health care providers working in nutrition. It continues to emphasise nutrition during pregnancy and the first two years of life, including breastfeeding for at least six months, and promotes a balanced healthy diet, both important for diabetes prevention. On the other hand, the lack of a specific focus on the nutritional management of overweight and obesity does not bode well for the path out of under-nutrition, which in South Africa so often results in over-nutrition and diabetes and associated diseases that follow later in life.

For the last decade the Department of Health has included a 'National Nutrition Week' in its annual calendar with the active collaboration of many partners including the Departments of Social Development and Education, UNICEF, the Consumer Goods Council South Africa, Consumer Education Project of Milk SA, Association of Dietetics in South Africa, Heart and Stroke Foundation SA, Nutrition Society of Southern Africa and Diabetes South Africa The purpose of the week is to educate South Africans to eat healthily and it focusses on a balanced diet.[22] The activities for 2012 included the launching of a pictorial 'SA Food Guide' representing food groups with pictures of typical foods consumed in the country. The relative amounts of food groups that should be consumed are shown in different sized circles in the Food Guide poster.

The government has recently promulgated a number of legislative measures that impact the food industry. Food labelling regulations, to protect the public against excessive and unrealistic claims often made in promotion of food products, came into effect in 2012. Nutritional labelling however remains voluntary unless health claims are made in which case strict criteria have to be met.

Regulations to compel the food industry to reformulate specific foods to ensure that some unhealthy products are limited in commercially

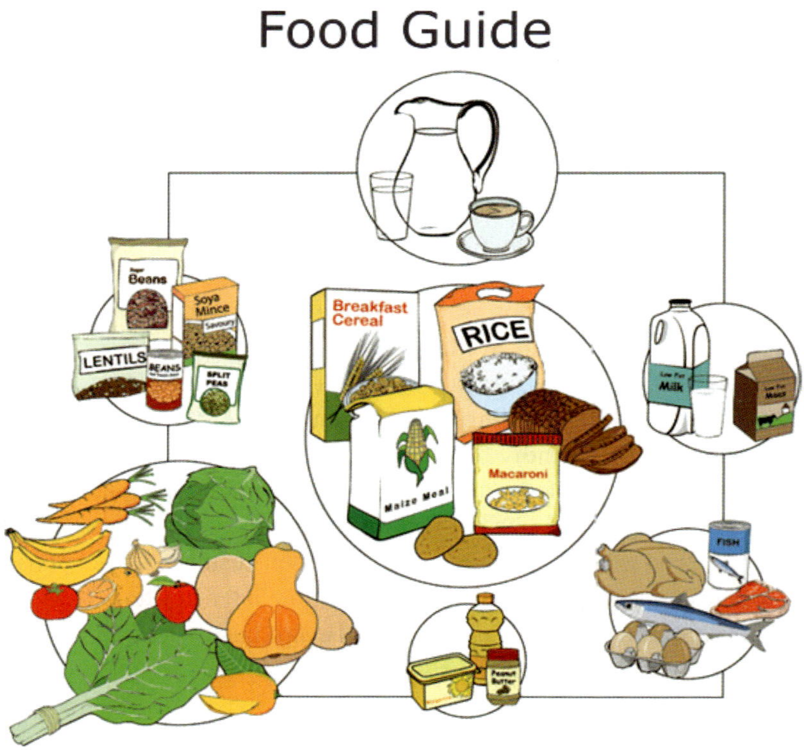

The SA Food Guide (reference: http://www.health24.com/Diet-and-nutrition/Nutrition-basics/Eat-healthier-with-the-news-SA-Food-Guide-20130318).

produced food have also been passed. For example, regulations limit the use of artificial trans fats to a maximum of 2% of oils or fat in all foods. A number of large food companies have voluntarily removed artificial trans fats from their products. In addition, a regulation relating to the reduction in salt content was published earlier this year (2013).[23,24]

1.2.3. *Other nutrition initiatives in South Africa*

Professional bodies and non-governmental organizations (NGOs) have engaged in a number of nutritional activities both independently and in collaboration with government departments. The Nutrition Society of South Africa along with the Association of Dietetics in South Africa and other stakeholders formulated the 'Food-based Dietary Guidelines' which aimed to promote healthy eating for all people in South Africa. These were widely promoted and formally adopted by the Nutrition Directorate of the National Department of Health in 2003. As mentioned earlier, the 'Food-based Dietary Guidelines' were revised in 2012.

In 2012, the Heart and Stroke Foundation of South Africa distributed 200,000 copies of a healthy cooking guide called 'Cooking from the Heart'.[25] The guide was developed by academicians and supported by industry. It demonstrates the principles of healthy eating and describes affordable recipes of popular foods that have been modified to ensure that they are healthier while remaining tasty. This book has proven to be very popular.

Many large food companies have been under pressure to improve the quality of their products. In response, some have developed corporate social responsibility programs that involve health and nutrition education. In addition, several 'Big Food' companies have taken voluntary action to stop the promotion of unhealthy foods to children. In 2009, the South African Pledge on marketing to children was established under the initiative of the Consumer Good Council of South Africa although the extent to which these pledges are being implemented is unclear.[11]

1.2.4. *Promotion of physical activity*

There have been many initiatives to promote physical activity over the past two decades, but no specific legislative action has been undertaken in this regard. Increasing physical activity was integral to promoting a healthy lifestyle as part of the restructuring of health care after 1994[26] and has been followed by a number of collaborative actions among public and private sector partners and tertiary institutions. In 2002, the South African government and their collaborators launched a 'Move for Health' campaign in line with the World Health Organisation's World Healthy theme of that year. The larger 'Healthy Lifestyles' campaign of 2004 of the National Department of Health resulted in the development of 'Vuka SA-Move for your health', a multi-organizational public-private collaborative on-going initiative.[27] The collaboration is comprised of health, sports and recreation, education governmental departments, five NGOs, four private sector companies and a tertiary institution and has received high level backing. It was presented in parliament and received wide television coverage and a consistent message promoting 30 minutes of physical activity on at least five days a week. The Minister of Health launched the campaign in May 2005 in Alexandra township, a high-population density and low socio-economic community and led a 4 km walk. A number of prominent physical activity workshops and a widely publicised international physical activity and public health course were offered in March 2007 under the umbrella of Vuka SA-Move for your health. Subsequently, there has been a sporadic implementation of programs and events linked to Vuka SA.

Until relatively recently, the promotion of physical activity in schools was one significant avenue that had been neglected. In November 2011, the national Departments of Basic Education and Sports and Recreation put forward a Memorandum of Understanding to promote an Integrated School Sport Framework.[28] This plans to make sports accessible during the school day to all children. An objective of the Department of Sports and Recreation South Africa is 'getting the nation to play'. A mass participation program mobilizing communities to take part in sporting activities has been implemented. This program arranges the 'Golden games,' a sports event for older adults and focusses on marginalised groups including women, children, youth, elderly, persons with disability and people living in rural areas.

The first draft of a National Physical Activity Plan was presented in 2012 after consultation with the relevant government departments and other stakeholders. A consultative workshop was planned for 2013 with a wider range of stakeholders and the completed plan will then be presented to the South African National Parliament.

1.2.5. *Tobacco control*

South Africa has pursued an active tobacco control policy for the last two decades. The success of these measures has ensured that tobacco use is the only diabetes risk factor to date to have reduced in prevalence. The legislation commenced with the introduction of written health warnings on cigarette packages and advertisements. This was followed by, separation of smoking areas in restaurants, banning tobacco advertising and the sale of tobacco to minors as well as prohibiting smoking in public places and steep increases in excise taxes resulting in increased real cigarette prices by 115% between 1993 and 2003.[4]

During the past decade, there has been further legislation to address loopholes utilised by the tobacco industry and smokers. Although the implementation of the law frequently leaves much to be desired, the smoking rates in the country has fallen from 34% in 1995 for adults >18 years and older[5] to approximately 23% in 2003.[29,30]

1.2.6. *Alcohol*

Alcohol control efforts have lagged behind those for tobacco, but are finally receiving serious attention. The Minister of Health has presented draft regulation to parliament proposing a ban of alcohol advertisements and of sports sponsorship by alcohol producing companies.[31] It is anticipated that if these regulations are passed and the glamorisation of alcohol use is stopped that it will reduce alcohol consumption significantly particularly in younger people. This should be an important measure to prevent or reduce diabetes.

1.2.7. *The vitality program of discovery health*

An innovative health promotion program is to be found from within the private health insurance sphere.[32] The voluntary, comprehensive, integrated, incentivized program enables accumulation of points on a tier system for health promotion activities such as health knowledge, assessment and screening and fitness-related activities. The status achieved allows members to claim discounts on services such as airline flights and purchases in shops. It also determines the extent of a cash rebate of up to 25% on the purchase of healthy foods at national supermarkets. Recent evidence demonstrates that activating this option was associated with the reporting of a reduction in the consumption of unhealthy foods and an increase in the intake of fruits, whole grain cereals and vegetables. Further, that activation of the highest rebate was associated with significantly lower levels of obesity. Yet despite increasing levels of participation in the physical aspects of the program, with concomitant lower subsequent hospital admissions and health claims, a majority of members still do not have beneficial use of the gym from a health perspective.

The applicability and generalisability of this program to the broader South African population require careful consideration. There are other examples of similar initiatives in this country and elsewhere. For example, Mexico and Brazil have used conditional cash payments for incentivizing certain behaviors while providing a cash incentive was successful for promoting HIV testing amongst men in South Africa.

2. HEALTH CARE DELIVERY LANDSCAPE IN SOUTH AFRICA

Public health policies to prevent prediabetes and diabetes are articulated by the National Department of Health and implemented by local government authorities. The National Department of Health also sets the policy and service delivery framework for treatment and secondary prevention which are implemented by provincial departments of health. Not surprising, the semi-federal system of government has resulted in a breakdown in implementation and monitoring of health policies and regulations.

Health care in South Africa is delivered by both public and private sectors.[33] Over 60% of South Africans receive all of their health care through the public health care system in which all primary level services and medications are free while in-hospital service charges are means tested. One-fifth of the population makes use of the private sector for outpatient primary care needs (GPs) which is paid for on an ad-hoc and out-of-pocket basis but continue to rely on public sector services for in-patient care and chronic medications. Only approximately 15% of South African residents are sufficiently covered through private medical insurance plans and receive all or most of their care via private GPs, specialists and hospitals. Given growing concern about the functioning and financial sustainability of the public health system, the National Health Insurance scheme (NHI) has been proposed and is expected to be phased in over the next 15 years (see Panel 2).[1,2,34]

There has not been any implementation of a screening program for diabetes or prediabetes outside of pregnancy. The health care provider assesses the risk for gestational diabetes (GDM) in women receiving

Panel 2: National Health Insurance (NHI) Scheme[31]:

The NHI aims for universal coverage by funding a comprehensive package of services for all South Africans from an integrated pool of public funds, sourced from general tax revenue and possibly additional taxes (such as a surcharge on taxable income and increased VAT). The scheme will increase funding for health care services particularly at the primary care level and in district hospitals. It will also enable purchasing of services from private providers where appropriate. There will be no co-payments. It is thought that through the financial protection provided by this scheme there will be a large increase in health services utilisation. Some members of private insurance schemes are likely to opt out of these schemes instead relying on their universal system entitlements, even those who choose to remain on private insurance will use some of their NHI entitlements.

antenatal care with a screening questionnaire. Women who are at high-risk are offered an oral glucose tolerance test and once diagnosed, are referred to tertiary care obstetric services for management. To date, no specific follow-up or care is given to women who are at increased risk but do not meet GDM diagnostic criteria, although women with GDM are referred for primary care postpartum.

The majority of those with diabetes attend crowded public sector primary care facilities for their management. In cities, larger facilities hold once or twice weekly specified diabetes clubs or clinics which about 50–70 people attend at a time because the diabetes burden is so great. Diabetes care includes attention to commonly associated chronic comorbidities such as hypertension and dyslipidaemia, but not for concurrent tuberculosis and/or HIV/AIDS care. This is about to change as there are new policy calls for the integration of care for chronic infectious diseases and NCDs. Despite the availability of national diabetes management guidelines, their implementation remains suboptimal. The reasons for this are many. One example is that although the guidelines include an annual measurement of glycated hemoglobin, but as the cost is so prohibitive, it is not done routinely or, in many instances, at all. Figure 3 shows the tiers

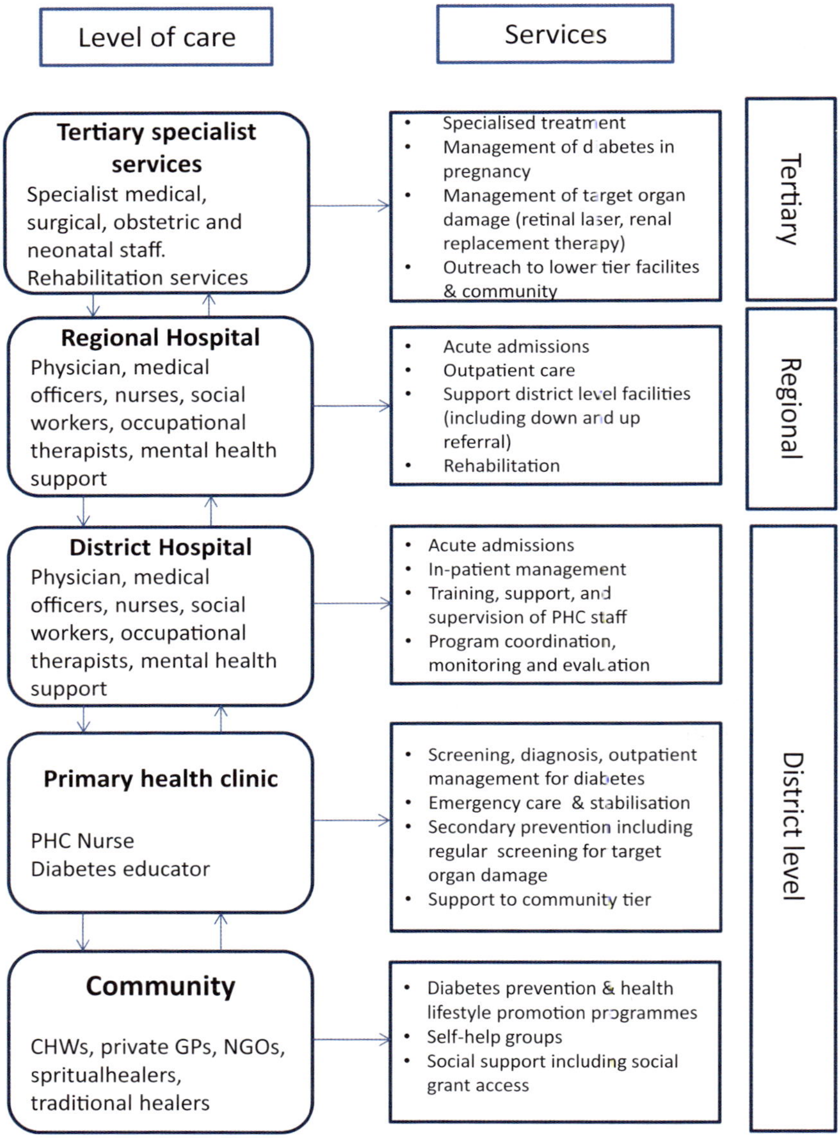

Fig. 3. Tiers of care for pre-diabetes and diabetes in the South African health care system (adapted from Ref. [35]).

of care available in the South African health care system as applied to the management of prediabetes and diabetes.[35]

3. CONCLUSIONS

Currently, considerable health care resources are consumed by the management of people with diabetes and its complications in the country, a situation that will only worsen in the future unless diabetes and prediabetes are prevented. Clearly, this a major challenge. It is hoped that the diabetes tide will turn with the emerging national focus on promoting a healthy lifestyle to reduce the impact of NCDs. Given the common coexistence of the different NCDs, it is appropriate that preventive strategies are directed at diabetes together with other chronic conditions. One planned initiative will be to call on the Department of Health to turn its attention to legislation directed at sugar-containing beverages.

REFERENCES

1. Mooney G, Gilson L. (2009) The economic situation in South Africa and health inequities. *Lancet* **374**: 858–859.
2. Coovadia H, Jewkes R, Barron P, Sanders D, McIntyre D. (2009) The health and health system of South Africa: Historical roots of current public health challenges. *Lancet* **374**: 817–834.
3. Mayosi BM, Flisher AJ, Lalloo UG, Sitas F, Tollman SM, Bradshaw D. (2009) The burden of non-communicable diseases in South Africa. *Lancet* **374**: 934–947.
4. Levitt NS, Steyn K, Dave J, Bradshaw D. (2011) Chronic noncommunicable diseases and HIV-AIDS on a collision course: Relevance for health care delivery, particularly in low-resource settings — insights from South Africa. *Am J Clin Nutr* **94**: 1690S–1696S.
5. Bradshaw D, Groenewald P, Laubscher R, Nannan N, Nojilana B, Norman R *et al.* (2003) Initial burden of disease estimates for South Africa, 2000. *South Afr Med J Suid-Afr Tydskr Vir Geneeskd* **93**: 682–688.
6. Bertram MY, Jaswal AVS, Van Wyk VP, Levitt NS, Hofman KJ. (2013) The non-fatal disease burden caused by type 2 diabetes in South Africa, 2009. *Glob Health Action* **6**: 19244.

7. Erasmus RT, Soita DJ, Hassan MS, Blanco-Blanco E, Vergotine Z, Kegne AP *et al.* (2012) High prevalence of diabetes mellitus and metabolic syndrome in a South African coloured population: Baseline data of a study in Bellville, Cape Town. *South Afr Med J Suid-Afr Tydskr Vir Geneeskd* **102**: 841–844.
8. Peer N, Steyn K, Lombard C, Lambert EV, Vythilingum B, Levitt NS. (2012) Rising diabetes prevalence among urban-dwelling black South Africans. *PloS One* **7**: e43336.
9. Tibazarwa K, Ntyintyane L, Sliwa K, Gerntholtz T, Carrington M, Wilkinson D *et al.* (2009) A time bomb of cardiovascular risk factors in South Africa: Results from the Heart of Soweto Study 'Heart Awareness Days'. *Int J Cardiol* **132**: 233–239.
10. Micklesfield LK, Lambert EV, Hume DJ, Chantler S, Pienaar PR, Dickie K *et al.* (2013) Socio-cultural, environmental and behavioural determinants of obesity in black South African women. *Cardiovasc J Afr* **24**: 1–7.
11. Igumbor EU, Sanders D, Puoane TR, Tsolekile L, Schwarz C, Purdy C *et al.* (2012) 'Big Food,' the Consumer Food Environment, Health, and the Policy Response in South Africa. *PLoS Med* **9**: e1001253.
12. Stuckler D, Nestle M. (2012) Big Food, Food Systems, and Global Health. *PLoS Med* **9**: e1001242.
13. Case A, Menendez A. (2009) Sex differences in obesity rates in poor countries: Evidence from South Africa. *Econ Hum Biol* **7**: 271–282.
14. Puoane TR, Tsolekile L, Steyn NP. (2010) Perceptions about body image and sizes among Black African girls living in Cape Town. *Ethn Dis* **20**: 29–34.
15. General Assembly of the United Nations [Internet]. [cited 2013 Oct 31] (Available at http://www.un.org/en/ga/president/65/issues/ncdiseases.shtml).
16. Brazzaville Declaration on NCD prevention and control in the WHO African region | GHD-NET [Internet]. [cited 2013 Oct 31] (Available at http://www.ghd-net.org/negotiations/un-summit-non-communicable-diseases/official-documents/brazzaville-declaration-ncd-prev)
17. Strategic Plan for the Prevention and Control of Non-Communicable Diseases 2013-17 — Health-e [Internet]. [cited 2013 Oct 31] (Available at http://www.health-e.org.za/2013/09/19/strategic-plan-prevention-control-non-communicable-diseases-2013-17/).
18. Mayosi BM. (2013) The 10 'Best Buys' to combat heart disease, diabetes and stroke in Africa. *Heart Br Card Soc* **99**: 973–974.
19. News, Health Systems Trust [Internet]. [cited 2013 Oct 31] (Available at http://www.healthlink.org.za/news/20040434)

20. The Primary Health Care Package for South Africa — Aa set of norms and standards [Internet]. [cited 2013 Nov 17] (Available at http://www.doh.gov.za/docs/policy/norms/full-norms.html)
21. Strategic Plan for Maternal, Newborn, Child and Women's Health (MNCWH) and Nutrition in South Africa [Internet]. [cited 2013 Nov 18] (Available at http://www.doh.gov.za/docs/stratdocs/2012/MNCWHstratplan.pdf)
22. Nutrition Week 2013 [Internet]. [cited 2013 Nov 17] (Available at http://www.nutritionweek.co.za/)
23. National Department of Health [Internet]. [cited 2013 Nov 18] (Available at http://www.doh.gov.za/healthtopics.php?t=Food%20Control&c=Legislation)
24. Tighter regulations for salt, tobacco use [Internet]. [cited 2013 Nov 18] (Available at http://www.sanews.gov.za/south-africa/tighter-regulations-salt-tobacco-use)
25. Cooking from the heart | heartandstroke [Internet]. [cited 2013 Nov 17] (Available at http://www.heartfoundation.co.za/cooking-heart)
26. A National Health Plan for South Africa [Internet]. [cited 2013 Nov 17] (Available at http://www.anc.org.za/show.php?id=257)
27. Kolbe-Alexander T, Bull F, Lambert EV. (2012) Physical activity advocacy and promotion: The South African experience. *South Afr J Sports Med* **24** [Internet]. [cited 2013 Nov 17] (Available at http://www.sajsm.org.za/index.php/sajsm/article/view/349)
28. Department of Sport and Recreation SA | Minister launches Integrated School Sport Framework [Internet]. [cited 2013 Nov 17] (Available at http://www.srsa.gov.za/pebble.asp?relid=1228)
29. Van Walbeek C. (2002) Recent trends in smoking prevalence in South Africa — some evidence from AMPS data. *South Afr Med J Suid-Afr Tydskr Vir Geneeskd* **92**: 468–472.
30. Peer N, Bradshaw D, Laubscher R, Steyn K. (2009) Trends in adult tobacco use from two South African Demographic and Health Surveys conducted in 1998 and 2003. *South Afr Med J Suid-Afr Tydskr Vir Geneeskd* **99**: 744–749.
31. National Liquor Authority [Internet]. [cited 2013 Nov 17] (Available at http://www.thedti.gov.za/business_regulation/nla_reports.jsp)
32. Lambert EV, Kolbe-Alexander TL. (2013) Innovative strategies targeting obesity and non-communicable diseases in South Africa: What can we learn from the private healthcare sector? *Obes Rev* **14**: 141–149.
33. The District Health System in South Africa: Progress made and next steps [Internet]. [cited 2013 Nov 17] (Available at http://www.doh.gov.za/docs/policy/dhsystem.html)

34. McIntyre D, Ataguba JE. (2012) Modelling the affordability and distributional implications of future health care financing options in South Africa. *Health Policy Plan* **27**: i101–i112.
35. Petersen I, Lund C, Bhana A, Flisher AJ. (2012) A task shifting approach to primary mental health care for adults in South Africa: Human resource requirements and costs for rural settings. *Health Policy Plan* **27**: 42–51.

Chapter 16: Prevention of Diabetes in Israel

*Avivit Cahn**,‡, Ronit Endevelt*† *and Itamar Raz*‡

1. INTRODUCTION

Preventive health care has become a vital aspect of medical practice. In recent decades, much focus has been placed on the prevention of the metabolic syndrome and its associated ailments in Israel and worldwide. In this chapter we describe the programs developed in Israel for the prevention of diabetes. The programs are directed at two levels:

1. *Whole population*: programs directed at the entire population aimed at (i) prevention and treatment of obesity, (ii) promoting physical activity and (iii) promoting healthy nutrition.
2. *High-risk populations*: screening programs for high-risk populations identifying undiagnosed diabetes and prediabetes, and development of interventions directed at diabetes prevention in these high-risk populations.

2. EPIDEMIOLOGY

The Israel National Health Interview Survey (INHIS-2) was conducted during the years 2007–2008 and included a representative sample of 10,331 participants aged 21 and above.[1] The overall prevalence of diabetes in Israel according to this survey is 8.3% [95% confidence interval (CI) 7.8–8.8%]. The estimated prevalence in the Jewish population is 8.2%, whereas in the

*Corresponding author. Email: Avivit@hadassah.org.il

† Director of Health Promotions, Maccabi Health Medical Services. Head, Health Promotion Stream, School of Public Health, Haifa University.

‡ The Diabetes Research Center, Hadassah Hebrew University Medical Center, Jerusalem, Israel.

Arab population it is 8.8%. These data are based on self-reported, physician-diagnosed diabetes. The INHIS-1, conducted during the years 2003–2004, noted a diabetes prevalence of 5.7% (95% CI 5.3–6.2%) thus displaying a clear upwards trend in disease prevalence.[2]

The major cause for the increasing diabetes rate in Israel, as well as worldwide, is the obesity epidemic which has been expanding at an alarming rate. The INHIS-2 found that 35.4% of the adult population was overweight and 15.4% was obese, compared to INHIS-1 which noted rates of 30.4% and 14.4%, respectively.

A recent survey in kindergarten children in central Israel found 15% of the children to be overweight.[3] A study of the BMI records of Jewish adolescents examined between the years 1967 and 2010 revealed that the prevalence of obesity has greatly increased during these years. In males, obesity prevalence had risen from 1.38% to 6.33% whereas in females a rise in obesity rates from 0.88% to 5.21% was observed. Average BMI rose from 21.44 kg/m^2 to 22.46 kg/m^2 for men and from 21.62 kg/m^2 to 22.15 kg/m^2 for women. The likelihood of obesity was higher among with low socioeconomic status or those belonging to minority groups such as Arabs and Ethiopian or Russian Jewish immigrants.[4]

3. PROGRAMS AIMED AT THE WHOLE POPULATION

In 1989, following the "Health for All" WHO initiative in 1984, Israel's Ministry of Health crafted its healthcare objectives for the year 2000. While these did not advance beyond the publication, they prepared the ground for the recent health initiative launched in 2006 with its final draft published at the end of 2011.[5] The initiative was termed: "Healthy Israel 2020" and encompassed multiple aspects of preventive medicine including oral health, occupational diseases and neonatal anemia. Twenty professional committees worked to evaluate disease burden, and define the program's objectives and quantitative targets for 2020. The committees included over 300 members who were senior professionals from government ministries, healthcare organizations, academia and other organizations. The methodologies of the committees included:

1. Review of older national recommendations where available.
2. An extensive scientific literature review for evidence-based interventions.

3. Identification and analysis of relevant data in Israel, including trends observed over the years.
4. A series of face-to-face meetings and extensive consultations with the electronic media to assist in deciding upon the most effective strategies.

Several committees focused on the "diabesity" (diabetes–obesity) epidemic and the major contributing factors to chronic non-communicable diseases in developed countries.

The professional committees' initial focus was on gathering data and evaluating disease burden. In several areas, information was limited and the 2020 goal was improve data collection to better ascertain the magnitude of the problem. In most fields, the experts defined realistic goals for year 2020 and suggested multiple strategies by which these goals may be attained.

Israel's national program complies with the "Health in All Policies" strategy for health governance and involved multiple coordinated projects of the different sectors.

The "Healthy Israel 2020" program included the following subcommittees:

(1) Prevention and treatment of obesity
(2) Promoting physical activity
(3) Promoting healthy nutrition

On November 28, 2011, the Israeli government unanimously accepted the national program for the promotion of a healthy, active lifestyle-based upon this initiative.[6]

In the following sections we will discuss the data and goals set by each sub-committee separately, and the strategies which are occasionally similar will be discussed together.

3.1. Physical Activity

The 20th century has been characterized by social and economic changes that led to a decrease in physical activity. These include improvements in motor-powered transport to the workplace, an expansion in the scope of sedentary employment and an increase in leisure activities of a sedentary nature such as watching television and using the computer. Physical inactivity contributes to disease burden, overuse of healthcare services, morbidity and mortality. The degree of physical activity performed by the individual is affected both by personal-behavioral factors and by social-environmental factors. Recent surveys indicate the Israeli population is not sufficiently physically active. In the 2013 survey conducted by the "Israel sport for all association," only a third of the surveyed population reported engaging in regular physical activity of at least 30 m at a time for at least three days a week. Women were engaged in less physical activity than men.[7] International guidelines for adults recommend engaging in aerobic physical activity of moderate intensity for 150 m a week, or 75 m a week of rigorous activity. The recommendation for children and adolescents is 60 m of moderate to intense aerobic physical activity on a daily basis.

In Israel, only 9.7% of the adult population and 17.4% of adolescents in 6th to 10th grades meet the aforementioned recommendations. Men and boys are generally more active than women and girls. The percent of Arab men and women meeting guidelines is much lower than that of the Jewish population (Table 1).

The "Healthy Israel 2020" program set out to increase the proportion of the population engaged in physical activity according to guidelines by 10–40% for the different segments of the population (Table 1). Different goals were set for different population groups based upon their baseline characteristics aiming to minimize current disparities. One of the likely underlying causes for lack of physical activity, in Israeli youth in particular, is the many daily hours spent watching television and using the computer. 35.9% spend at least four hours daily watching television while 28.9% play computer games for the same duration each day. A decrease by 20% in the proportion of adolescents watching television for 2 hr or more is an additional goal.

3.2. Prevention and Treatment of Obesity

Overweight and obesity have reached epidemic proportions in Israel and worldwide. The prevalence of obesity and overweight in Israel is similar to that in other Western countries. In general, obesity rates are higher among women than men, though overweight is more prevalent among

Table 1. Current proportions of sub-populations exercising adequately, and the 2020 target.

Subpopulation	% Currently Meeting their Goal	2020 Goal (%)	% increase
Adolescents (11–17 year olds)			
Recommendation: 60 daily minutes of moderate or vigorous intensity physical activity			
Jewish boys	18.6	23.3	25
Jewish girls	7.0	9.5	35
Arab boys	34.4	37.8	10
Arab girls	19.6	24.5	25
Adults —			
Recommendation: moderate intensity physical activity for at least 150 m per week or vigorous intensity exercise for at least 75 m per week			
Jewish men and women	9.6	11.5	20
Arab men	3.1	3.9	25
Arab women	2.7	3.5	30
Seniors —			
Recommendation: moderate intensity physical activity for 150 m per week			
Jewish men and women	18.5	22.2	20
Arab men	3.6	4.5	25
Arab women	0.7	1.0	40

men. In the Western world, as well as in Israel, obesity is more prevalent among those in lower socioeconomic strata.

Baseline obesity rates and recommended 2020 goals are shown in Table 2. The committee further recommended measurement of waist circumference in future surveys as a better predictor for developing the metabolic syndrome.

3.3. Promoting Healthy Nutrition

MABAT-1 (Matzav Briut ve-Tzuna) is a survey conducted during 1999–2001 in the adult Israeli population aged 25–64.[8] The survey included questions regarding eating habits, food content, fluid intake and alcohol consumption. According to this survey, the median intake of energy from fat in the average Israeli's diet is 32% of total caloric intake. Saturated fats comprise 9% of the Israeli's mean caloric intake. The percentage of the population exceeding recommended fat levels is currently unknown and should be assessed in future surveys. The mean daily percentage of calories from protein is within the range of 15–20% according to the MABAT-1 survey. The median consumption of fiber was 15 g per day which is lower than the recommended 25 and 38 g per day for women and men, respectively. Israelis consume an average of 2.5 ± 2.1 servings of vegetables a day and 2 ± 1.7 servings of fruits. The percentage of the population consuming less than the recommended three servings of vegetables and two servings of fruits a day is unknown.

The health objectives for year 2020 were defined as follows:

- Increase the contribution and variety of dietary fruits and vegetables Reduce consumption of calories from solid fats and added sugars.
- Ban importing, production and sale of foods rich in trans fats by the year 2013 which should not be replaced with saturated fats. Foods high in trans or saturated fats should be clearly labeled.
- Reduce the sugar content in processed foods by 15% by year 2020. Sugars, of all kinds, should be clearly labeled on all products.
- A national program to reduce salt consumption is to be initiated in 2012.

Table 2. Baseline obesity rates and the 2020 goal.

Subpopulation	Baseline Prevalence of Obesity (%)	Target Prevalence of Obesity (%)	% Change
Jewish men	12.3	11.1	10
Jewish women	13.8	12.4	10
Arab men	16.8	14.3	15
Arab women	17.7	15.1	15
Boys, grade 6	13.7	12.3	10
Girls, grade 6	8.0	7.2	10
Boys, grade 10	13.8	12.4	10
Girls, grade 10	4.8	4.3	10

3.4. Suggested Strategies for Achieving the 2020 Goals

The "Healthy Israel 2020" committees focused on data collection, goal setting and suggested strategies for attaining these goals.

The operational principles suggested by all committees include:

1. Joint operation by the Ministries of Health, Education, and Culture and Sports.
2. Operation of programs modeled on similar plans implemented worldwide and proven cost-effective.
3. Establishment of cooperation between governmental and private bodies with pooling of resources.
4. On-going monitoring throughout the programs evaluating their effectiveness as well as cost-benefit ratio.
5. Special attention to subpopulations attempting to reduce inequities in disease burden and disease control.

The suggested programs targeted multiple domains aiming to encompass as many aspects of daily life as possible including:

1. Local authorities — municipalities and communities
2. Workplaces
3. Educational system
4. Health care system
5. Industry
6. Media and social marketing
7. Legislation

3.4.1. *Local authorities: municipalities and communities*

Regular engagement in physical activity depends considerably on the environment in which one resides, accessibility of relevant facilities and the importance physical activity has in the community. Municipalities and community centers have a pivotal role in encouraging active lifestyles. The recommendations for municipalities included:

1. Creating community programs for encouraging physical activity. These include competitions held at community centers, local sports events and yearly marathons. Local marathons have been held in Tel

Aviv and around the Sea of Galilee. An official international marathon was first held in Jerusalem on March 2011 and yearly since.

2. Increasing accessibility of places in which physical activity can be undertaken. This includes construction of walking paths, physical activities facilities and ensuring access to existing facilities. Dozens of municipalities have already created walking paths and more are being constructed. Outdoor exercise facilities are built alongside these paths.
3. Urban planning that brings residential areas closer to schools, stores and workplaces encouraging citizens to walk rather than drive. Provide continuity, safety and convenience of sidewalks and streets.
4. Posting signs next to stairs to encourage their use instead of elevators.

3.4.2. *Workplaces*

Most adults spend a majority of their time at their workplaces. These should encourage a healthy active lifestyle by:

1. Providing a healthful menu. Standards should be set for defining the minimum recommended intake levels of healthy nutrients and the upper limits of nutrients which may be harmful in excess.
2. Increasing awareness and motivation of employers through health promotions and financial incentives to increase physical activity in their employees. These include provision of on-site facilities to perform physical activity along with facilities such as lockers, showers, and bicycle racks. Some workplaces already hold competitive and non-competitive physical activities.

3.4.3. *The educational system*

1. Increase weekly time allocated to physical activity with emphasis on raising awareness of the importance of health promoting physical activity. Today, all grades up to the 12th are required to provide two weekly hours of physical education.
2. Include education for a healthy lifestyle in the school curriculum.

3. Involve the family and/or community in programs encouraging adoption of a healthy lifestyle for the entire family. Encourage parents to supervise the nutrition and level of activity of their children. Promote daily family meals, which present an opportunity for parents to set an example of eating a balanced diet.
4. Maintain a high level of skill among physical education teachers.
5. Encourage walking and cycling to school while observing appropriate safety rules.
6. Implementation of a healthy lifestyle program at kindergartens and schools. This program addresses multiple issues including physical activity, healthful nutrition, etc.
7. Expand and improve infrastructures for physical activity for students, faculty and staff at higher education institutes.
8. Limit the sales of low nutritional foods and drinks and increase the availability of healthy foods in cafeterias and vending machines.

3.4.4. *Healthcare system*

In Israel, the National Health Insurance Law, enacted in 1994, required that all citizens be registered in one of four health plans: Clalit, Maccabi, Meuchedet or Leumit. The health plans are obligated to provide preventive, ambulatory and inpatient care for their members.[9] As very few people switch their health plan every year (1–1.5% per year),[10] the health plans have an incentive to invest in preventive medicine. Prevention of obesity and diabetes is of leading importance in all health plans, though not all aspects of prevention are covered by State Health Insurance Law.

Recommendations for health plans include:

1. Regular monitoring of BMI in the general population.
2. Provide incentives to encourage behavioral changes in patients including subsidies provided by the government to the health plans encouraging participation in workshops focusing on better nutrition, eating habits and/or encouraging physical activity.
3. Individual counseling on physical activity with the assistance of skilled professionals. The intervention includes behavioral prescriptions, activity planning and education tracking.

4. Increase the proportion of health care practitioners who receive theoretical and practical training on providing counseling for physical activity during their primary training.

3.4.5. *Industry*

Cooperation between the government, legislative body and industry may yield resolutions and eventually laws which may promote healthy nutrition while considering the limitations imposed by industry. The recommendations include:

1. Reduce the cost of healthy products (e.g., fruits, vegetables, low fat milk products, whole grains and whole wheat bread).
2. Eliminate or reduce discounts given to manufacturers of "unhealthy foods".
3. Reduce portion size of food sold in marketing chains and restaurants.
4. Comprehensive nutritional labeling of ready to eat or cooked foods sold in food chains and served in restaurants.
5. Encourage the marketing of relatively low density foods.

3.4.6. *Media and social marketing*

Multiple, ongoing consultations with the media have led to these recommendations:

1. Public information campaign using mass media adapted to specific target audiences encouraging physical activity.
2. Limit advertisement of food with low nutritional value during children's viewing hours and prime time.
3. Encourage use of positive role models to encourage consumption of healthy foods.

3.4.7. *Legislation*

1. Amend the provision in the Fitness Institutes Law which currently requires individuals interested in training at fitness gyms to

provide a medical clearance form so that it would suffice for the applicant to submit a health declaration form which would be renewed annually.

2. Limit the sales of foods high in trans fats.
3. Special budgets for HMO's dedicated to health promotion.
4. Limit advertisement of foods with low nutritional value during prime time.
5. Including fruits and vegetables as refreshments covered by tax deductions and not just coffee and pastries benefiting from this. This will enable private and governmental companies to serve healthy refreshments during staff meetings and lead to adoption of healthier eating habits.

4. EXAMPLES OF ON-GOING PROGRAMS IN ISRAEL

4.1. The Israeli Forum of a Healthy Lifestyle

The Forum's goals are to encourage leading a healthy lifestyle at the personal, municipal and national levels.[11] The Forum achieves its goals by a combination of publicity and action engaging governmental institutions, local municipalities and business corporations aiming to create a significant change in the community's agenda and priorities. The Forum is led by Prof. Itamar Raz, head of the Israeli National Council on Diabetes, and its members include physicians, parliament members, mayors and leading figures in Israeli society as well as organizations and corporations involved in health and food industries.

One of the forum's initial programs was to create a "healthy city" in the city of Ashdod. Multiple programs were enacted in order to create a meaningful change in public awareness of a healthy lifestyle. These included:

- Improving the accessibility of physical activity facilities as well as opening multiple outdoor exercise facilities.
- Creating walking paths and cycling lanes throughout the city.
- Programs for special populations including Ethiopian immigrants and the ultra-orthodox population.

- Dedicated programs for all age groups: kindergartens, schools, students, army conscripts, workplaces and retirees.
- Combined activities for parents and children on Fridays in the city's public parks and playgrounds.

The city of Ashdod served as an example for additional cities in Israel much due to the mayor's dedication and cooperation with the project.

The forum additionally promotes legislation by keeping the legislative body informed of the current health status of the Israeli population and maintaining health topics high on the parliament's and governments' agenda. Digital media and social networks are additional tools utilized by the forum to promote knowledge and increase awareness to the hazards of an unhealthy lifestyle and the risks associated with obesity and diabetes. The forum supports leading organizations in their attempts to create a healthy environment such as the Israeli Defense Force, universities or large corporations.

4.2. BINA Program and the Year of an "Active and Healthy Lifestyle" in the Educational System

A pilot interventional program for promoting a healthy lifestyle was operated during the school year 2009–2010 in 23 schools and kindergartens throughout the country encompassing different cultural and ethnic groups in Israel.[12] The purpose of the pilot was to evaluate the feasibility of this program and its success rate. The program was directed at three levels: school, kindergarten, family, and community (leisure time). A steering committee monitored the program, defined its goals and contents, and resolved problems as they arose.

The goals of the program included promoting healthy nutrition and physical activity during leisure time and limiting time spent on the computer or watching television.

The principles of the program were:

- Creating a health promoting environment in the educational institutions and community centers.
- Creating commitment to the program's goals by all those involved.

- Involving students, parents, teachers, school staff members, and local authorities in building the program and defining its goals.
- Integrating the health promoting program into the school curriculum.
- Practical sessions, enabling the children to directly experience the recommended nutritional intake and physical activities.
- Continuous monitoring of the program while quantifying measures of success or failure.

The program was implemented in two stages: an initial stage, which included education of staff members and preparation of educational materials, and a second stage when the program was implemented.

The intervention program lasted 6–8 months. No significant change in BMI was observed possibly because of the short duration of the intervention. Questionnaires and interviews with school staff members revealed their significant role in the establishment of the program and in conveying the program's theme to the students. The program served as the basis for the subsequent program operated in schools.

The school year 2011–2012 was declared as the year of "active and healthy lifestyle".[13] Eighty-five schools responded to the Ministry of Education's call to join yearly activities and become a "health promoting school". These schools received a financial grant and were guided by the Ministry of Education's local committee throughout the year. During this year the schools focused on transforming the educational environment into one that promotes a healthy lifestyle. Health issues were integrated in multiple classes during the year granting the students knowledge and skills required in order to adopt a healthy lifestyle. Moreover, the information conveyed did not remain theoretical but was incorporated in numerous school activities, including sports, cooking lessons, art exhibitions, competitions and community programs. The topics discussed included:

- Principles of a balanced nutrition
- Food pyramid
- Content of the food we eat
- Learning to read food labels
- Wise consuming

- The "Healthy" sandwich
- Importance of eating a family meal together
- Limiting ingestion of sweets and soft drinks
- Drinking water
- Culture, heritage and nutrition
- Importance of physical activity
- Incorporating physical activity into everyday life

The purpose of the program was to lead to fundamental behavioral changes in children and to reach out to their families and community. Therefore, many activities encouraged active participation by the parents and other family members.

In each school, one staff member was elected to lead the program and to represent the school to authorities and other external parties. The program leader was required to undergo a training course of 30 hr led by the Health Department in the Ministry of Education. The leader's role was to create a comprehensive multi-level, multi-year program including operational plans as well as modes of measurement and assessment of the program's efficacy.

The Ministry of Education composed a document of health standards which defined the skills and contents of the program to be assessed including questionnaires completed at the onset of the program and at its termination. Specific programs were developed for different age groups and sectors including the Arab population and the ultra-orthodox population addressing different cultural needs. Each school had the autonomy to create a program most suitable to its needs, however, all schools were required to report their activities and quantify their success rates.

Following that year, the Ministry of Education encouraged schools to maintain the health-oriented atmosphere created. Additional schools that wished to be defined as "Health Promoting" were required to submit a document to the local authority summarizing their yearly strategies and outcomes. The best schools would receive recognition as "health promoting" as well as economic incentives.

For the school year 2013–2014, the Ministry of Education defined three levels (three stars) for a "health promoting school" depending on the school's commitment to the program. Thus, a one star school is one in which the principal and the health promoting staff member incorporate health contents in at least three subjects and at least three age groups and are in touch with the local health promoting staff of the Ministry of Education. A two star school extends the health promoting programs to at least five subjects and to all age groups as well as involving parents and community in health promoting programs occasionally throughout the year. A three star school meets the above criteria and additionally is extensively involved in the community in long-term meaningful programs (i.e., in nearby kindergardens, schools or old age homes). Furthermore, a three star school attempts to share its experiences with other schools and educational facilities. Quantitative assessment of the program is an inseparable component of becoming a three star school.

During the school year 2011–2012, schools were encouraged to remove vending machines selling soft drinks and unhealthy foods from their campuses and sell only foods of high nutritional value. This was later reinforced by the CEO of the Ministry of Education regarding the content of foods sold in school vending machines as well as cafeterias and catering services.[14] These issues will hopefully be incorporated into Israeli law in the near future.[15]

4.3. The Israel Healthy City Network

The Israel Healthy City Network was founded in 1990 as part of the International Healthy Cities Network led by the World Health Organization.[16] The primary goal of the network is to put health high on the social, economic, and political agenda of city governments. Disease prevention, health promotion, minimizing the inequality in health, and dealing with risk factors for non-communicable diseases and injuries are additional goals.

There are currently 29 cities and four regional authorities in the network. The network has recently published a guide for the transformation of a city to a "healthy active city". The principles include:

- Cooperation between the local authority and other public, individual and voluntary sectors involving leading figures from the municipality in all stages of program development.

- Collection of information regarding population needs and habits, understanding barriers to regular participation in physical activity and how to overcome them (e.g., cost, difficult access).
- Basing programs on WHO recommendations as well as consulting local experts and the local population.
- Creating city infrastructure which promotes physical activity — easing the accessibility of schools, parks, shopping places, and workplaces thus encouraging the population to walk or cycle, other than to drive. This refers both to improving facilities in existing neighborhoods and planning new physical-activity oriented facilities.
- Each program should follow the following steps: setting goals and ways to measure their attainment, definition of priorities, modes of action, pricing and fund raising.

Examples for programs include:

- Constructing walking lanes and outdoor exercise facilities.
- Installing parking facilities for bicycles next to high schools and workplaces.
- Local sport competitions.
- A "walking school-bus" — forming a walking group to and from school for children accompanied by an adult.
- Sport classes in community centers for populations with special needs.
- A local blog or social media which sends reminders to participants to join in regular physical activity.

4.4. Ethiopian Immigrants: "Tene Briut" Program

The Jews of Ethiopia arrived in Israel in two main waves of immigration, the first in 1984–1985 and the second in 1991. The dramatic transition from Ethiopian rural living conditions to a modern urban lifestyle brought on a drastic change in the immigrants' morbidity profile. While there was a significant reduction in various types of infectious diseases, there was an increase in the prevalence of chronic non-communicable diseases. BMI rose from 17–19 kg/m^2 to 24 kg/m^2 and, together with a decline in fitness, a sharp increase in the prevalence of type 2 diabetes was observed from 0% to 0.4% on arrival to Israel, to 17% after residing in the country for 10 years.

These data led to the foundation of "Tene Briut" — an interventional program for the Ethiopian immigrant population in Israel.[17,18] This program aimed to familiarize the Ethiopian population with concepts of chronic diseases in general and diabetes in particular, preventive behavior, and preventive medicine. The program is implemented mainly by Ethiopian-Israeli medical and paraprofessionals and its activities consist of sessions that take place in a community setting.

The model was developed in several stages. The early stages focused on learning about the community from non-medical professionals (e.g., welfare and absorption workers, teachers) and from members of the community and initial gathering of information via a questionnaire based study on beliefs, perceptions, and attitudes to health and chronic diseases. Later, a steering committee was set up, composed of members of the community, government representatives, health care providers, academic and philanthropic organizations. The program was initially operated by a non-Ethiopian physician and later a group of Ethiopian immigrant nurses were trained to become Health Trustees and gradually took over running the organization.

The main goals of the program were to:

- Enhance awareness and capacity of health care providers caring for the Ethiopian community.
- Provide members of the Ethiopian immigrant community with new concepts regarding health care and information about patients' rights.
- Document health care needs of the population.
- Influence the agenda of medical professionals and decision makers.

The program developed instructional materials suited to the immigrants' cultures and beliefs and addressed many topics including the traditional Ethiopian diet and Israeli foods combining them to create a balanced diet, physical activity as well as detecting, diagnosing, preventing and treating diabetes. As most adult immigrants were illiterate, information was disseminated using educational movies combining the traditional story teller format with music, dance, and drawing. Print media was also created. The program is on-going assessment to ensure the issues and materials presented are relevant and understood.

The program's activities included:

- Developing a booklet for health care professionals on food and nutrition discussing the nutritional value of traditional Ethiopian food.
- Lectures in the community setting. At the end of some sessions, blood glucose was tested to send the message that there is no stigma attached to diabetes.
- Cooking classes.
- A monthly radio "healthy program."
- A medical telephone interpreting service has been implemented in clinics and hospitals since 2007.

Tene Briut is now a non-governmental organization working in collaboration with local and/or national organizations aiming to promote the health of the Ethiopian immigrant community in Israel.

5. SCREENING AND TREATING PREDIABETES

The purpose of diagnosing prediabetes is to identify the segment of the population at increased risk for the development of both diabetes and cardiovascular disease (CVD) so that interventions (lifestyle and pharmacologic) can be initiated.

In 2008, the National Council on Diabetes presented a plan, targeting high-risk populations, in order to prevent their progression to diabetes.[19] The program was based upon risk stratification of the population according to age, BMI, fasting plasma glucose, triglyceride level and family history of diabetes (Table 3). Those in whom the risk for progression to diabetes is calculated to be over 10% in the upcoming six years were to comprise the intervention group, and receive counseling regarding possible preventive measures.

The intervention will focus on lifestyle modification with predefined targets, including:

- Weight loss of 5–7% in those who are overweight or obese
- Reduction of the fat content of calories to less than 30% and saturated fat to less than 10%

Table 3. Six-year risk of developing diabetes according to data from the Israeli Diabetes Research Group.[20] The shaded areas indicate increased risk (>10%) for developing diabetes.

Family history	BMI (kg/m²)	Age	Triglycerides (mg/dL*)	Fasting plasma glucose mg/dL (mmol/l)				
				<80 (<4.4)	81–90 (4.5–5)	91–99 (5.0–5.5)	100–109 (5.5–6.0)	110–125 (6.1–6.9)
No	<25	<45	<150	<1	<1	<1	1.5	6
			≥150	<1	<1	2	3	10
	25–30	<30	<150	<1	<1	<1	2	5
			≥150	<1	1	3	4	10
		30–45	<150	<1	1.5	2	2.5	14
			≥150	1	2	3	5	18
	≥30	<30	<150	0	<1	3	5	6
			≥150	0	2	3	10	12
		30–45	<150	0	2.5	3	6	15
			≥150	0	2.5	4	9	25

(Continued)

Table 3. (*Continued*)

Family history	BMI (kg/m²)	Age	Triglycerides (mg/dL*)	<80 (<4.4)	81–90 (4.5–5)	91–99 (5.0–5.5)	100–109 (5.5–6.0)	110–125 (6.1–6.9)
Yes	<25	<45	<150	<1	<1	1	3	11
			≥150	<1	<1	4	5	15
	25–30	<30	<150	<1	<1	1	4	12
			≥150	<1	1	3	6	15
		30–45	<150	2	2	3	6	20
			≥150	3	4	6	10	30
	≥30	<30	<150	0	<1	3	8	40
			≥150	0	2	5	15	50
		30–45	<150	0	2	5	10	40
			≥150	0	5	10	30	50

*150 mg/dL = 1.7 mmol/L.

- Increased intake of dietary fiber
- 150 m of exercise per week

High-risk patients were to be referred for six sessions delivered by a multidisciplinary team, including physicians, nurses, physiotherapists or physical educators, dietitians, and psychologists or social workers.

The program has not yet been initiated by any of the four health plans in Israel due to budgetary restrictions, and possibly larger investment in programs aimed at the whole population.

A new venture has recently been proposed by the National Council of Diabetes, and as it includes funding sources it stands a better chance of being implemented. It is based upon a pilot interventional program conducted by Macabbi Health Services – the second largest Health Maintenance Organization in Israel – operated in the Sharon region in 2006.[21]

The Sharon diabetes prevention initiative was based upon the principles of the American DPP with the goal of reducing weight, blood glucose, LDL and HbA1c by dietary modifications structured on the MedDiet[22] and physical activity. Patients included in this program were considered prediabetic if their fasting plasma glucose was between 110 and 125 mg/dL (6.1–6.9 mmol/L), or the 2-hr post-load glucose value was 140–199 mg/dL (7.8–11 mmol/L) during an OGTT.

The aim of the intervention was to modify the participants' dietary habits mainly by adoption of the low calorie MedDiet, changing eating behaviors and increasing physical activity. Patients diagnosed with prediabetes were invited through their family physicians to join the interventional program. 223 enrolled and were divided in two groups, one receiving individual and the other group counseling. The latter consisted of groups of 12 men and women, had ten meetings over a period of six months with a trained dietician, a social worker, a general practitioner, and a physical activity consultant in addition to a "walking group" twice weekly. The agenda included benefits of MedDiet, planning nutritional behavior and mindful eating, and importance of physical activity. Individual counseling consisted of eight meetings over a six months period with a trained dietician in addition to a "walking group" twice weekly. The agenda was the same as for the group treatment.

Both interventions were highly effective in delaying and preventing the development of diabetes with only 39% of patients developing diabetes within seven years in both intervention groups. No significant differences in diabetes development or glucose levels were observed between the two groups possibly indicating that it is the content of the intervention which matters and not its mode of delivery. Since group counseling costs 50% less than individual counseling, the former will be implemented in the future.

The proposed diabetes prevention program is composed of two parts:

1. Diabetes prevention in a high-risk population having impaired fasting glucose or impaired glucose tolerance.
2. Creating a change at the urban level, both in diabetes prevention and in encouraging a healthy lifestyle for the entire population. The city of Nazareth will be a pilot for this program.

5.1. Diabetes Prevention in a High-Risk Population

5.1.1. *Identification of a population at high-risk for development of diabetes*

- Generation of a prediabetes registry which will include patients with at least two measurements of either fasting plasma glucose level exceeding 100 mg/dL (5.5 mmol/L) or HbA1c 5.7–6.4 %, or 2-hr post–load glucose level of 140–199 mg/dL (7.8–11 mmol/L) during an OGTT.
- Distribute a health questionnaire via websites of individual health plans, waiting rooms, clinics and pharmacies encouraging high-risk individuals to have their blood glucose levels measured. Those with one abnormal value will be referred for an additional test in order to confirm the diagnosis of prediabetes.

High-risk individuals are defined as having at least three of the following:

(1) Overweight: BMI >25 kg/m^2
(2) Age: >40

(3) Family history of diabetes
(4) Triglycerides: >250 mg/dL (2.8 mmol/L)
(5) Personal history of gestational diabetes mellitus

5.1.2. *Interventional program for high-risk individuals including:*

- Increasing awareness to the risk of progression to diabetes in the health plans' websites and information systems.
- Individualized information regarding balanced nutrition, physical activity and weight loss will be available in electronic files which can be accessed independently.
- On-line telephone service will be available for those unable to reach the clinic but want personal guidance and support in lifestyle modification.
- Individuals in the prediabetes registry will be personally contacted by the nurse in their region and invited to participate in a lecture regarding prediabetes.
- Group therapy, in a similar format to that in the pilot study, will be offered to all those in the prediabetes registry. It will include 6–8 structured sessions regarding proper nutrition, weight loss, exercise, and stress reduction.
- Health employees will be compensated for every high-risk individual they recruit to the on-going prevention programs.
- Walking groups and cooking classes will be available.

5.2. Diabetes Prevention in Nazareth

The Arab population in Israel has a high prevalence of diabetes, overweight and obesity due to reduced awareness of the importance of weight control and regular physical activity. A recent survey conducted by the Israeli Diabetes Society revealed that 80% of the Arab population consumes high fat (>5%) dairy products and red meat regularly. Additionally, 40% do not eat vegetables daily.

In order to exert a significant change in this population, personnel who are aware of the unique cultural issues of Arab society as well as barriers to accepting counseling, must be trained to work whilst respecting their traditional codes. The operating principles are similar to the aforementioned, however, special funds must be dedicated for:

- Training of staff from within the community.
- Increasing awareness of community directors and religious leaders to the risks of an unhealthy lifestyle.
- Empowerment of Arab woman — cooking and exercise classes.
- Assistance in purchase of medications and medical equipment.

REFERENCES

1. Israel National Health Interview Survey INHIS-2 (2012) 2007–2010: Selected Findings, **331**. Israel Center for Disease Control, Ministry of Health Publication.
2. Israel National Health Interview Survey INHIS-1 (2006) 2003–2004: Selected Findings, **294**. Israel Center for Disease Control, Ministry of Health Publication.
3. Pinhas-Hamiel O, Bar-Zvi E, Boyko V, Reichman B, Lerner-Geva L. (2009) Prevalence of overweight in kindergarten children in the centre of Israel: association with lifestyle habits. *Child Care Health Dev* **35**: 147–152.
4. Meydan C, Afek A, Derazne E, Tzur D, Twig G, Gordon B, Shamiss A. (2013) Population-based trends in overweight and obesity: A comparative study of 2,148,342 Israeli male and female adolescents born 1950–1993. *Pediatr Obes* **8**: 98–111.
5. Lev B, Rosenberg E, Shohat T. (2000) Healthy Israel (Available at https://extranet.who.int/nutrition/gina/sites/default/files/ISR%202011%20Health%20Behaviors.pdf, accessed 9 October 2013).
6. http://www.sela.pmo.gov.il/PMO/Secretarial/Decisions/2011/12/des3921.htm (accessed 9 October 2013).
7. Israel sport for all association, 2013 survey (Available at http://www.isfa.co.il/2013.pdf, accessed 9 October 2013).
8. The first Israeli health and nutrition survey. Part 2 (Available at http://www.old.health.gov.il/download/pages/mabat2.pdf, accessed 9 October 2013).
9. http://www.health.gov.il/LegislationLibrary/Bituah_01.pdf (accessed 9 October 2013).
10. Shmueli A, Bendelac J, Achdut L. (2007) Who switches sickness funds in Israel? *Health Econ Policy Law* **2**: 251–265.

11. The Israeli forum for a healthy lifestyle (Available at https://www.facebook.com/optimisticside, accessed 9 October 2013).
12. The BINA program for a healthy lifestyle for children in Israel. Summary. January 2011.
13. http://cms.education.gov.il/EducationCMS/Units/Mazkirut_Pedagogit/Briut/ShnatBriut.
14. http://cms.education.gov.il/EducationCMS/applications/mankal/arc/sg3ak2_2_61.htm.
15. www.knesset.gov.il/privatelaw/data/18/3732.rtf (accessed 9 October 2013).
16. http://www.healthycities.co.il/upload/infocenter/info_images/01082011052914@peilut10-11.pdf (accessed 9 October 2013).
17. Jaffe A, Guttman N, Schuster M. (2007) The Evolution of the Tene Briut Model: Developing an Intervention Program for the Ethiopian Immigrant Population in Israel and its Challenges and Implications. Appropriate Health Care by Culturally Competent Health professionals International Workshop Report. In Leon E(ed) *The Israel National Institute for Health Policy and Health Services Research*, pp. 121–142.
18. www.tene-briut.org.il (accessed 9 October 2013).
19. The National program for the prevention of type 2 diabetes. The national council of diabetes, The Israeli Diabetes Association, Febuary 2008.
20. Tirosh A, Tekes-Manova D, Israeli E, Pereg D, Shochat T, Kochba I *et al.* (2005) For the Israeli Diabetes Research Group. Normal fasting plasma glucose levels and type 2 diabetes in young men. *N Engl J Med* **353**: 1454–1462.
21. Endevelt R, Peled R, Azrad A, Kowen G, Valinsky L, Heymann AD. Diabetes Prevention Program in a Mediterranean Environment: Individual or Group Therapy? *An Effectiveness Evaluation.* Submitted for publication
22. Bach-Faig A, Berry EM, Lairon D, Requant J *et al.* (2011) Mediterranean diet pyramid today. Science and cultural updates. *Public Health Nutr* **14**: 2274–2284.

Chapter 17: Diabetes Prevention in Australia: The Challenges of Scaling-up and Rolling-out Programs

Philip Vita, Prasuna Reddy†, Amy Timoshanko‡ and Stephen Colagiuri§*

1. INTRODUCTION

Diabetes is Australia's fastest growing chronic disease, with an estimated 280 Australians developing this condition every day. The total number of Australians currently with diabetes and pre-diabetes is estimated at 3.2 million.[1] If current trends continue, by 2031 there will be 3.3 million Australians with type 2 diabetes. It is one of the most challenging public health problems.[2]

Australia has a diverse population of 22 million people spread over a huge land mass equivalent to the size of Europe, divided into seven administrative regions (States and Territories). New South Wales and Victoria are the most populous states. More than a quarter of Australians are born overseas. Life expectancy is high (average 74 years), but

*Corresponding author. Sydney Medical School Boden Institute of Obesity, Nutrition & Exercise, Medical Foundation Building K25, The University of Sydney, NSW, 2006, Australia. Email: philip.vita@sydney.edu.au.

†Faculty of Health and Medicine The University of Newcastle Bloomfield, Campus, Orange NSW 2800 Australia. Email: prasuna.reddy@newcastle.edu.au

‡Prevention and Health Promotion, Diabetes Australia, Victoria, 206 Queensberry St, Carlton, Victoria, 3053, Australia. Email: atimoshanko@diabetsvic.org.au

§Professor of Metabolic Health, Sydney Medical School Boden Institute of Obesity, Nutrition & Exercise, Medical Foundation Building K25, The University of Sydney, NSW, 2006, Australia. Email: stephen.colagiuri@sydney.edu.au

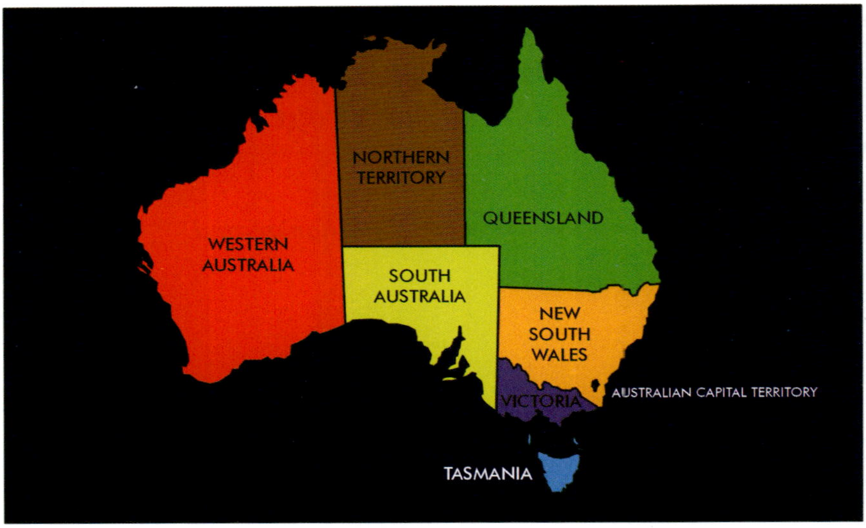

modernization and industrialization have led to a reduction in physical activity and an increase in the consumption of energy-rich foods. Lifestyle diseases such as type 2 diabetes are increasing rapidly, and lead to an array of adverse outcomes.

The Australian Diabetes, Obesity and Lifestyle study (AusDiab) was the first national Australian, longitudinal, population-based study established to examine the prevalence and incidence of diabetes and its complications.[3] The study, began in 1999, when 11,247 adults (aged 25 years and above) were recruited from the general community. It found that the prevalence of diabetes was 7.4% and had doubled in two decades. An additional 16.3% had prediabetes — either impaired glucose tolerance (IGT) or impaired fasting glucose (IFG). People of Southern European, South Asian, Middle Eastern and Aboriginal backgrounds were at higher risk of developing diabetes. Moreover, living in the most socially-disadvantaged areas of Australia doubled the risk of developing diabetes.

The potential to prevent or delay type 2 diabetes in high-risk individuals by lifestyle intervention has been unequivocally established ('proof of concept'); however, most landmark studies conducted exclusively in primary care settings used intensive, individualized interventions, which would be difficult to roll-out as population-wide programs.[4] The challenge is to translate this evidence into feasible, sustainable and effective community-based programs that can be scaled-up and rolled-out more broadly in existing health and community systems.

Moving from scientific discovery to population-wide implementation requires a series of steps, each building upon the achievements of the previous, from basic research to diffusion of interventions.[5] It took several years for international evidence to influence research, policy and practice in Australia. In this chapter, we describe the Australian experience over the past decade highlighting the challenges and key learning implementing national, statewide and regional programs.

2. BUILDING THE CASE

In Australia, Victoria has been leading the way, and has built on several small scale diabetes prevention programs including the Greater Green Trial (GGT),[6] Ballarat Diabetes Prevention Study[7] and the Healthy Living Course.[8] In all of these studies, screening and recruitment took place exclusively in the primary health care (PHC) setting.

2.1. Greater Green Trial (GGT)

The GGT conducted from 2004 to 2006, adapted the GOAL program from Finland to an Australian context. The cohort study recruited 237 individuals 40–75 years of age with moderate or high-risk of developing type 2 diabetes to a structured group program with six 90-m sessions delivered during an eight months period by trained nurses. Main outcome measures taken at baseline, three, and 12 months included weight, height, waist circumference, fasting plasma glucose (FPG), lipids, blood pressure, measures of psychological distress and general health outcomes. At 12 months participants' mean weight was significantly reduced by 2.52 kg and waist circumference by 4.17 cm. Blood glucose, lipids and diastolic blood pressure showed significant improvement. This study demonstrated that a type 2 diabetes prevention program using lifestyle intervention is feasible in PHC settings with a lesser reduction in risk factors than was observed in clinical trials and provides emphasis for a national approach for addressing this issue.

Several years later, a qualitative evaluation conducted in individuals who completed the GGT assessed the degree to which they had sustained program strategies and identify contributing factors. There was relatively good self-reported maintenance of diabetes risk reducing behaviors. Moreover, family and local community support contributed to sustained motivation after the program was completed. It was recommended that behavior modification programs should incorporate strategies to ensure that family and local community support are strengthened.

2.2. Ballarat Diabetes Prevention Pilot

The Ballarat Diabetes Prevention Pilot study (2007–2008) investigated the effect of a low-resource-intensive modification program on diabetes risk and compared home-based and gym-based resistance training in a sample of 122 participants.[4] A quasi-experimental two-group study was undertaken in 122 participants at high-risk of developing diabetes, 36.9% had IGT or IFG at baseline. The intervention included a 6-week group self-management education program, a gymnasium-based or home-based 12-week resistance training program, and a 34-week maintenance program. FPG and 2-hr plasma glucose, blood lipids, blood pressure, body composition, physical activity, and diet were assessed at baseline and one-year follow up. There were significant improvements in mean 2-hr plasma glucose and FPG. This intervention significantly reduced diabetes risk to a degree comparable to that of other low-resource-intensive lifestyle modification programs and more intensive interventions applied to individuals with IGT. However, effects of home-based and gymnasium-based resistance training did not differ significantly.

2.3. Healthy Living Course

The Healthy Living Course (HLC) was a randomized control trial which began in 2006.[8] It was designed to evaluate the effectiveness of a 6-months, group-based diabetes prevention program, The HLC assessed whether participation in the program led to changes in modifiable risk factors for type 2 diabetes in a high-risk population. Individuals designated at high-risk for diabetes by their general practitioners (GPs) were screened using an Oral Glucose Tolerance Test (OGTT) to determine eligibility. Three hundred and seven participants with pre-diabetes were assigned to an intervention or a put on waiting list and received standard care from their GP (control group) with the knowledge they would receive the intervention 6-months later, in an approximate 2:1 ratio. Biochemical, anthropometric and self-reported behavioral, cognitive and mood variables were compared between baseline and follow-up either at the end of the educational/support-based lifestyle program or at the end of the 6-months waiting list period. The analyses revealed that the intervention group significantly improved their diabetes knowledge, motivation to change, attitude, healthy eating and activity levels and showed significantly greater reductions in weight, body mass index, waist circumference, diastolic blood pressure and FPG in comparison with controls. The intervention group also changed their diagnostic status from prediabetes to non-diabetes at a greater rate than the control group (43% vs 26%) who received standard care from their GPs.

2.4. Leadership and Political Support

Australia is governed by a federated system in which health policy and service delivery is provided by a mixture of Australian, State, and Territory governments. There is a universal health care system funded by the Australian Government under Medicare. There is also a complementary private health care system. PHC is primarily coordinated and funded by the Australian Government under Medicare while treatment services are principally delivered by State and Territory governments. Diabetes prevention programs in Australia have a brief history in Australia.

Leaders of the Australian, State and Territory governments meet regularly as the Council of Australia Governments (COAG) to discuss public policy of national significance including health care reform. One of the concerns raised through the Australian Health Ministers' Council in 2005 was the impact chronic disease was having on the productivity and longevity of the workforce. The National Public Health Partnership undertook economic modeling of diabetes prevention and the Australian

Government Productivity Commission undertook analyses of the impact of chronic disease (including diabetes) on workplace productivity in Australia. Results of these economic analyses, accumulating scientific evidence of effectiveness of diabetes prevention internationally and the results of local translation research projects, such as the (GGT), all strengthened the case for a national policy on diabetes risk reduction.

In April 2007, COAG commissioned the development of national standards for lifestyle modification programs and the development of the Australian Diabetes Risk Assessment Tool (AUSDRISK). The AUSDRISK was released on 1 July 2008.[9] It is a ten-item questionnaire that assesses a person's risk of developing type 2 diabetes within the next five years. Items are based on the following risk factors: age, gender, country of birth, family history of diabetes, history of high blood pressure, smoking status, fruit and vegetable intake, physical activity levels, and waist circumference. A score equal to or above 12 on AUSDRISK is currently considered high-risk.

Also, as part of the (COAG) reform agenda, three very distinct initiatives were implemented in Australia to prevent type 2 diabetes under the umbrella of the Australian Better Health Initiative. A national program, the Australian Government Lifestyle Modification Program, a State program, Victorian program (*Life!*), and a regional translational project, the Sydney Diabetes Prevention Program.

3. THE AUSTRALIAN GOVERNMENT LIFESTYLE MODIFICATION PROGRAM

3.1. The Program

The National Program targeting 40–49 year old Australians at high-risk of type 2 diabetes was funded through Australian Government funds and Medicare to reimburse GPs for screening and referring patients. The National program was administered by the Australian General Practice Network (AGPN) through the 111 Divisions across Australia. Divisions of General Practice are voluntary associations funded by the Australian Government that supported practices to implement health promotion, early intervention and prevention strategies, chronic disease management, medical education and workforce support. They are the gateway for working with GPs. National Standards for the accreditation of Lifestyle Modification programs to prevent diabetes became available in 2008 and were used by the AGPN to accredit programs that GPs could refer eligible patients. An AUSDRISK score of ≥15, excluding diabetes with an OGTT and medical clearance to undertake moderate to vigorous physical activity from a GP, determined eligibility for those in the specified age range. The preferred program was called *Reset your Life* that consisted of seven group sessions held over a 6–8 months period with an intensive phase of 4 months. The three-year program was launched on 1 July 2008 with a target of 150,000 participants.

3.2. Barriers and Enablers

There were a range of system implementation barriers including poor coordination, short lead times, lack of resources to market and promote the initiative, insufficient reimbursement to providers of lifestyle modification programs, and the inherent difficulties involved in screening and recruiting patients in the PHC setting. In 2009, the AUSDRISK score for eligibility was reduced to ≥12 but this had little impact on referral rates. The requirement to exclude diabetes was a significant barrier reported by staff in the Divisions supporting the program. In addition, there was additional instability during this period as the PHC system was undergoing reform with 111 Divisions being amalgamated into 61 Medicare Locals with an increased agenda to engage with allied health professionals.

3.3. Results and Outcomes

In late 2010, approximately 4,000 patients had been screened and less than 500 had enrolled in a program. As a consequence, the initiative was discontinued in early 2011 as a stand-alone program with no formal evaluation. The Australian Government has subsequently incorporated diabetes prevention into a chronic disease management and prevention program.

4. VICTORIAN PROGRAM: *LIFE!*

4.1. The Program

The *Life!* program began in Victoria in 2007 with a phased roll-out of a statewide program targeting adults at high-risk of diabetes aged 50 years and over.[10] The age range was chosen to ensure there was no overlap with the Australian Government program. It was funded by the Victorian Government and coordinated by Diabetes Australia-Victoria for an initial four-year period (2007–2011) focusing entirely on diabetes prevention and in 2012 was extended with additional funding (2011–2015) to address both diabetes and cardiovascular disease. The program achieved steady state recruitment into the second year of implementation and is the largest group-based diabetes prevention program conducted in Australia. Key factors contributing to the successful implementation of the program are multiple referral pathways for systematic recruitment that included direct community engagement, work place promotion and linkages with general practice, a centralized referral service that supports participants through the referral process, integrated social marketing activities, referral initiatives, and development of a network consisting of accredited providers and trained facilitators that specialize in diabetes prevention.

Life! was developed based on the Finnish Diabetes Prevention Study, the GGT and the HLC. The program delivers three interventions: group-based courses conducted in community settings across Victoria, individual telephone health coaching and the Road To Good Health (RTGH) course for Aboriginal or Torres Strait Islanders. Underlying objectives of all *Life!* interventions are for participants to learn strategies and receive support to change behavior and reduce risk of developing a chronic disease. *Life!* applies health behavioral change theory (Health Action Process Approach), individual goal setting, and coaching or group support to encourage participants to adopt a healthy diet and an active lifestyle. The *Life!* Course and RTGH are group-based interventions. The RTGH consists of six sessions over an eight months period whereas the *Life!* course involves a face-to-face initial session, four intensive fortnightly sessions, and a follow-up session at six months. Telephone coaching occurs over a three months period.

4.2. Barriers and Enablers

Barriers to program implementation include slow recruitment during the initial program phase resulting in an over capacity of trained facilitators, finding the right balance for data collection and evaluation, complicated referral process with different national and local programs, inadequate payment model to cover the cost of face-to-face recruitment, differences across health provider systems and resources available to deliver the *Life!* Program. On-going development of the program has overcome these barriers and involved tailoring course structure to include an individual one-to-one initial session with a *Life!* facilitator, modifying course materials and the workbook to ensure that it is suitable for people of low literacy and culturally diverse backgrounds, development of on-line training and web community to support the work force, creation of a course DVD to ensure consistency of information presented to each group, development of a workbook and activities for telephone health coaching participants.

Raising awareness of both the problem and prevention actions that can be taken has been crucial to the implementation of the *Life!* Program. Community awareness raising initiatives, targeted engagement and development of local referral networks are priorities for sustainable recruitment to the program. A central referral team was established to contact and support participants through the referral process. Engagement strategies and campaigns were developed to support systematic risk assessment using the AUSDRISK tool and recruitment to the program. Four main referral pathways were established: (1) Local community recruitment by our workforce; (2) Primary care engagement and patient referral initiatives; (3) Social marketing campaigns designed with a clear call-to-action response resulting in self-referrals; (4) Referrals through workplaces and the WorkHealth — the Victorian Government's worker health check program which provided over 500,000 Victorian workers with a workplace-based health check from 2009–2013.[a] Other important factors for successful implementation of the program have been the development of an on-line system to coordinate delivery and provide direct database access to facilitators, primary care engagement including GPs, health service provider recruitment and accreditation, and health professional recruitment, training and development. Additionally, feedback from facilitators and participants have highlighted the importance of retaining specialist facilitators for sessions on diet and physical activity as it provides credible advice that motivates and guides participant goals.

4.3. Results and Outcomes

The *Life!* Program is evaluated using a systematic framework which identifies the program's effectiveness, reach, adoption, implementation and maintenance over time. The program is delivered statewide with 314 health service organizations accredited as *Life!* providers across regional Victoria and metropolitan Melbourne. Development and support of the specialized workforce is on-going with 382 health professionals trained to deliver the *Life*! Program. Over 40,000 people at high-risk have been referred to the program which has good reach with a high proportion of lower income and education levels participating. There is an 85% completion rate for the intensive phase of the group course whereas 54% complete telephone health coaching.

Significant weight (1.4 kg) and waist circumference reduction (2.4 cm) occurred after completion of the intensive phase of the *Life!* Course which lasted two months. By the end of the eight months *Life!* Course the average weight and waist circumference reduction was significant, 2.2 kg and 3.5 cm, respectively. Similarly, telephone health coaching participants reported significant reduction in weight and waist circumference of 2.7 kg and 4.1 cm, respectively, by the final health coaching call. The following quote from a *Life*! Course participant demonstrates the impact of the program on the lives of participants:

> *"...The course helped me make small lifestyle changes ... I've lost about seven kilos but the numbers aren't important to me, rather it is how I feel, I feel fitter and much happier now ..."*

5. SYDNEY DIABETES PREVENTION PROGRAM

5.1. The Program

The Sydney Diabetes Prevention Program (SDPP) was a lifestyle modification program targeting people aged 50–65 years at high-risk of diabetes in central and southwestern Sydney.[11] It was funded by the New South Wales (NSW) Ministry of Health and was a partnership between the Sydney Local Health District, University of Sydney, Australian Diabetes Council and three Divisions of General Practice. The NSW Government chose to fund a translational study adapting a 12-months lifestyle modification intervention delivered through PHC settings based on successful interventions in the Finnish and US Prevention Programs, rather than a rolling-out a statewide program.

The AUSDRISK tool was used to identify people at high-risk (risk score ≥15) of future diabetes. These subjects were offered a lifestyle modification program (the 'Program') administered by Lifestyle Officers (LO), trained allied health professionals, which included one individual and three 2-hr group sessions of intensive behavioral intervention to increase physical activity, reduce fat and saturated fats, increase fiber, and reduce weight. Participants unable to attend groups were offered an alternative individual module, three health-coaching sessions conducted over the phone. All participants were then offered three monthly telephone health coaching calls (at 3, 6 and 9 months) which delivered on-going lifestyle advice and then a final face-to-face 12-months review. The goals of the Program were to:

- increase physical activity to at least 210 m per week of at least moderate intensity
- reduce daily fat intake (≤30% total energy)
- reduce daily saturated fat intake (≤10% of total energy)
- increase daily fibre intake (≥15 g/1000 kcal per day)
- reduce body weight by 5%

The aim of this translational study was to examine the feasibility of screening and recruiting people at high-risk of developing diabetes in the PHC setting and assess the acceptability and efficacy of a moderately intensive lifestyle modification intervention to prevent or delay diabetes.

5.2. Barriers and Enablers

The SDPP found that it was feasible to screen and recruit high-risk participants using an Australian validated risk tool. However, engaging and supporting the PHC setting to screen and refer participants required considerable effort highlighting the challenges in providing prevention activities in a setting which is structured and remunerated to predominately focus on providing episodic care. In addition, the screening and referral processes were complex and required several steps including identifying high-risk individuals, formally excluding prevalent diabetes and providing medical clearance before referral to the LO. While the screening could be done by PHC staff, excluding diabetes, providing medical clearance and completing the referral form required involvement of the GP. Excluding diabetes required measurement of FPG and implementation of Australian guidelines that included an OGTT in those with an elevated fasting glucose[12] which proved to be a significant barrier.

During the course of this study, HbA_{1c} was accepted as a diagnostic criterion for diabetes[13] and was incorporated into the screening and recruitment process streamlining and increasing referral rates. It is also worth noting that the AUSDRISK tool was only officially adopted for general use on July 1, 2008 and hence, was not in routine practice in the primary care setting when screening and recruitment for this study began. Research staff spent considerable time working with the PHC settings to facilitate screening and recruitment strategies. Anecdotal reports from LO's suggested that a 'whole of practice' approach in which at least one PHC staff was given the responsibility and rewarded for screening patients seemed more likely to be effective. The SDPP experiences suggested that primary care systems and structures were not configured to readily undertake identification of high-risk individuals or to facilitate participants engaging in prevention activities of this nature.

5.3. Results and Outcomes

Two hundred and twenty GPs were recruited who screened 4,055 patients of whom 1,983 (49%) where found to be at high-risk of developing diabetes during the two year recruitment period 2008–2010. Of these, 1,238 participants began the 12 months program. At baseline, the mean age was 58.8 years, 63% were female, and the mean body mass index was 31.6 kg/m^2. There was a significant weight reduction of 2 kg in the 850 participants who completed the 12-months follow-up accompanied by improvements in diet (reduced total and saturated fats, and increased fiber intake) and physical activity. There were also significant reductions in waist circumference (2.6 cm) and total cholesterol. Diabetes risk reduction was estimated to be 30%, consistent with similar trials.

SDPP participants were more likely to be women, highly educated, have higher incomes, and be non-smokers compared to the general population. This is consistent with other diabetes prevention programs.[14] Diabetes prevention programs need to consider how to specifically target recruitment strategies that increase participation by males, smokers, those socioeconomically disadvantaged and other under-represented high-risk groups.[15]

The SDDP demonstrated the feasibility and effectiveness of developing and implementing a community-based lifestyle modification diabetes prevention program with participants screened and referred in the PHC setting.

6. DISCUSSION

In Australia, many lessons have been learned from attempts to scale-up diabetes prevention programs from small implementation trials to national initiatives. These experiences suggest that much remains to be improved especially engagement of the PHC setting and extending initiatives community-wide. The ill-fated Australian government program highlighted the need for more evidence on appropriate planning and the implementation processes. Not withstanding, all programs found it challenging to screen and recruit participants. The Australian Government program and SDPP recruited exclusively in the PHC setting with limited success, whereas *Life!* has been successful in implementing additional strategies including social marketing, workplace screening and facilitator-led recruitment.

The AUSDRISK tool, designed for use by the public as well as health care professionals, is a powerful tool of identifying those at risk for developing type 2 diabetes. A national consensus currently considers that a score equal to or above 12 is considered high-risk. However, the requirement to exclude diabetes by blood tests remains an inherent barrier although the use of HbA1c for this purpose appears to simplify this task.

Reducing barriers to determine eligibility for participation in prevention programs is urgently needed.

Evidence-based diabetes prevention programs which target high-risk participants can reduce the risk for diabetes. However, structural barriers exist that continue to make screening and recruitment difficult particularly in those who may benefit the most. Systematic changes are required in PHC before the real benefits of diabetes prevention programs can be realized.

The increasing recognition that social disadvantage plays an important role in developing chronic diseases such as diabetes, extends preventive interventions beyond strictly the medical setting, engaging social and political communities as well. Fortunately, the *Life!* Program has been able to recruit participants from lower socio-economic backgrounds. Nonetheless, policy and environmental interventions that reduce the obesogenic environment are needed to increase the chances for success of prevention programs. Both a high-risk and population health approaches that complement each other are needed.

Type 2 diabetes can be prevented or delayed through lifestyle modification with the challenge of translating this approach into cost-effective community programs. The evidence for lifestyle modification is compelling so we are knowledgeable as to what is required to reduce progression to type 2 diabetes. However, determining the optimal method for persuading those who could benefit the most to take action is lacking. In addition, it is necessary to develop more flexible programs that can be delivered by several modalities including the phone and internet. The NSW Government has invested in an evidence-based telephone health (Get Healthy) coaching service as its primary method to support its prevention activities (https://www.gethealthynsw.com.au).

Efforts in Australia have increased the evidence base towards effective community-based programs but the influences on program uptake and retention are still not well understood. There is still a need for an increase in implementation science to inform policy and practice in order to 'scale-up' and roll-out community-wide diabetes prevention programs in Australia. Moreover, advocacy strategies are crucial to increase political will across all levels of government and to obtain bi-partisan support. There has been a recent call-to-action for a renewed national approach to diabetes prevention advocating for a national roll-out of the *Life!* Program which unfortunately has fallen on deaf ears (http://www.letspreventdiabetes.org.au).

In the last decade, the US, Finland, and other European countries have been leading the way in scaling-up and rolling-out diabetes prevention interventions. In these countries, led by ambitious governments and collaborations between policy makers, researchers, private providers (health insurers and delivery agents) and practitioners, innovative approaches have been applied and a global approach has been recommended.[16,17]

Tackling the increasing diabetes epidemic will require integration of primary care and public health initiatives targeting both high-risk individuals and the general population if Australia is to be successful in reducing the growing burden of diabetes.[18]

REFERENCES

1. Australian Institute of Health and Welfare (2012) *Diabetes: The facts.* Canberra, Australia.
2. Beaglehole R *et al.* (2011) Priority actions for the non-communicable disease crisis. *Lancet* **377**: 1438–1447.
3. Tanamas SK, Magliano DJ, Lynch B, Sethi P, Willenberg L, Polkinghorne KR, Chadban S, Dunstan D, Shaw JE. (2012) *The Australian Diabetes, Obesity and Lifestye Study.* Baker IDI and Diabetes Institute,. Melbourne, Australia.
4. Gillett M *et al.* (2012) Non-pharmacological interventions to reduce the risk of diabetes in people with impaired glucose regulation: A systematic review and economic evaluation. *Health Technol Assess* **16**: 1–236.
5. Schwarz PEH, Albright AL. (2011) Prevention of type 2 diabetes: The strategic approach for implementation. *Hormone Metab Res* **43**: 907–910.
6. Laatikainen T *et al.* (2007) Prevention of type 2 diabetes by lifestyle intervention in an Australian primary health care setting: Greater Green Triangle (GGT) Diabetes Prevention Project. *BMC Public Health* **7**: 249–256.
7. Payne WR *et al.* (2008) Effect of a low-resource-intensive lifestyle modification program incorporating gymnasium-based and home-based resistance training on type 2 diabetes risk in Australian adults. *Diabetes Care* **31**: 2244–2250.
8. Moore SM *et al.* (2011) Can the onset of type 2 diabetes be delayed by a group-based lifestyle intervention? A randomised control trial. *Psychol Health* **26**: 485–499.

9. Chen L *et al.* (2010) AUSDRISK: An Australian type 2 diabetes risk assessment tool based on demographic, lifestyle and simple anthropometric measures. *Med J Australia* **192**: 197–202.
10. Reddy P *et al.* (2011) Life! in Australia: Translating prevention research into a large-scale intervention. *The Br J Diabet Vascular Disease* **11**: 193–197.
11. Colagiuri S, Vita P, Cardona-Morrell M, Singh M, Farrell L, Milat A *et al.* (2010) The Sydney Diabetes Prevention Program: A community-based translational study. *BMC Public Health* **10**: 328–335.
12. Colagiuri S *et al.* (2009) *National Evidence based Guideline for the Case Detection and Diagnosis for Type 2 Diabetes*. Diabetes Australia and the NHMRC, Canberra, Australia.
13. World Health Organisation (2010) Report of a World Health Organisation consultation: Use of glycated haemoglobin (HbA1c) in the diagnosis of diabetes mellitus. *Diabetes Res Clin Practice* **93**: 299–309.
14. Ali MK, Echouffo-Tcheugui J, Williamson DF. (2012) How effective were lifestyle interventions in real-world settings that were modeled on the Diabetes Prevention Program? *Health Affairs* **31**: 67–75.
15. Laws RA *et al.* (2012) Diabetes prevention research: a systematic review of external validity in lifestyle interventions. *Am J Preventive Med Corresponding* **43**: 205–214.
16. Green LW, Brancati FL, Albright A. (2012). Primary prevention of type 2 iabetes: Integrative public health and primary care opportunities, challenges and strategies. *Family Practice* **29**: i13–i23.
17. Bergman M *et al.* (2012) Diabetes prevention: Global health policy and perspectives from the ground. *Diabet Management* **2**: 309–321.
18. Vita P, Colagiuri S. (2012) A strategic approach to diabetes prevention: How much evidence is required before we act? *Diabet Management* **3**: 1–4.

Chapter 18: Prediabetes and Diabetes Prevention Initiatives in Turkey

M. Temel Yilmaz and Sehnaz Karadeniz†*

1. INTRODUCTION

Turkey is among the countries in the world where the number of people with diabetes is increasing rapidly, since its unique location at the crossroads of Asia, Europe, and the Middle East has influenced the lives and nutritional cultures of the region throughout history. Accelerated technology and modernization have negatively impacted individual's lifestyle and have been largely responsible for the increase in the incidence of diabetes. Although Turkey signed the St. Vincent Declaration in 1989, the Kos Declaration in 1993, and the Istanbul Commitment in 1999, a national diabetes policy has only recently been developed. The centralized structure of the health care system and the inefficiency of this system in meeting the needs of a rapidly increasing population in a large country have played a major role in this delay.

2. DIABETES AS A HEALTH CONCERN IN TURKEY

2.1. The Demographics of the Turkish Population

The population of Turkey (74 million) with 1.1 percent of the world's population ranks 18th in size among 187 countries in the world. According

*Corresponding author. Istanbul University, Istanbul Medical Faculty, Division of Endocrinology and Metabolism, Turkey. Email: dr.mtyilmaz@gmail.com

†Istanbul Science University, Medical Faculty, Department of Ophthalmology, Turkey

to projections for 2050, the world population will exceed 9 billion and Turkey is estimated to rank 19th with a population of 94 million 585 thousand.[1] The population growth rate of Turkey during 2010–2015 will approximate 1.3 percent and rank 92nd in the world. During the period 2045–2050, Turkey is expected to rank 109th with a population growth rate of 0.2 percent.[1] According to the World Bank data, the life expectancy at birth in Turkey has been steadily improving from 67.4 years in 1990 to 71.0 years in 2000 and to 74.3 years in 2010.[2]

The median age in Turkey is 28.9 years compared to 29.2 years in the world according to 2010 estimates. In this respect, Turkey is 80th among 186 countries. In 2050, it is predicted that the median age of the world's population will be 38, and that of Turkey 40.2.[1] Turkey is 128th among 186 countries with a crude death rate of 6.3 per thousand compared to 8.2 per thousand in the world according to estimates for the period 2010–2015.[2] According to the World Health Organization (WHO) estimates, Turkey's total health expenditure is 6.7% of GDP and the expenditure on health is 12.8% of total government expenditure.[3]

2.2. Environmental Factors and Lifestyle

In recent years, especially in urban areas, traditional foods have been replaced by foods high in carbohydrates and saturated fats. Fast food is becoming the most preferred nutrition style among children and adolescents. This food is rich in unsaturated fatty acids but poor in fiber and vitamins A and C, and increases the risk of developing obesity, non-communicable diseases like cardiovascular disorders, and diabetes.

The principal foods in Turkey are bread and other grains. 44% of the daily caloric intake is derived from bread alone and 58% from bread and other grains. Over the years, consumption of bread, milk-yogurt, meat and meat products, fresh fruits, and vegetables has decreased and the consumption of legumes, egg, and sugar increased. Although the amount of fat did not differ significantly, more vegetable oil is being used.[4,5] Fruit and vegetable/salad consumption, according to the Health Survey carried out by the Turkish Statistical Institute in 2012, is described in Tables 1 and 2.[6]

There are various estimates regarding physical activity of the Turkish population. According to the results of the Turkey Demographic and

Table 1. Percentage of individual fruit consumption in Turkey by residence, 2012 (at and over the age of 15 years).[6]

Frequency of fruit consumption	Total (%)	Urban (%)	Rural (%)
Twice or more a day	9.8	10.5	8.4
Once a day	44.4	46.8	39.0
Less than once a day, but at least 4 times a week	22.0	21.2	23.8
Less than 4 times a week, but at least once a week	16.1	14.9	18.9
Less than once a week	6.6	5.6	9.0
Never consumed	1.0	1.1	0.9

Source: Turkish Statistical Institute, Health Survey 2012. Publication Number 4117. Ankara, 2013.

Table 2. Percentage of individual vegetables and salad consumption in Turkey by residence, 2012 (at and over the age of 15 years).[6]

Frequency of vegetables/salad consumption	Total (%)	Urban (%)	Rural (%)
Twice or more a day	13.0	12.9	13.2
Once a day	51.8	55.0	44.7
Less than once a day, but at least 4 times a week	21.3	20.3	23.5
Less than 4 times a week, but at least once a week	10.4	9.0	13.7
Less than once a week	3.1	2.5	4.6
Never consumed	0.4	0.4	0.4

Source: Turkish Statistical Institute, Health Survey 2012. Publication Number 4117. Ankara, 2013.

Health Survey in 2003, about 20% of the population over the age of 18 years has a sedentary lifestyle and only 16% pursue low activity levels. Only 64% of the population over the age of 18 years engages in weekly physical activity of 150 minutes or more.[4,5] According to the World Health Organization Global Health Observatory Data on physical activity in 2008, a crude estimate of insufficient activity in those over the age of 15 is 54.6% with an age-standardized estimate of 56%.[7]

2.3. Prevalence of Diabetes

The Turkish Diabetes Epidemiology Study (TURDEP-I), a nationwide cross-sectional population-based survey, carried out between 1997 and

1998 in 24,788 randomly selected persons aged 20 years or older showed a 7.2% crude prevalence rate of Type 2 diabetes (T2D) with a 6.7% prevalence of impaired glucose tolerance (IGT) in the adult population. In this survey, glucose tolerance was classified according to WHO recommendations on the basis of 2-hr glucose values.[8] Extrapolating these results to the last population census from the State Institute of Statistics of Turkish Republic at that time, nearly 2.6 million adults may have diabetes and another 2.4 million, IGT.[8]

TURDEP-I findings suggest an upward trend of diabetes prevalence much beyond the projections of 7.2% for the year 2025 published in 1998.[9] Additionally, TURDEP-I found that 22% of adults have general obesity (defined as BMI ≥30 kg/m^2). The mean BMI in women was 27.45 kg/m^2 and in men, 25.47 kg/m^2.[8] This study also noted that about 32% of people with diabetes are unaware of their diagnosis and that diabetes and IGT were more common among women than in men. Diabetes and IGT were higher in urban than rural subjects. Multiple logistic regression analysis indicated that increasing age, BMI, waist-to-hip ratio (WHR), hypertension, and familial diabetes in both sexes, education in men, and living in the south in women were associated with diabetes.[8]

The prevalence of central obesity based on the WHR was 19% but when calculated according to waist girth, it was 34%. Central obesity was defined as WHR ≥1.0 in men and ≥0.85 in women or waist girth in women ≥88 cm and in men ≥102 cm. The mean waist girth and WHR in the survey population were 87.20 cm and 0.81 in women and 90.03 cm and 0.88 in men, respectively.[8] The overall frequency of hypertension was 29%, hypertension being defined as systolic blood pressure ≥140 mmHg and diastolic blood pressure ≥90 mmHg.[8]

About 12 years after TURDEP-I, the Turkish Epidemiology Survey of Diabetes, Hypertension, Obesity and Endocrine Disease (TURDEP-II) was conducted in the same 540 centers covered in the previous survey. TURDEP-II included 26,499 randomly sampled adults aged 20 years and older.[10] In this survey, the crude prevalence of diabetes was 16.5% (if the same diagnostic definition at the time of the TURDEP-I was applied, diabetes prevalence was estimated at 11.4%). 45.5% of the survey population had newly diagnosed diabetes and 54.5%, previously known diabetes. The crude prevalence of prediabetes was 30.8% (isolated-impaired fasting glucose (IFG), isolated-IGT, and combined IFG+IGT were 14.7%, 7.9%, and 8.2% respectively). As in TURDEP-I, diabetes was more common in women than men and in the urban than the rural populations. In both sexes, age, BMI, and hypertension, and additionally in women, low education and living environment were independently associated with an increased prevalence of diabetes.[10]

36% of the survey population was obese and another 37% overweight (defined as BMI between 25-29.9 kg/m^2). The mean BMI was 29.2 kg/m^2 in women and 27.4 kg/m^2 in men. The prevalence of central obesity based on waist girth was 54%. Obesity and central obesity were more common in women than men, whereas being overweight, was more prevalent among men. The mean waist girth and WHR in the survey population were 92.8 cm and 0.85 in women and 97.1 cm and 0.92 in men.[10] Compared to TURDEP-I, the rate of increase for diabetes was 90%, IGT 106%, obesity 40%, and central obesity 35%. During the past 12 years, mean height increased by 1 cm in both sexes while weight increased by 6 kg in women and 8 kg in men, waist circumference increased by 6 cm in women and 7 cm in men, and hip circumference increased by 7 cm in women and 3 cm in men.[10]

According to the results of the prospective TEKHARF study based on the cohort followed from screening during 1997-98 until 2004-05, diabetes prevalence in Turkey was estimated at 11% of the population aged ≥35 years, with an incidence of 11.7 expressed per 1,000 person-years. This corresponded to an annual incidence of 300,000. A peak was reached in the age group 60-69 years with a prevalence of 20%, after which it declined to 15%. There were no significant differences between both sexes. While Southeast Anatolia and the Black Sea regions had above-average prevalences, Eastern Anatolia and the Aegean regions exhibited the lowest prevalence.[11] The data demonstrate that the diabetes growth rate in Turkey is higher than that in Europe and has already exceeded projections for 2030. The situation is the same for IGT as shown in Tables 3 and 4.[12,13] The main factors for this include the growing percentage of the elderly population and lifestyle changes, in particular eating habits and physical activity levels.

No surveys exist that investigated the incidence of Type 1 diabetes (T1D) on a national scale. The incidence of T1D in Turkey among

Table 3. Diabetes cases in 2000 and projections for 2030 in the WHO European Region and Turkey.[12]

	2000	2030
Europe	33,332,000	47,973,000
Turkey	2,920,000	6,422,000

Source: WHO. (http://www.who.int/diabetes/facts/world_figures/en/index4.html).

Table 4. Estimate for diabetes prevalence in 2011 and projection for 2030 in Turkey.[13]

	2011	2030
Diabetes cases	3,502,270	5,920,810
DM national prevalence	7.40%	9.5%
DM comparative prevalence(WHO standard)	8.12%	8.09%
IGT cases	3,161,700	4,833,090
IGT national prevalence	6.68%	7.79%
IGT comparative prevalence (WHO standard)	7.07%	6.99%

Source: *IDF Diabetes Atlas*. 5th Edition. International Diabetes Federation, 2011. (http://www.idf.org/atlasmap/atlasmap).

children aged 0-14 years is estimated at 3.2 per 100,000 children in 2009.[14] In Istanbul, the reported prevalence of T1DM is 0.67/1,000. According to this study, the prevalence of T1D in primary, secondary, and high schools were 0.46/1,000 vs 0.16/1,000, 0.57/1,000 vs 0.34/1,000, and 0.92/1,000 vs 0.69/1,000, respectively.[15] A recently published study carried out in Diyarbakir, one of the largest cities in the south-east region of Turkey, the overall annual incidence of T1D was reported as $7.2/10^5$ in the 1–14 year age group.[16]

2.4. Chronic Complications and Mortality

In the Turkish Diabetes Chronic Complications Trial, carried out in 27 diabetes centers in Turkey, the mean duration of diabetes was 9.8 years in the group with T1D ($n = 213$) and the HbA1c = 9.6%; the same parameters were 9.9 years and 8.5% in patients with T2D ($n = 1876$). In T1D and

T2D patients, the prevalence of neuropathy was 30.4% vs 48.1% and for retinopathy, 28.5% vs 31.5%, respectively.[17]

A cross-sectional observational study was carried out in 44 centers in Turkey to determine the level of glycemic control. A total of 2358 adult patients with diabetes who were treated for at least 3 months were included. The majority of patients had T2D (94%). The mean age was 55.7 ± 12.1 years. Patients had been diagnosed with diabetes for 9.1 years, and were treated for 6.9 years. In total, 69% had HbA1c ≥7% and the mean HbA1c level was 8.0%, 42.7% were obese, and 39.7% overweight. Dyslipidemia and hypertension were present in 77% and 88% of subjects, respectively. A total of 49.7% of patients reported paresthesias and 26.6% the presence of retinopathy.[18]

A multicenter, cross-sectional study revealed that the prevalence of retinopathy was 31% among 2362 subjects from 14 centers. In patients diagnosed under the age of 30 years, 31% of those with T1D and 28% of those with T2D had diabetic retinopathy. In those diagnosed at or older than 30 years of age, the same parameters were 51% and 23%, respectively. In patients diagnosed under the age of 30 years, the longer duration of diabetes and male gender were identified as important risk factors.[19] The prevalence of diabetic retinopathy was higher in a study carried out in a Diabetes Outpatient Clinic in Istanbul (42.8%) in 1,702 patients with mean duration of diabetes of 9.6 years.[20]

The IDF Diabetes Atlas of 2013 reports that globally 5.1 million deaths are attributable to diabetes in the population aged 20–79 years. The estimate for Turkey is 59,786.[21] According to the Turkey Burden of Disease Study 2004, diabetes ranks eighth, with 2.2% among the number of deaths by major disease groups. By gender, diabetes is the 8th leading cause of death in men and 7th in women. With regard to the burden of mortality, of twenty leading diseases by gender, diabetes ranks 16th in men and 8th in women in years of life lost (YLL).[22]

2.5. Economic Burden

Diabetes imposes a large economic burden on individuals, national health care systems, and countries. According to the Diabetes Atlas data, an estimated average of USD 866 per person with diabetes was spent on treating and managing the disease in Turkey in 2013.[21] According to the findings of the DiabCost study that was conducted in Turkey in 1993, the direct annual cost of an individual with diabetes who experiences no complications approximates USD 400 whereas the cost estimate is 4 times as much for those with the presence of complications.[23]

3. NATIONAL DIABETES PREVENTION INITIATIVES

3.1. St. Vincent Declaration in 1989 and Istanbul Commitment in 1999

A major European initiative for the fight against diabetes was started in St Vincent, Italy, and a meeting was organized during October 10-12, 1989 with the participation of representatives from government health departments and patients' organizations from 52 member European countries meeting with diabetes experts under the aegis of the WHO Regional Offices for Europe and the International Diabetes Federation (IDF), European region. Objectives were agreed upon to offer a high quality of life to patients with diabetes and to minimize diabetes-related complications, with the eventual signing of the St. Vincent Declaration. All countries signing the declaration formally pledged themselves to achieve the goals set in the Declaration, to develop their national diabetes programs and to take decisive action in implementing this program. Turkey signed the declaration in 1991.

At the 10th Anniversary Meeting of the St. Vincent Declaration in Istanbul in 1999, a follow-up meeting was organized to review the progress made. All stakeholders associated with diabetes, representatives of governments of all European countries, representatives of WHO, EURO, and IDF Europe declared that the current situation was distant from achieving the goals set in the St. Vincent Declaration. Turkey and other European countries and the diabetes associations re-committed themselves to taking urgent and decisive action, to set local achievable goals, and to establish targets towards common high standards of care for people with diabetes.[24]

3.2. Diabetes Prevention and Control Programs of the Ministry of Health

The Ministry of Health has been implementing the Health Transformation Program since 2003 and radical changes have occurred both in the provision and financing of health care services. Health promotion and public health education activities are mainly the responsibility of the Ministry of Health's General Directorate of Primary Health Care Services. The General Directorate of Primary Health Care Services develops policies and prepares plans for public health education activities on preventive health services and prevention of obesity and chronic diseases, among others.[25] Diabetes, Hypertension and Obesity Centers were established as pilots and studies have been started for regulating Diabetes Centers.

Turkey signed "the European Charter on Counteracting Obesity" at the WHO European Ministerial Conference on Counteracting Obesity which was held in Istanbul in 2006 and "the European Heart Health Charter" in 2007. In 2008, the Ministry of Health put into practice the "Prevention and Control Program for Cardiovascular Disease in Turkey, Strategic Plan and Action Plan for the Risk Factors" which is an integrated, community-based program focused on three main risk factors: tobacco, obesity, and physical activity.[4,26]

"Obesity Prevention and Control Program of Turkey" was prepared with the aim of strengthening the intersectoral actions for the prevention of obesity. An Action Plan for 2010–2014 has been prepared which provides political will and determination at national and local levels, informing the public of preventive health services regarding obesity, adequate and balanced diet, physical activity, diagnosing and treating obesity, and monitoring studies in this domain.[4]

3.2.1. *Diabetes Prevention and Control Program*

In response to findings that diabetes has been growing beyond initial projections, the Ministry of Health in 2009 has started to develop an updated strategy to combat diabetes risk factors and complications. On April 17, 2009, an Advisory Council Meeting was held, presided over by the Undersecretary of Health, where the basic operational framework was set for the "Preparatory

Workshop for Diabetes Prevention and Control Program of Turkey Action Plan." A workshop was held in Ankara during February 15-20, 2010, in two phases, three days each, involving a total of 16 working groups. On March 9, 2010, the program was developed in Ankara during the "Diabetes Prevention and Control Program of Turkey Review Meeting."[23]

The "Diabetes Prevention and Control Program Action Plan (2011-2014)" was launched in 2011.[23] The objective of the plan was to ensure early diagnosis and treatment of diabetes — an important source of mortality and burden of disease — while raising public awareness of the risk factors and reducing the frequency of diabetic complications to WHO target levels for a healthier life in Turkey. Integrated community-based programs for preventing chronic diseases constitute a significant component of the diabetes prevention and control program. The plan covers risk factors and their prevention, organization, work force planning and education, rehabilitation, treatment and home care, surveillance and research, funding and inter-sectoral collaboration, and prospective considerations for diabetes prevention and control.[23]

Goals include public education about diabetes, undertaking initiatives to drive permanent behavioral changes towards risk factors, early diagnosis of diabetes and preventing its progression, effective treatment, prevention of diabetic complications, rehabilitative services for diabetes, and, through effective surveillance, ensuring that individuals enjoy a high quality of life.[23]

The Prevention and Control Program of Cardiovascular Diseases, Obesity Prevention and Control Program, Diabetes, Prevention and Control Program executed by the Ministry of Health are of considerable significance in terms of being society-based programs and representing crucial milestones for protecting public health. Accomplishments of these programs require the support and coordinated efforts of all sectors and organizations.

3.3. Program for Improving Multisectoral Health Responsibility

As of 2011, the "Program for Improving Multisectoral Health Responsibility" was started through a protocol concluded between the Ministry of Health and University of Duzce and with the support of the Ministry of Development. The aims of the program are to mobilize parties through a multisectoral health responsibility approach and to strengthen public health functions. The program is composed of 13 components with "Food Safety and Healthy Nutrition" and "Improving the Management of Non-Communicable Diseases" among them. The "Food Safety and Healthy Nutrition" component aims to ensure healthy nutrition by achieving water and food safety, improving the quality of staple foods and water, and raising awareness of consumers through evidence-based data. One of the focus areas of the "Improving the Management of Non-Communicable Diseases" component is to develop evidence-based, cost-effective multisectoral health interventions for the prevention, early diagnosis, treatment, and rehabilitation of chronic diseases.[27]

In its Strategic Plan 2013–2017, the Ministry of Health, set as an objective in the area of multisectoral health "to take effective action on social determinants of health by centralizing health into all policies."[28]

3.4. Diabetes and Prevention Programs of Non-governmental Organizations (NGOs)

3.4.1. *Southeastern Anatolia Diabetes Support Project — GAPDIAB*

Elevated diabetes prevalence was observed in Southeastern Anatolia.[8,11] Social factors including difficulties in availability and accessibility to health care, economic difficulties compared to other regions, migration from peripheral settlements to big cities all have a negative influence on chronic conditions like diabetes. These circumstances led to the development of a regional project, Southeastern Anatolia Diabetes Support Project (GAPDIAB) which was launched in November 2000.

The project, a civilian initiative coordinated by the Turkish Diabetes Foundation, brought together more than 30 institutions (including six regional Universities) and organizations (including the Turkish Medical Association, Diabetes Nursing Association, Turkish Dietetic Association, Turkish Pharmacists Association, and others). The project was also supported by the Ministry of Health.

The overarching targets of the project were:

- Diabetes patient education
- Update on diabetes care and treatment for HCPs (physicians, nurses, and dieticians) with courses and meetings

- Raising public awareness about diabetes and organization of public meetings and wide distribution of informative materials
- Establishment of Insulin Support Units (ISU) to meet the insulin need of patients under the age of 18 years who are not covered by the social security system

Local Coordination Boards have been established to carry out these activities in their provinces.

The principal importance of this project was that diabetes was put on the agenda in this region as an important public health issue. The number of Diabetes Centers and their annual capacity have increased. Besides, physicians, nurses, and dieticians participated in the courses. A close collaboration was established between regional universities, other hospitals and stakeholders in the region. Diabetes patients organizations have been established in several cities as individual organizations or mostly as branches of the nationwide "Living With Diabetes Association." This project may serve as a good model for the implementation of the St. Vincent Declaration.[29–31]

Other regional projects followed including the Cukurova Diabetes Support Project (CUKUROVADIAB) launched in 2002 and the Eastern Anatolia Diabetes Support Project (DOGUDIAB) in 2003.

3.4.2. *Diabetes 2020: Vision and Targets — Turkey Project*

In spite all of the efforts, Turkey was among the countries which did not have a National Diabetes Plan to combat diabetes until 2009. In 2009, 24 non-governmental organizations came together for the "Diabetes 2020: Vision and Targets — Turkey" (referred to as D2020) to develop a national diabetes strategy. D2020 aims to evaluate problems and suggest solutions regarding prevention, care, and follow-up of diabetes and related complications, and to develop a roadmap to reach specific targets by 2020 with a multidisciplinary and participatory process. D2020 is carried out under the auspices of the Ministry of Health and coordinated by the Turkish Diabetes Foundation. The WHO, EURO, and the IDF Europe supported this project and were represented on the International Advisory Board.[32]

Working Groups were established by the representatives of the governmental and non-governmental stakeholders. The project is planned in three phases. A workshop on the "Current Situation and Problems in Diabetes" was organized in 2009. Another workshop focused on "Fighting against Diabetes in Turkey, Targets for the year 2020 and Development of Strategies" was held in 2010. The discussions and recommendations of the relevant working groups were comprehensively documented after each workshop.[5,32,33]

A final report including the roadmap was published in December, 2010.[34,35] D2020 as a civil initiative, served as a resource and gave support to studies of the "National Diabetes Prevention and Control Program" which has been launched by the Ministry of Health.[23] The third phase of the project is the yearly follow-up of implementation of programs, achievements, and the emerging problems between the years 2011 and 2020. The follow-up reports are a source of reference and in this way contribute to the effectiveness of the programs.

D2020 is a new approach which may serve as a model for strengthening the fight against diabetes. The civil platform established in this model supports government institutions for the development and implementation of National Diabetes Programs and ensures the maintenance of an independent follow-up mechanism in the process. This will contribute to the development of more effective methods for solving problems.

3.4.3. *Diabetes Parliaments*

Diabetes Parliaments bring together all diabetes stakeholders and provides the opportunity to directly communicate problems and concerns with the decision-makers — the Presidency of the Republic of Turkey, Parliament Members from the Commission of Health, Family, Labor and Social Affairs of the Grand National Assembly of the Republic of Turkey, the Ministry of Health, and other governmental institutions. The Diabetes Parliaments, coordinated by the Turkish Diabetes Foundation, has been convening regularly since 2011. After each session, the discussions about diabetes prevention policies, health care services, patients' rights, accessibility and availability of medicines and medical devices, discrimination against people with diabetes, and improvements since the last Diabetes Parliament are comprehensively published.[36–38] In this way, the Diabetes Parliaments serves also as a civil initiative to follow-up and contribute to the success of implementing the national diabetes policies.

3.4.4. *Diabetes in School Program*

The prevalence of obesity in the 6-16 year age group has increased from 5% to 10.5% (16.3% in the high-income group) in the last 8 years in Turkey.[39]

The Turkish Diabetes Foundation and Living With Diabetes Association, a nationwide patients' organization, in 2004 surveyed 100 schools in Istanbul to investigate the type of foods served in the canteens, and the time allocated for breakfast and/or lunch. The results were submitted to the Ministry of National Education and the Ministry of Health. Chips and fast foods, chocolates, and sugar-sweetened beverages were available in all school canteens but milk was sold only in 45% of them and salad in only 3.4%. In primary schools, a lunch break of 45–60 minutes was allocated in 63% of those surveyed whereas in secondary schools, 78% reported lunch breaks of 30–45 minutes.[40]

In order to prevent obesity in adulthood, healthy choices and physical activity should become part of "lifestyle in childhood and puberty. The survey results were not promising for the future. In December 2007 and March 2008, the Ministry of National Education issued two circulars followed by the last in July 2011 in order to regulate food and beverages sold in school canteens.[41,42] In 2010, the Turkish Pediatric Endocrinology and Diabetes Society in cooperation with the Ministry of National Education and Ministry of Health started the Diabetes Program at School.

The objectives of this program are:

- Raise school community and teacher awareness about T1D and ensure early diagnosis of T1D and decrease frequency of diabetic ketoacidosis,
- Provide better care for children with diabetes
- Create a healthy nutrition attitude among school children
- Raise awareness about obesity

In 2011, a one-day training meeting was organized across Turkey, which included teachers, government officials, and pediatric diabetes and obesity experts. By the end of 2011, over 7.5 million students, and nearly 600,000 teachers were trained in 25,000 schools. To the credit of the program, 30 teachers who had undergone diabetes training helped detect diabetes in 40 children.[39]

3.4.5. *"Balanced Nutrition" Education Project*

This Program was started by the Sabri Ulker Food Research Institute Foundation in collaboration with the Ministry of Education's Elementary Schools General Directorate and carried out under the auspices of the Ministry of Education. The aim is to develop healthy nutritional habits in children at the primary school level and thus contribute to their mental and physical well-being in the long-term. School children aged 8-10 years, their parents, and teachers fall within the scope of this project.

"Training for Teachers" was realized as the first step of the project. Teachers are also provided "Balanced Nutrition" materials (presentations, messages, handbook, handouts, and booklets). The project is carried out in pilot schools on a "weekly one hour" basis throughout the school year for a total of 32 hours. The project assessment is done through a "self-check" questionnaire. The project has reached 20,000 students in 2011-2012 and 400,000 students in the 2012-2013 school years. The aim is to reach 1,000,000 school children and their families by the end of the 2013-2014 school term.[43]

3.4.6. *'Let's Stop Diabetes!' Project*

The Turkish Diabetes Foundation carried out a Diabetes Awareness Survey in 1000 people over the age of 18 years in 81 provinces from all regions in Turkey. According to its results, diabetes awareness is 37% among the population, and 17% of participants stated that there was at least one person with diabetes at home. These results led to a new strategic approach to this problem. In 2011, the nationwide "Let's Stop Diabetes!" Project has been started under the auspices of the Presidency of the Turkish Republic and coordinated by the Turkish Diabetes Foundation. The objectives of this project is to promote a healthy lifestyle in all living spaces during the next 3 years. This is organized as a modular project, each focusing on one target group: pregnant women/women planning pregnancy, school children, university students, people at work, families, general public, and people with diabetes.

Several programs are run under each module, the main components of which are:

- Awareness and educational programs for promoting a healthy lifestyle,
- Programs for promoting physical activity and regular sports,
- Activities for the nationwide improvement of dialogue between patients with diabetes and strengthening patients' organizations.

"Diabetes Education Delivered by Peer Advisers — DAKE" is one of the main programs in this module.[44–46]

3.4.7. *Diabetes Education Delivered by Peer Advisers: DAKE*

From the time of diagnosis, patients with diabetes should take responsibility for and be actively engaged in the management of their disease. Therefore, diabetes education has to be delivered not only at the time of diagnosis but must be continued throughout an individual's lifetime. It is debatable whether health services have or will ever have a large enough workforce to cope with the demands related to the explosion in the number of people with diabetes. Questions remain about the potential for widespread implementation and maintenance of care, despite the promise offered by diabetes education programs. Therefore, involving peer advisers in diabetes education could complement services provided by health care professionals.

The DAKE program is designed to reach people with diabetes via peer educators within 3 years starting in November 2011 in 23 Turkish cities. The program carried out under the auspices of the Presidency of the Turkish Republic and coordinated by the Turkish Diabetes Foundation is supported by the World Diabetes Foundation and has reached more than 15,000 people thus far. Aside from diabetes education and optimizing outcomes, the goals of this project are to increase locally the social relations between patients, and establish or strengthen patients' organizations which will, at the end, serve to place diabetes on the agenda and raise awareness to the public.[45,46] The project, in light of its focus on self-management and peer involvement, has the potential to demonstrate a relevant approach towards realizing progress in the achievement of health care objectives in relation not only to diabetes, but to other chronic conditions as well.

3.5. Diabetes Guide

In Turkey, the Health Transformation Program has been implemented since 2003. Strengthening primary health care and coodination with family medicine are priorities for this program.[2]

Both the Turkish Diabetes Foundation and the Society of Endocrinology and Metabolism of Turkey have published a diabetes guide.[47–49] These guidelines have been widely distributed in Turkey. Also, meetings are organized in collaboration with the primary care organization in Turkey, and coordinated by the Turkish Diabetes Foundation.

4. THE FUTURE OF DIABETES PREVENTION IN TURKEY

The implementation of the Diabetes Prevention and Control Program with support from governmental and non-governmental institutions in order to reach the following targets — as mentioned in the Program — is very important for the future of diabetes prevention in Turkey.[23]

Goal 1. Educating both healthy and at-risk individuals on diabetes prevention, and raising their awareness level.

Action Steps

1. Develop standardized “Diabetes Education Modules” for use in healthy lifestyle programs aimed at various societal strata, mainly high-risk groups.
2. Identify and educate the population at-risk for developing diabetes.
3. As part of raising public awareness, identify appropriate role models for diabetes (e.g., political leaders, opinion leaders, scientists, artists, members of the media) and hold campaigns to communicate specific messages to the public through these role models using catch-phrases.
4. Hold health promotion events using visual and audio aids.

5. Use both printed and visual media effectively to raise awareness in the public, particularly among at-risk groups.
6. Raise public awareness of gestational diabetes and improve collaboration with other health care specialists.
7. Educate pregnant women who are at risk of developing diabetes using a monitoring program (Pregnancy Risk Monitoring Program).
8. Publish and regularly update a webpage for Diabetes Prevention and Control Program of Turkey on the Ministry of Health website.

Goal 2. Advocating inclusion of more and effective education on diabetes and prevention in formal curricula on healthy living.

Action Steps

1. Advocate inclusion of diabetes in healthy living programs, in social studies and science textbooks in primary education.
2. Promote active participation of students in World Diabetes Day activities.
3. Encourage students to take part in community activities on diabetes.
4. Develop educational aides for diabetes at schools.

Goal 3. Instilling and sustaining lifelong adequate and balanced diets, regular physical activity, and preventing obesity.

Action Steps

Effectively implement the "Healthy Nutrition and Physical Activity Program of Turkey (2010–2014)" which sets forth the goals and strategies for combating obesity.

Goal 4. Preventing risk of developing diabetes in the prediabetic population.

Action Steps

1. Create a suitable environment for individuals with IFG and IGT to join Lifestyle Programs (LSPs) for weight control and regular physical exercise.
2. Support pharmaceutical treatment of persons who have combined glucose intolerance (CGI) and additional risk factors as an adjunct to LSP.
3. Implement a Pregnancy Risk Monitoring Program to prepare women (for pregnancy) with pregestational diabetes.

Goal 5. Ensuring early detection of diabetes.

Action Steps

1. Integrate descriptors in the Family Practice Information System (FPIS) and Hospital Information System (HIS) to identify persons with prediabetes, and ensure collection of descriptor information on a regular basis.
2. Create relevant screening programs.
3. Ensure that pregnant women diagnosed with GDM are evaluated for permanent diabetes at week 6 after delivery, and followed up thereafter on a yearly basis (Postpartum Care Protocol).

5. CONCLUSION

Diabetes is a growing health concern in Turkey beyond what has been predicted. To reverse the alarming rise in diabetes, we have to combat the lifestyle evolved in the 21st century. We strongly believe that much has been done in recent years to fight diabetes and yet, much more needs to be done.

We should be empowering individuals to make healthy choices. Aside from regulatory and/or legislational policies, we should be innovative in finding ways to promote a healthy lifestyle — healthy eating and engaging in physical activity — in order to change established habits.

This can only be achieved by political commitment and implementation through the collaboration of governmental institutions with non-governmental stakeholders, an effort which should not only be maintained but also strengthened. Non-governmental institutions serve not only to increase awareness about diabetes and implementation of programs but also to follow-up the process which will contribute to its success.

REFERENCES

1. Republic of Turkey, Turkish Statistical Institute, TurkStat. Demographic structure of Turkey and its future, 2010–2050. Press Release No: 13140 (11.07.2012) (http://www.turkstat.gov.tr/PreHaberBultenleri.do?id=13140).
2. World Health Organization Regional Office for Europe. Turkey Health System Performance Assessment 2011, Executive Report. World Health

Organization, 2012 (http://www.euro.who.int/en/health-topics/Health-systems/health-systems-governance/publications/2012/turkey-health-system-performance-assessment-2011).

3. World Health Organization Regional Office for Europe. Core health indicators in the WHO European Region 2013. Special focus: Noncommunicable diseases. (http://www.euro.who.int/__data/assets/pdf_file/0005/172724/Core-Health-Indicators-in-the-WHO-European-Region-2012-Eng.pdf).
4. Ministry of Health of Turkey, General Directorate of Primary Health Care, Obesity Prevention and Control Program of Turkey (2010–2014). Publish Number 773. Ankara, Turkey. Kuban Matbaacılık Yayıncılık, 2010 (http://www.beslenme.gov.tr/content/files/home/obesity_prevention_and_control_program_of_turkey_2010_2014.pdf).
5. Diyabet 2020: Vizyon ve Hedefler-Türkiye. Türkiye'de Diyabet Profili. Diyabet bakım, izlem ve tedavisinde mevcut durum değerlendirmesi. Çalıştay Raporu, 2009.
6. Turkish Statistical Institute. Health Survey 2012. Publication Number 4117. Turkish Statistical Institute, Ankara, 2013.
7. World Health Organization. Global Health Observatory Data Repository. Physical inactivity: Physical inactivity by country (http://apps.who.int/gho/data/node.main.A893?lang=en).
8. Satman I, Yilmaz T, Sengül A *et al.* (2002) The TURDEP Group. Population-based study of diabetes and risk characteristics in Turkey. *Diabetes Care* **25**: 1551–1556.
9. King H, Aubert RE, Herman WH. (1998) Global burden of diabetes, 1995–2025. Prevalence, numerical estimates, and projections. *Diabetes Care* **21**: 1414–1431.
10. Satman I, Omer B, Tutuncu Y *et al.* (2013) Twelve-year trends in the prevalence and risk factors of diabetes and prediabetes in Turkish adults. *Eur J Epidemiol* **28**: 169–180.
11. Onat A, Hergenc G, Uyarel H, Can G, Ozhan H. (2006) Prevalence, incidence, predictors and outcome of type 2 diabetes in Turkey. *Anadolu Kardiyol Derg* **6**: 314–321.
12. World Health Organization. Country and regional data on diabetes. (http://www.who.int/diabetes/facts/world_figures/en/index4.html).
13. *IDF Diabetes Atlas*. 5th Edition. International Diabetes Federation, 2011 (http://www.idf.org/atlasmap/atlasmap).
14. *IDF Diabetes Atlas*, 4th Edition. International Diabetes Federation, 2009.
15. Akesen E, Turan S, Güran T, Atay Z, Save D, Bereket A. (2011) Prevalence of type 1 diabetes mellitus in 6–18-yr-old school children living in Istanbul, Turkey. *Pediatric Diabetes* **12**: 567–571.

16. Demirbilek H, Özbek MN, Baran RT. (2013) Incidence of type 1 diabetes mellitus in Turkish children from the Southeastern Region of the country: A regional report. *J Clin Res Pediatr Endocrinol* **5**: 98–103.
17. Yılmaz MT, Karadeniz Ş, Sargın M, Büyükbeşe A, and the Turkish Diabetes Chronic Complications Study Group. Chronic complications in longterm type 1 and type 2 diabetic patients with comparable duration of diabetes and poor glycemic control: Turkish Diabetes Chronic Complications Trial — TUDIC results 1. The World Congress on Controversies in Obesity, Diabetes and Hypertension (CODHy). 26–29 October 2006, Berlin, Germany. Program and Abstracts 54-A, 2006
18. Oğuz A, Gedik O, Hatemi H *et al.* (2008) Glycemic control of Turkish adult diabetic patients. *Turk JEM* **12**: 50–54.
19. Taş A, Bayraktar M, Erdem Ü *et al.* (2005) Diyabetik hastalarda retinopati sıklığı ve risk faktörleri. *Gulhane Med J* **47**: 164–174.
20. Karadeniz ZS, Yilmaz MT. (2007) Duration of diabetes and prevalence of diabetic retinopathy: Istanbul Diabetic Retinopathy-IDRS results 1. Diabetes & Metabolic Syndrome. *Clin Res Rev* **1**: 43–48.
21. *IDF Diabetes Atlas*. 6th Edition. International Diabetes Federation, 2013 (http://www.idf.org/diabetesatlas).
22. Ministry of Health, Refik Saydam Hygiene Center, School of Health. Turkey burden of disease study 2004. MoH Publication No: 701. SPH Publication No: SB-HM-2007/11. Aydoğdu Ofset Matbaacılık San. Ve Tic. Ltd. Şti., Ankara 2007 (http://ekutuphane.tusak.gov.tr/kitaplar/turkey_burden_of_disease_study.pdf).
23. Turkish Republic, Ministry of Health, General Directorate of Primary Health Services. Diabetes Prevention and Control Program. Action Plan (2011/2014). Ministry of Health Publication No 816. Ankara 2011.
24. St.Vincent Declaration and Istanbul Commitment (http://www.idf.org/regions/EUR/landmarkdocuments).
25. Tatar M, Mollahaliloğlu S, Şahin B, Aydın S, Maresso A, Hernandez-Quevedo C. (2011) Turkey: Health system review. *Health Systems in Transition* **13**: 1–186. (http://www.euro.who.int/__data/assets/pdf_file/0006/158883/e96441.pdf).
26. Turkey Health Transformation Program Evaluation Report (2003–2010). Ed. R. Akdağ. T.C.Sağlık Bakanlığı Yayın No: 839. 2011 (http://ekutuphane.tusak.gov.tr/kitaplar/turkey_health_transformation_program_evaluation_report_(2003_2010).pdf).
27. Ministry of Health. Implementing Health 2020: Strengthening multisectoral-responsibility for health in Turkey. Background paper for Technical Briefing, WHO Europe 63rd Regional Committee, Çeşme, İzmir, Turkey. 2013 (https://euro.sharefile.com/download.aspx?id=sfa097437524481eb).

28. Ministry of Health of Turkey. "Health for all..." Strategic Plan 2013–2017. Ministry of Health Publication No:896, 2012 (http://sbu.saglik.gov.tr/Ekutuphane/kitaplar/stratejikplaning.pdf).
29. Yilmaz MT. (2001). Turkey responds to St. Vincent. *Diabetes Voice* **46**: 32–33.
30. Southeastern Anatolia Diabetes Project GAPDIAB. Turkish Diabetes Foundation, 2011.
31. Southeastern Anatolia Diabetes Project GAPDIAB. First Activity Report. Turkish Diabetes Foundation, 2011.
32. Diabetes 2020. Vision and Targets-Turkey. Executive Summary. Turkish Diabetes Foundation, 2011.
33. Diyabet 2020: Vizyon ve Hedefler-Türkiye. Türkiye'de Diyabette Çözüm Yolları. Çalıştay Raporu 2010. Türkiye Diyabet Vakfı, 2010.
34. Diyabet 2020: Vizyon ve Hedefler-Türkiye. 2010–2020 Ulusal Diyabet Stratejisi, Sonuç Dokümanı. Türkiye Diyabet Vakfı, 2010.
35. "Diabetes 2020". International Diabetes Federation-Europe. The European Diabetes Newsletter 2011, No 21, 2011, p.5 (http://www.idf.org/webdata/docs/idf-europe/IDF%20E%20Newsletter%2021%200.pdf).
36. Diyabet Parlamentosu. Birinci Oturum. Diyabetli Hasta Hakları. 19 Kasım 2011. Türkiye Diyabet Vakfı, 2011.
37. Diyabet Parlamentosu. İkinci Oturum. Diyabetli Hasta Hakları. 24 Mart 2012. Türkiye Diyabet Vakfı, 2012.
38. Diyabet Parlamentosu. Üçüncü Oturum. Türkiye Büyük Millet Meclisi. 14 Kasım 2012. Türkiye Diyabet Vakfı, 2012.
39. Hatun S, Özcan Ş. (2013). National programme in Turkey. Diabetes at School. *Diabetes Voice* **58**: 21–23.
40. Diyabetle Yaşam Dergisi. Türkiye Diyabet Vakfı, 2004.
41. T.C.Milli Eğitim Bakanlığı İç Denetim Birimi Başkanlığı. Okul Kantinleri Süreci İç Denetim Raporu. 28 Aralık 2010–2010/11 (http://icden.meb.gov.tr/digeryaziler/Okul_Kantinleri_ic_denetim_2010_11.pdf).
42. Republic of Turkey, Ministry of National Education. (http://mevzuat.meb.gov.tr/html/1782_41.html).
43. "Yemekte Denge". Sabri Ülker Dıda Araştırma Enstitüsü Vakfı. (http://www.yemektedenge.com).
44. "Let's stop diabetes". International Diabetes Federation-Europe. The European Diabetes Newsletter 2011, No 22, 2011, p.6 (http://www.idf.org/sites/default/files/idf-europe/IDF%20E%20Newsletter%2022%20f.pdf).
45. Diyabeti Durduralım. Birinci Yıl 2012. Türkiye Diyabet Vakfı, 2013.

46. Diyabeti Durduralım. İkinci Yıl 2013. Türkiye Diyabet Vakfı, 2013.
47. Ulusal Diyabet Kongresi Konsensus Grubu. Diyabet Tanı ve Tedavi Rehberi. Güncellenmiş Yeni Baskı. Türkiye Diyabet Vakfı yayını. Portakal Basım Matbaacılık San. Tic. Ltd.Şti, 2011.
48. Ulusal Diyabet Kongresi Konsensus Grubu. Diyabet Tanı ve Tedavi Rehberi. Üçüncü Baskı. Türkiye Diyabet Vakfı yayını. Armoni Nüans Baskı Sanatları, 2013.
49. Türkiye Endokrinoloji ve Metabolizma Derneği. Diabetes mellitus ve komplikasyonlarının tanı, tedavi ve izlem kılavuzu-2013. Yenilenmiş 6. Baskı. Miki Matbaacılık ve San. Tic. Ltd. Şti., Ankara, 2013.

Chapter 19: Prediabetes and Diabetes Prevention Initiatives in Siberia, Russia

Mikhail Voevoda[*,†,‡,††], *Olga Sazonova*[‡], *Galina Simonova*[†], *Yuri Nikitin*[†], *Eugene Shubnikov*[†], *Diana Denisova*[†], *Marina Fomicheva*[†,§] *and Elena Dergacheva*[§]

1. INTRODUCTION

Russia is a huge country with territory which can fit several other countries. Russia has a common health policy and health care system but various regions of Russia may have different regional diabetes prevention programs details of which are not always known. We cannot describe all of these in this chapter, however, we will be able to reflect and present initiatives of the Russian government and the Ministry of Health of Russia in diabetes prevention. We will describe the detailed initiatives in Siberia, the Eastern part of Russia. Incidentally, the first diabetes prevention programs, the World Health Organization's (WHO) first population-based studies in Russia and first children's diabetes epidemiologic surveys in Russia were conducted in Eastern Russia — in the City of Novosibirsk. A diabetes registry was organized with the assistance of Dr. Jaakko Tuomilehto in 1989 and a diabetes prevention program is on-going with the collaboration of Dr. Peter Schwarz.

[*] Corresponding author. Email: mvoevoda@ya.ru

[†] Federal State Budgetary Institution "Institute of Internal and Preventive Medicine" of the Federal Agency of Scientific Organizations (IIPM FASO), Novosibirsk, Russia.

[‡] Novosibirsk State Medical University, Russia.

[§] State Public Novosibirsk Region Health Agency "Regional Centre for Medical Prevention", Russia.

[††] Novosibirsk State University, Russia.

The Asian part of Russia comprises 2/3 of the Russian Federation and its population approximates 26 million people. In addition to the Caucasoid population, Siberia is home to more than 30 predominantly Mongoloid aboriginal ethnic groups which include the Yakuts, Buryats, Tuvinians, Chukchi, Altay and several other small nationalities. Although the information is fragmentary, the prevalence of diabetes mellitus (DM) in Siberia based on available data, especially in its eastern segment, is lower than in the European portion of the country. Among the indigenous Mongoloid population, the prevalence of diabetes and its risk factors, including the metabolic syndrome, is lower than that of Caucasoid inhabitants of Siberia.

2. PREVALENCE OF DIABETES IN SIBERIA

Data on the prevalence of DM (number of individuals with DM per 100,000 individuals) in all administrative regions of Siberia and the Far East in 2008 is presented in Fig. 1. The highest levels of DM morbidity recorded are in the south-western regions of Siberia, in the Omsk and Novosibirsk regions and the Altai Territory and accordingly, among the Far East regions, in Magadan, the Jewish Autonomous Region, and the Republic of Sakha (Yakutia). Standardized by age and gender, DM is less prevalent in the Siberian and Far Eastern federal districts than in Russia in general and its European segment (Fig. 2).[1–5]

Until recently, diabetes was relatively rare among natives of the Siberian regions.[6,7] Specialists of the Institute of Internal Medicine revealed only two cases of diabetes in the early 1980s in the Chukchi Autonomous District. The absolute number of patients with diabetes in the Chukchi Autonomous District increased from 2 in 1983 to 12 in 1992. Epidemiological surveys carried out in the Chukotka region in 1990s, showed that the prevalence of diabetes in the indigenous population approximated 1%, and 2.5% in the Caucasoid population in the 25-64 year age group (Fig. 3).[5,8–10] A similar pattern was observed later in the epidemiological survey of residents in Yakutsk; in the 45-65 year old population, diabetes was found in 4.2% among the Yakuts, and in 9.7% among Caucasians. T.I. Ryabova[11] examined three indigenous ethnic groups

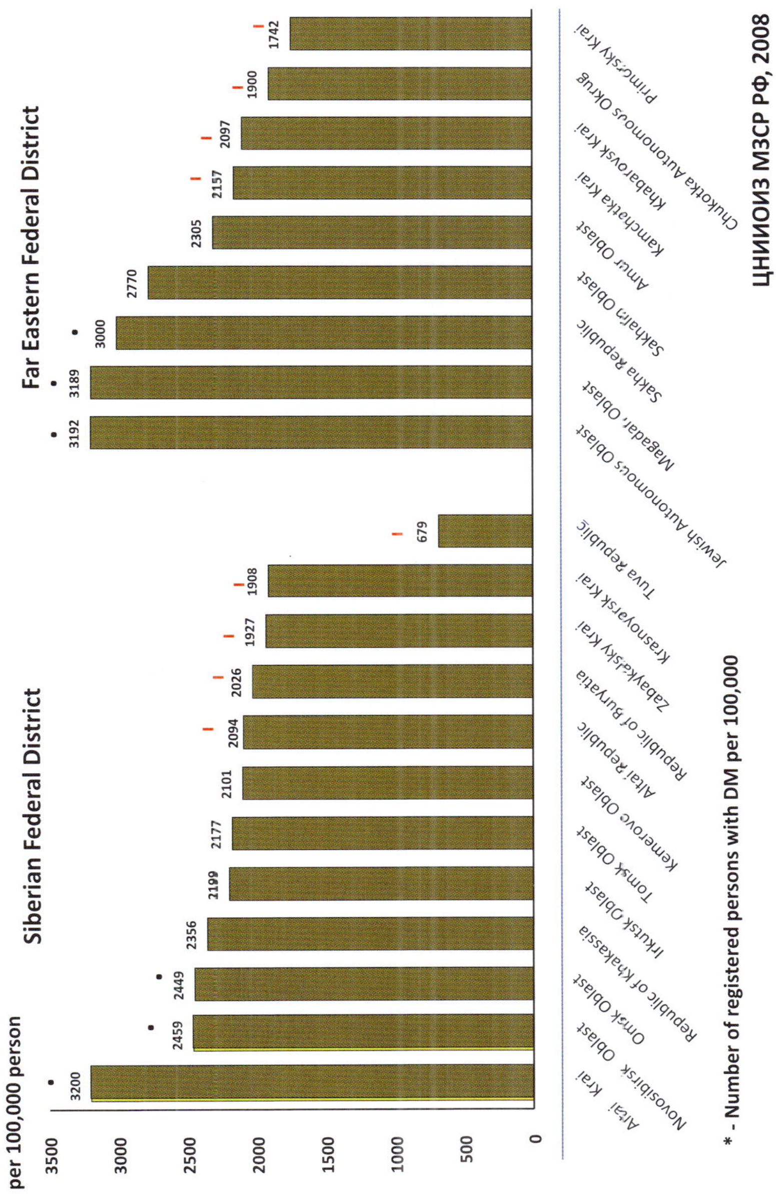

Fig. 1. Prevalence of DM in different administrative regions of Siberia and Far East (2008 Г.).

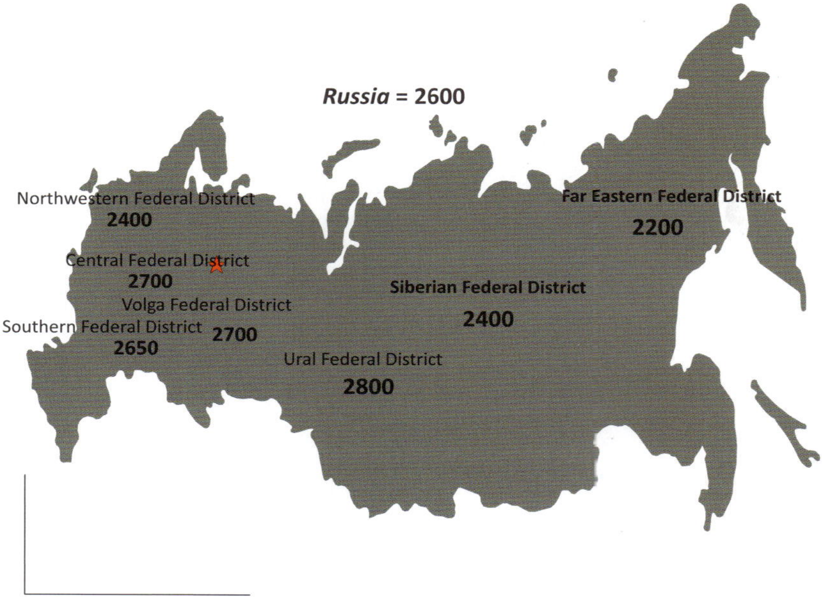
Russia = 2600
Northwestern Federal District
2400
Central Federal District
2700
Volga Federal District
2700
Southern Federal District
2650
Ural Federal District
2800
Siberian Federal District
2400
Far Eastern Federal District
2200

Fig. 2. Prevalence of DM in adult population of Russian Federal Districts (per 100,000).

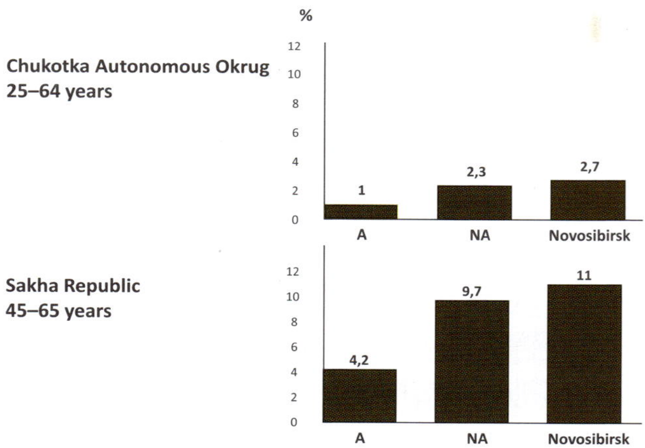

Fig. 3. Prevalence of DM in aboriginal (A) and non-aboriginal (NA) populations of Siberia and Far East.

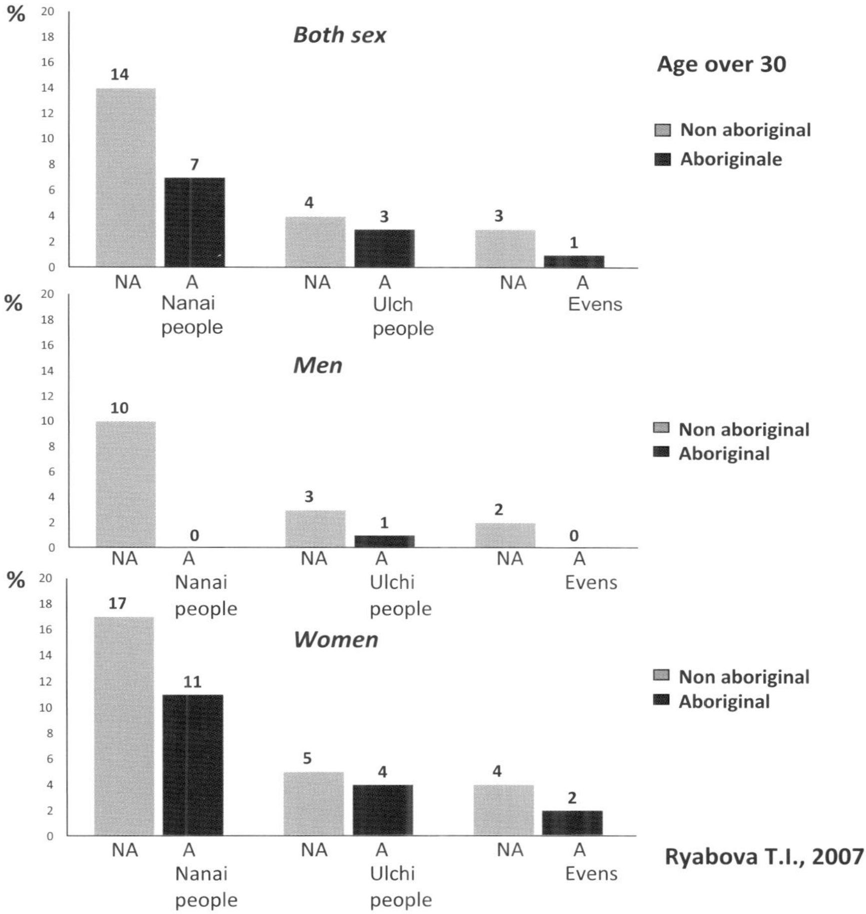

Fig. 4. Prevalence of Type 2 DM in residents of Khabarovsk Krai.

(Nanai, Ulchi, Evens) in different zones of the Khabarovsk region in order to compare the prevalence of diabetes in the aboriginal and non-aboriginal populations in these regions (Fig. 4). Diabetes occurred significantly less frequently in the aboriginal groups of both sexes than in non-aboriginals.

Type 1 diabetes occurs in the Asian part of Russia 10-15 times less frequently than type 2 diabetes. Its prevalence in separate administrative units of Siberia and the Far East is shown in Fig. 5. The highest levels

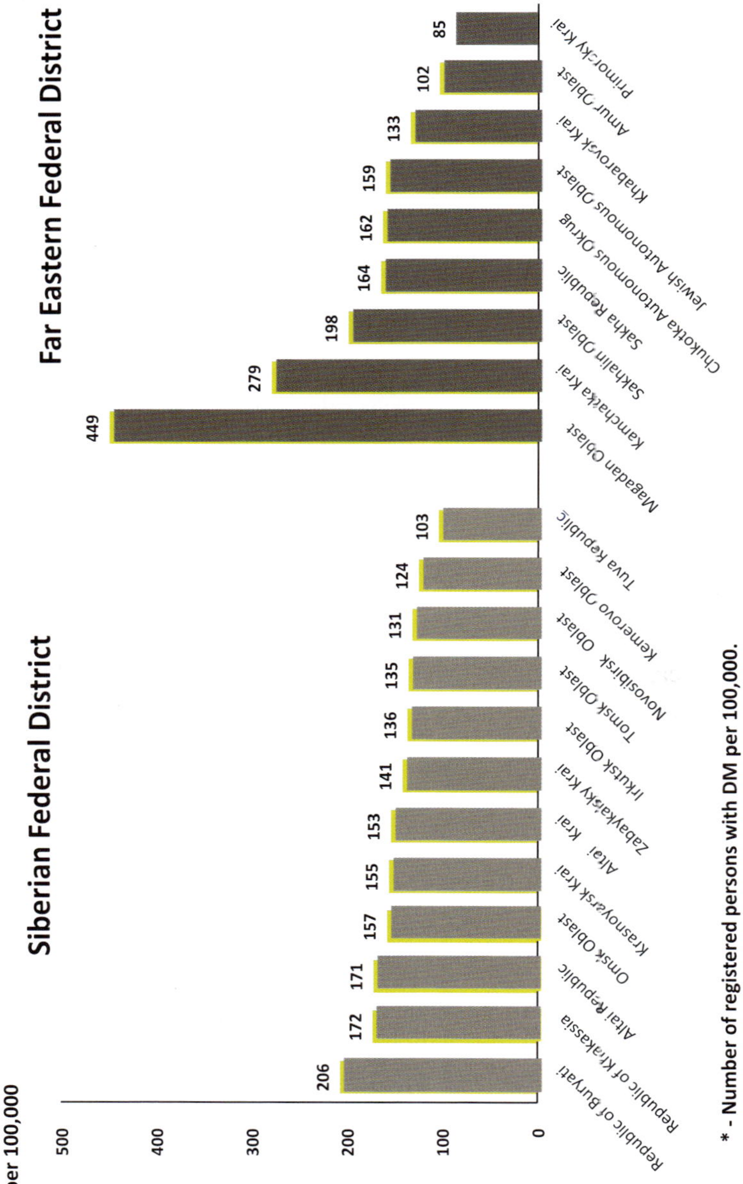

Fig. 5. Prevalence of Type 1 DM in different administrative regions of Siberia and Far East.

were reported in the Far Eastern Federal Districts, in particular in the Magadan and Kamchatka regions — 449 and 279 per 100,000, respectively. Highest rates of type 1 diabetes in the Siberian Federal District was observed in the Republics of Buryatia, Khakassia and Altai, but it was much lower than in the aforementioned regions of the Far East — 206, 172 and 171 cases per 100,000, respectively. When comparing official statistics of the distribution of type 1 diabetes in the European and Asian parts of Russia, a pronounced West-East "gradient" was noted.

3. EPIDEMIOLOGICAL STUDIES OF DIABETES IN SIBERIA

A representative sample of 3233 people aged 25–64 years was surveyed in two administrative districts of Novosibirsk in 1988–1989 within the framework of the WHO international project "Monitoring trends of morbidity and mortality from cardiovascular diseases and their underlying causes" (MONICA), with a total population of about 350,000 people. This major industrial city, was selected by WHO experts as a collaborating center of the MONICA project (Project Coordinator — Pr. Yu. P. Nikitin). Disorders of carbohydrate metabolism were detected using a standard oral glucose tolerance test. The prevalence of diabetes in the population of both sexes aged 25-64 years was 2.6%. In the female population, it was twice as high (3.5%) as in men (1.8%). In age subgroups 25-44 years, the prevalence of diabetes showed no significant gender differences. Diabetes was diagnosed 1.5-2 times more frequently in women 45 years and older than in men. It was identified for the first time in 35% of cases during this screening.[12] It should be noted that carbohydrate metabolism impairment including diabetes, according to WHO criteria in 1999, was diagnosed in 10.7% of the population of Novosibirsk (7.2% in men and 14.3% in women). In 1995, the prevalence of diabetes based on a single-stage epidemiological study in the same population was 3% (2.3% in men and 3.2% in women). In both sexes, the prevalence of diabetes at screening was 1.3% in 1988 and 1.6% in 1995.

Between 2002 and 2005, the Novosibirsk epidemiological study was conducted to estimate the prevalence of diabetes, its risk assessment, and the frequency and levels of risk factors including the metabolic syndrome. This research was carried out in the framework of the international project — "HAPIEE" ("The determinants of cardiovascular disease in Eastern Europe: A multicenter cohort study"). A representative sample of 9,190 people of both sexes aged 45–69 years was surveyed. The study protocol included an assessment of the socio-demographic data, blood pressure and anthropometric measurements (height, weight, waist circumference), certain biochemical parameters including total cholesterol, triglycerides, HDL-cholesterol, fasting blood glucose as well as other measurements.

The prevalence of diabetes in the Novosibirsk population based on fasting hyperglycemia [>126 mg/dL (7 mmol/L)], and history of diabetes was 11.4%. In the 45–69 year age range, there was no statistically significant gender difference in the incidence of diabetes (females 11.1%, men 11.7%). The mean level of fasting glucose in the overall population in both sexes was 108 mg/dL (6.0 mmol/L). On this basis, the Novosibirsk population can be described as a population at a high-risk of diabetes. Only 43% of patients with DM were aware of their diagnosis. Of these, only 5% were not treated. However, among patients with DM, only 18.6% were effectively treated with fasting blood glucose levels below 110 mg/dL (6.1 mmol/L). Thus, in 6.5% of the population aged 45-69 years, diabetes was diagnosed for the first time at screening. This again emphasizes the need to control fasting glucose levels in a healthy population to prevent progression.[5]

4. PREDIABETES IN SIBERIA

Individuals with impaired fasting glucose and impaired glucose tolerance in context of the insulin resistance syndrome are at high-risk for diabetes. These premorbid, often asymptomatic conditions comprise prediabetes. Among the residents of Novosibirsk 45-69 years of age, fasting glucose was studied in 9,157 individuals, including 4,171 men and 4,986 women using two criteria for impaired fasting glucose: ≥110 mg/dL (6.1 mmol/L) and ≥100 mg/dL (5.6 mmol/L). Fasting glucose levels ≥110 mg/dL (6.1 mmol/L) and <126 mg/dL (7.0 mmol/L) were detected in 19.4% of men and 17.2% of women. Fasting glucose levels ≥100 mg/dL (5.6 mmol/L) and <126 mg/dL (7.0 mmol/L) were detected in 46% of men and in 42.8% of women. Glucose levels exceeding ≥126 mg/dL (7.0 mmol/L) were diagnosed in the male population in 10.2% of cases and in 9.7% of women. If those with previously established diabetes who were reported to be normoglycemic at screening are considered, the prevalence of diabetes in the Novosibirsk population was 11.1% and 11.7% in men and women, respectively.

The prevalence of diabetes was higher in women up to 55 years of age and in the male population in older age groups. In both sexes, the frequency of diabetes in the younger sub-groups was 2-3 times lower than in the 65-69 year sub-group; the proportion of women was 56.8% and men 44.2%. Nearly 29% of men and 27% of women 45-69 years old had high fasting glucose levels ≥110 mg/dL (6.1 mmol/L) or diabetes. Our data suggest that the Siberian urban population should be classified as a high-risk population.

There is every reason to expect a further increase in the prevalence of diabetes in Siberia if significant efforts are not undertaken to correct the major behavioral risk factors for diabetes such as an unhealthy diet and lack of physical inactivity, which are directly related to the high prevalence of excess weight and obesity in the population. The prevalence of overweight in the study population was 61% in men and 82% in women, and obesity, 20.7% and 47%, respectively. High prevalence of the metabolic syndrome and its individual components was observed in Novosibirsk with increased fasting blood glucose levels in 29% of subjects, blood pressure >130/85 in 75%, and abdominal obesity in 43%. The frequency of abdominal obesity according to NCEP ATP III criteria (2001) was higher in women (59%) than in men (24%).

One of the main tasks in primary prevention of the metabolic syndrome and other disorders of carbohydrate metabolism, diabetes and cardiovascular complications is detection of abdominal obesity in the population — a very sensitive screening marker of insulin resistance associated with high level of diabetes and cardiovascular disease risk factors. Several publications have shown that waist circumference cut points, associated with an elevated risk for metabolic disorders, are variable in different populations and ethnic groups. This is reflected in several of the existing definitions of the metabolic syndrome. A number of studies of the metabolic syndrome in south-east Asia, have established that waist circumference cut points for the Mongoloid population is considerably lower than for the

Caucasoid population in Europe and the United States. In a consensus document on the metabolic syndrome of the International Diabetes Federation, the National Heart, Lung, and Blood Institute (United States), the American Heart Association, the International Society for Atherosclerosis and the International Association for the Study of Obesity identified clear research priorities in this area: "We need long-term prospective studies to develop more accurate cut points of waist circumference of various ethnic groups, especially for women".[13]

Waist cut-off points for the metabolic syndrome were 94 cm in men and 91 cm in women and for diabetes, 97 and 95 cm, respectively. It is evident from these results that the female population in Western Siberia has different waist cut-points associated with metabolic syndrome and diabetes. In Novosibirsk, male waist cut points are equal to the IDF criteria proposed for the male Caucasoid population, >94 cm.[5,14]

In conclusion, it should again be noted that long-term monitoring of the incidence and prevalence of diabetes in Siberia shows a significant average two-fold increase in a 10-15-year period. The latter basically refers to type 2 DM. As for type 1 diabetes, type 2 diabetes is detected in Siberia less frequently than in the European part of the country. Among the indigenous (native) inhabitants of Siberia and the Far East, the prevalence of both types of diabetes remains lower (as in previous years) than among the Caucasian population living in the same localities. Epidemiological screening enabled identification of undiagnosed diabetes in addition to reported cases, the former exceeding the latter.[5,14]

The very disappointing data reflecting worsening of the epidemiological situation with respect to DM were obtained during the study of children and adolescent population in Novosibirsk. There is a growing incidence of obesity among children and adolescents. The results of consecutive screening examinations have shown that since 2003, the incidence of elevated body mass index (BMI) in teenagers began to increase affecting more boys, from 4% in 1999 to 11% in 2003 ($p < 0.001$) up to 13% in 2009, than girls (4.3%, 5.2% and 8.5% in 1999, 2003 and 2009, respectively). Coincident with this, there was an increase in the average hip circumference (in both genders), waist circumference (in boys), and the average level of fasting blood glucose levels (in both sexes) in adolescents. The progressive increase in type 2 diabetes and an increase in the frequency of overweight and obesity in children and adolescents of Novosibirsk further reflect unfavorable trends in cardiovascular risk in the general population and point to the urgent need for large-scale preventive measures.

As overall trends in diabetes prevalence in Siberia are very similar to other developed populations, it is important that genetic association studies also demonstrate similar results for the Siberian population of Caucasian origin. In particular, the association of type 2 DM with specific genetic markers (rs9939609 of gene FTO, rs7903146 of gene TF7L2, rs10811661 of gene CDKN2A/B and rs2237892 of gene KCNQ1) characteristic for an increased risk of developing type 2 diabetes, were studied in Novosibirsk. This case-control study included 170 subjects, 45-69 year old residents, with confirmed type 2 diabetes and/or increased blood glucose levels exceeding 200 mg/dL (11.1 mmol/L). The control group was matched for age and sex (276 individuals with normal glucose levels). This study has been completed but not yet published.

5. DIABETES PREVENTION IN RUSSIA AND SIBERIA

The rapid and unprecedented increase in diabetes prevalence requires that Russia, like most countries in the world, identify an immediate solution for this problem. Therefore, on 7 October 1996, the Russian government approved the specialized federal program (SFP) DM, which became part of the federal program Prevention and Control of Social Diseases as of 2002. Among the main objectives defining the SFP program DM were organizing diabetes services and prevention of diabetes and its complications, providing individuals with diabetes modern and effective treatments, providing Russian professions with effective diabetes care information based on common international standards for the reduction of diabetes complications, and reduction of mortality and life expectancy of individuals with diabetes. The successful implementation of SFP is clear as at this time more than 100 regional diabetes centers equipped with modern facilities were created in Russia, specialized clinics were opened for patients with diabetic foot problems, diabetic retinopathy and nephropathy as well as for pregnancy complicating diabetes. Special classes for patients (adults, children, parents) were established in these newly-created diabetes centers and clinics. Patients with diabetes have an assured supply of oral medication including insulin, and equipment for self-monitoring. Disabled patients are assured of receiving medication for treating diabetic complications. As a result, over the last 5 years mortality of type 1 diabetes has decreased 4-5-fold, and 2-3-fold in those with type 2 diabetes. The average life expectancy of patients with type 1 diabetes has increased 6 years for men and 10 years for women and for those with type 2 diabetes, 7 years for men and 6 years for women over the past 10 years.[15]

6. STATE REGISTRY OF DIABETES MELLITUS

One of the undeniable achievements of the SFP was the creation of the State Registry of Diabetes Mellitus (SRDM), which united the work of 84 regional registries. Currently, SRDM is a unified information and analytic system permitting compilation of detailed and timely records for each patient. It provides monitoring, analysis and forecasting, planning and calculation of the need for antidiabetic drugs at different administrative levels. According to SRDM, over the last 10 years, the number of diabetic individuals in Russia has increased by more than one million. In 2012, 3,268.871 individuals with diabetes were registered and the forecast for 2030 anticipates an increase to 5.4 million.[16] The growth is mainly due to type 2 diabetes. Therefore at present, the primary prevention of diabetes is an extremely urgent task for the Russian health care system in addition to further improving diabetes patient care. It should be noted that the national guidelines for diabetes pays considerable attention to identifying diabetes risk factors and determination of type 2 diabetes risk and recommends the use of screening questionnaires, in particular "FINDRISC" which is well-established in international studies.

7. HEALTH CENTERS

Considerable hope for implementing the State policy on promoting a healthy lifestyle in the population and prevention of major social diseases, including diabetes, is placed on the newly established "Health Centers" (for children and adults). The priority national project "Health" was introduced in 2013 to actively screen the population 18 years and older for risk factors of chronic disease including diabetes. The Health Center examination includes obtaining a history, counseling in nutrition, lifestyle and exercise in addition to testing and providing treatment. All examinations and treatments are carried out within the framework of compulsory health insurance. A complete clinical examination (initial and follow-up) may also be performed in other health-care facilities in the community. Thus, Russia is now prepared to combat diabetes.

8. FROM THE HISTORY OF THE STUDY OF DIABETES MELLITUS IN SIBERIA

Initial studies on the epidemiology of DM in Siberia were conducted by the Institute of Internal Medicine, Siberian Branch of the Russian Academy of Medical Sciences, under the guidance of Prof. Yu. P. Nikitin in the early 1980s. For the first time in these studies, methodology of the WHO was used to survey the population of typical districts of Novosibirsk on the prevalence of chronic disease risk factors and diabetes prevalence. At about the same time, the registry of DM in the adult population of the city was established improving case registration, analysis of diabetes risk factors, social determinants, quality of treatment, complications and disease outcome. In 1989, another registry was created at the Institute of Internal Medicine as part of the international WHO program "Diamond", — the first Russian registry of diabetes in children, which was active from 1989 to 1999, until the project Diamond was completed. Since the termination of the international project, the Novosibirsk children's case registry has still continued. The methodology and experience was used as the basis for the creation of the now existing territorial Novosibirsk City diabetes registry, which, since 2002, has become an integral part of the State Register of Diabetes.

Since 2000, the city Novosibirsk territorial registry of diabetes widely employed public health authorities for organization of care to patients with diabetes and is still the basis of various scientific studies. So, based on combining databases of two children's registries, it became possible to study type 1 diabetes in the pediatric population of Novosibirsk. It was found that the incidence of diabetes in children of Novosibirsk is similar to that of other large Russian cities such as Moscow and St. Petersburg, but exceeds the national average by 1.8-fold. Over the past three decades, the incidence of type 1 diabetes in children of Novosibirsk increased 2.8 times; standardized indicators, taking into account age and sex, in these time periods were 6.05, 8.3 and 17.0 per 100,000 of the childhood population. The greatest increase in incidence was observed in young children, 12.85% in those up to the age of 4 years and 13% for those 5-9 years, compared to 7.1% from the ages of 10-14 years.[17,18]

Given that Novosibirsk is a major industrial city with high levels of man-made environmental pollution, we analyzed the association between levels of air pollutants with diabetes morbidity in different parts of the city. A significant association was found between high concentrations of the inhaled toxins formaldehyde and nitrogen dioxide with a higher incidence of type 1 diabetes in children and adults as well as a higher incidence of type 2 diabetes. Another area for implementation of the regional diabetes registry database relates to hereditary forms of diabetes. Adding to the database regarding family history has allowed us to identify and highlight familial forms of the disease, in particular, to identify families with MODY 2 diabetes and determine methods for treatment. Using the registry database together with population-based screening of representative samples of the population, 45-69 years old (international study "HAPIEE") has allowed us to establish sufficient data for developing a specific Siberian and first Russian-specific diabetes risk scale.

Practical implementation of the diabetes registry data and creation of regional diabetes centers allowed the achievement of positive outcomes during the last 7 years namely, a reduction in the incidence of diabetes complications, mortality and increased life expectancy of patients with diabetes. In accordance with the registry data, the frequency of diabetic retinopathy in patients with type 1 diabetes decreased by 10.83% and diabetic nephropathy by 6.8%. In those with type 2 diabetes these were reduced by 21.78% and 11.35%, respectively. The relative number of deaths from terminal chronic renal failure in patients with type 1 diabetes decreased 2-fold and in patients with type 2 diabetes, 1.8-fold. Death rates from acute myocardial infarction in patients with type 2 diabetes decreased 1.8-fold and acute cerebral circulatory disorders 1.4-fold. The average age of death in patients with type 1 diabetes has increased from 41.92 ± 1.84 to 51.74 ± 2.55 years and in patients with type 2 diabetes from 71.18 ± 0.38 to 73.24 ± 0.31 years.[19]

9. INTERNATIONAL COOPERATION

One of the initiatives in Novosibirsk in the primary prevention of diabetes is a joint Russian–German project, which was developed in the framework of cooperation between the Ministry of Health of the Novosibirsk region and Saxony and established in 2010. This project is supported over the next two years by the Health Department of the Ministry of Social Affairs and Consumer Protection Saxony and supported to date by the Department of Social Policy of the Novosibirsk government. The Novosibirsk diabetes prevention project was based on the "Praedias" program, successfully implemented and introduced into clinical practice in Germany. In 2011-2012, teaching materials for medical specialists and patients have been adapted to Russian circumstances. The kit includes educational materials about diet, physical activity, body weight control, energy consumption. In total, 12 medical specialists were trained as prevention program managers and successfully passed the exam. Currently, the diabetes prevention program is included in the target program of Novosibirsk "Healthy City". The "FINDRISC" questionnaire is used by Health Centers as well as during public city events. More than 3,000 people completed the "FINDRISC" questionnaire during public city events. Individuals at high-risk were detected in 22.7% of those screened, very high in 3.6%, average degree of risk in 18.1%, and impaired glucose tolerance in 5.3%. Those with impaired glucose tolerance were directed to the City Diabetes Center, whereas those with risk factors received advice on nutrition, physical activity and suggested treatment in health centers. An unexpected problem for implementing prevention programs was the lack of motivation and willingness of most of the population to participate. In this regard, the media is constantly informing the public about diabetes and prevention measures. Currently, the health centers have trained 122 individuals with risk factors for diabetes.

REFERENCES

1. Suncov YI, Bolotnaya LL, Maslova OV, Kazakova IV (2011) Epidemiology of diabetes mellitus and its prevalence prognosis in Russia Federation. *Diabetes Mellitus* **1**: 15–18. (in Russian)

2. Shishkina NS, Suncov YI, Bolotskaya LL *et al*. (2005) Prevalence of diabetes mellitus of type 2 (screening data). *Diabetes Mellitus* **2**: 7–9. (in Russian)
3. Dogadin SA, Kriganovskaya EV, Vinogradova SV *et al*. (2004) Results of diabetes mellitus screening in Krasnoyarsk. *Diabetes Mellitus* **1**: 7–10. (in Russian)
4. Suplotova LA, Suncov YI, Kretinina LN, Belchikova LN. (2005) Results of diabetes mellitus complications screening in Tumen Region. *Diabetes Mellitus* **2**: 10–13. (in Russian)
5. Nikitin YP, Voevoda MI, Simonova GI. (2012) Diabetes mellitus and metabolic syndrome in Siberia and in the Far East. *Annals of the Russian Academy of Medical Sciences* **1**: 66–74.
6. Burlak SI. (1982) Prevalence of diabetes mellitus in inhabitants of Kamchatskii region and its risl factors. *Endocrinology* **5**: 17–22. (in Russian)
7. Orechov KV. (1982) Medical-biological aspects of health researches in people of Extreme North. *Healthcare System of Russian Federation* **1**: 7–12. (in Russian)
8. Yuong TK, Schraer CD, Shubnikoff EV, Szathmary EJ, Nikitin YP. (1992) Prevalence of diagnosed diabetes in circumpolar indigenous populations. *Int J Epidemiol* **21**: 730–736.
9. Nikitin YP, Salechova GI, Simonova GI, Shubnikov EV, Kotyt EV. (1995) Diabetes mellitus in adults and children of Siberia and Extreme North. Problems of health in Extreme North. Novosibirsk: *Nauka*. **1995**: 71–73. (in Russian)
10. Nikitin YP. ed. (1995) Problems of health in the North Region in new economical conditions. Novosibirsk: *Nauka*. **1995**: 147. (in Russian)
11. Ryabova TI. (2007) Prevalence of type 2 diabetes mellitus in dominating aboriginal groups of Amur basin. *Diabetes Mellitus* **4**: 7–10. (in Russian)
12. Nikitin YP, Stepanov EG, Shubnikov EV. (1989) Diabetes mellitus and impared glucose tolerance test in Siberian regions. *Bulletin of Siberian Branch of Russian Academy of Medical Science* **5**: 12–16. (in Russian)
13. Alberti KGMM, Eckel RH, Grundy SM, Zimmet PZ, Cleeman JI, Donato KA, Fruchart J-C, James WPT, Loria cm and Smith SC, Jr. (2009) Harmonizing the metabolic syndrome: A joint interim statement of the International Diabetes Federation Task Force on Epidemiology and Prevention; National Heart, Lung, and Blood Institute; American Heart Association; World Heart Federation; International Atherosclerosis Society; and International Association for the Study of Obesity. *Circulation* **120**: 1640–1645.
14. Simonova GI, Mustafina SV, Pechenkina EA. (2011) Prevalence of metabolic syndrome in Siberia: Population survey in Novosibirsk city. *Bulletin of Siberian Branch of Russian Academy of Medical Science* **31**: 100–106. (in Russian)

15. Dedov II, Shestakova MV. eds. Diabetes mellitus: Diagnosis, treatment, prevention. *Moscow: Medical News Agency*: 808. (in Russian)
16. Dedov II. (2012) Diabetes Mellitus — the most dangerous challenge to the world community. *Bulletin of the RAMS* **1**: 7–13. (in Russian)
17. Shubnikov EV, Podar T, Tuomilehto J, Nikitin YP. (1992) Low Incidence of Childhood IDDM in District of Novosibirsk (Russia). *Diabetes Care* **15**: 915–917. (in Russian)
18. Shubnikov EV, Sazonova OV, Simonova GI, Nikitin YP. (2011) Dynamics of type 1 diabetes morbidity in children of Novosibirsk City. *Vestnic Novosibirsk State University. Series: Biology, Clinical Medicine* **9**: 73–77. (in Russian)
19. Sazonova OV, Nikiforov OA, Selivanova SV, Hachatrjan AD, Kuznetsova NG. (2011) Diabetes mellitus of Novosibirsk, Russia: Incidence, complications. *Vestnik Novosibirsk State University Series: Biology and Clinical Medicine* **9**: 33–37. (in Russian)

Chapter 20: Prediabetes and Diabetes Prevention Initiatives in Latin America (LA)

Rafael Gabriel, Clicerio González-Villalpando†, Patricio López-Jaramillo‡, Tania Acosta§, Ruy López Ridaura||, Ramfis Nieto-Martínez**, Jaakko Tuomilehto†† and Pablo Aschner‡‡*

1. EPIDEMIOLOGY OF PREDIABETES (PD) IN LATIN AMERICA (LA)

1.1. Prevalence

The number of people with diabetes in LA has been increasing faster than the population at-risk in the last decade (almost 200% vs 24% increase)

*Corresponding author. Head Unidad de Epidemiología Clínica, Instituto de Investigación IdiPAZ, Red de Investigación Cardiovascular (RIC); Member of IBERCARMEN-CYTED Network, Hospital Universitario La Paz, Universidad Autónoma de Madrid, Madrid, Spain. Email: rafael.gabriel@salud.madrid.org

†MACP Investigador Unidad de Investigación en Diabetes y Riesgo Cardiovascular, Centro de Investigación en Salud Poblacional; Member of IBERCARMEN-CYTED Network, Instituto Nacional de Salud Pública, Mexico City, Mexico.

‡Director de Investigación, Desarrollo e Innovación Tecnológica Director Clínica de Síndrome Metabólico, Prediabetes y Diabetes; Fundación Oftalmológica de Santander-FOSCAL, Facultad deMedicina, UDES, Bucaramanga, Colombia.

§Instituto de Investigación IdiPAZ, Hospital Universitario La Paz. Universidad Autónoma de Madrid, Spain; Member of IBERCARMEN-CYTED Network Centro de Investigación en Salud, Barranquilla, Colombia.

||Instituto Nacional de Salud Pública, Mexico; Red de Investigación Cardiovascular (RIC), Instituto IdiPAZ, Hospital Universitario La Paz, Universidad Autónoma de Madrid, Madrid, Spain.

**Associate Professor, Universidad Centro-Occidental "Lisandro Alvarado"; Director, Unidad Cardiometabólica 7, Barquisimeto, Venezuela.

according to the data provided periodically by the *IDF Atlas*.[1] At present, the mean prevalence of diabetes in LA approximates 10% with the number varying between 14% in Mexico and above 12% in the Dominican Republic to 7% in Peru. According to the IDF 2012 estimates, there are 41 million people with diabetes and approximately a similar number of people with impaired glucose tolerance (IGT) in South America/Central America/Caribbean countries.[1] The CARMELA study[3] demonstrated that the prevalence of diabetes is not very different among the main cities in the region, demonstrating that Lima (Peru) had the lowest prevalence (4.4%) and Mexico City the highest (8.9%). On the other hand, there is a considerable difference in diabetes prevalence within a country between urban and rural settings. A recent study in Peru showed a more than two-fold difference between the prevalence of diabetes in the coastal urban population (8.2%) and people living in suburban areas in the sierra and the jungle (4.5% and 3.5%, respectively).[4] An even bigger difference (almost five-fold) has been found comparing an urban and a rural population in Colombia (7.4% and 1.4%, respectively).[5] These differences may be attributed to lifestyle changes occurring with urbanization, such as a more sedentary life with decreased physical activity, physical fitness, and dietary changes towards more elaborated products with higher sugar (particularly sweet beverages) and lower fiber content, resulting in increased body weight.

Although in some countries such as Argentina, Uruguay, and Venezuela, more than 90% of the population is already urban, in most of the LA countries, urbanization is still evolving. There are still countries in Central America like Guatemala, Honduras, and Nicaragua where more than 40% of the population is rural. These data indicate that interventions to avoid unhealthy lifestyle changes and to preserve some of the dietary habits in

††Professor, Centre for Vascular Prevention, Danube-University Krems, Krems, Austria; Red de Investigación Cardiovascular (RIC), Instituto de Investigación IdiPAZ, Hospital Universitario La Paz; Member of IBERCARMEN-CYTED Network, Universidad Autónoma de Madrid, Madrid, Spain; King Abdulaziz University, Jeddah, Saudi Arabia.

‡‡Associate Professor, Universidad Javeriana, Director of Research — Hospital Universtario San Ignacio; Scientific Subdirector — Asociación Colombiana de Diabetes; Member of IBERCARMEN-CYTED Network, Bogotá, Colombia.

populations migrating to cities may constitute an important prevention strategy. The indigenous Amerindian population is a group at particularly high-risk for T2D. The latter represents more than 5% of the total population in Honduras, Nicaragua, Panama, Ecuador, and Peru, and more than 40% in Guatemala and Bolivia. For example, the Mapuches and Aymaras in Chile had the lowest prevalence of Type 2 diabetes (T2D) in the world (less than 1%), but the prevalence increased to 8.2% and 6.9% respectively in those who had moved from a rural to an urban environment.[6] Recently, a striking 28.2% prevalence was found in the Brazilian Xavante indigenous population which has undergone important changes in the nutritional and health profile.[7]

Strategies to avoid the adverse impact of a Westernized lifestyle in these communities are necessary.

The prevalence of diabetes may be five to six times higher in those above 60 years of age compared with the third decade of life. Of importance, the age pyramid is changing rapidly in our region. In 2010, the proportion of the population aged 60 years and over was 9.8% and the aging index was 3.4%. Low socioeconomic status is another risk factor for diabetes worldwide and some studies have shown that this is also true in LA.[1,8] Reducing socioeconomic inequities will lead to decreased diabetes prevalence.[9] Obesity is also epidemic in LA, with many countries reporting that 50% or more of the adult population is overweight, particularly women. Approximately one-third of the adult population has the metabolic syndrome according to the most recent definition using regional cutoffs for waist circumference (WC) to diagnose visceral adiposity (94 cm for men and 90 cm for women).[10] As observed in other regions, abdominal obesity (AO) is a cardio-metabolic risk factor in LA.[11] Obesity and the metabolic syndrome are major risk factors for diabetes and lead to IGT. The number of people with IGT is presenting an additional challenge in LA for prevention which can be very effective in this group.[1] For example, the prevalence of IGT in Mexico is 12% of the adult population.[12]

The high prevalence of T2D and prediabetes observed in many areas of LA for instance in Mexico, and in ethnic groups such as Amerindians, might also be related not only to Native American genetic admixture but also to Spanish genetic admixture. Data from a comparative analysis of four population-based epidemiological surveys conducted in two Mexican-origin and two European-origin samples provided data relevant to this question. A comparison of two Mexican-origin populations from Mexico City and San Antonio (Texas) showed that age- and sex-adjusted prevalence of prediabetes (IGT or IFG) was lower in Mexico than in San Antonio (18.2 vs. 22.2%, $p < 0.05$). Between the two European-origin populations, the prevalence of prediabetes was lower in San Antonio non-Hispanic whites than in Spain (13.6 vs. 17.0%, <0.008), but differences were attenuated by adjustment for body mass index (BMI) or after stratification by education. In logistic regression analyses, prediabetes was associated with Mexican ethnic origin after adjusting for age, education, BMI, and waist-to-hip ratio. This study concluded that the prevalence of prediabetes in Spain was intermediate between that in Mexican-origin populations and non-Hispanic whites in San Antonio. Although the higher degree of Native American admixture is a major contributor to the higher rates of prediabetes in Mexico, a partial contribution of Spanish admixture to diabetes susceptibility among Mexican-origin populations cannot completely be ruled out.[13]

Published investigations, exploring the genetic and environmental determinants of T2D, have estimated that approximately 30% of the excess in prevalence of T2D seen in the Mexican-American population in Texas could be explained by environmental factors,[14] showing the great impact of social and economic determinants on T2D risk. This finding will need to be considered in perspective with the recently identified novel genetic variant occurring with substantially higher frequency in patients with T2D with Amerindian ancestry. This discovery was performed using a very extensive GWAS approach. It was estimated that this might account for a higher genetic susceptibility to T2D seen in the Mexican population.[15] The differences in frequencies of common genetic variants of SLC16A11 located at chromosome 17p13.1, may be responsible for 27% of the higher disease burden of T2D in Mexican and LA populations. Individuals with T2D and who carry the risk haplotype develop the disease 2.1 years earlier and at a BMI 0.9 kg/m^2 lower than non-carriers. The odds ratio (OR) of T2D estimated in young individuals (≤45 years) was significantly higher than in older individuals. These clinical elements have been recognized previously and constitute a very important concept for public health implications. T2D in Mexico, in at least 25% of cases, is a disease of younger adults. Preventive efforts will need to take this fact into consideration.[16]

1.2. Progression from Normal Glycaemia to PD, incidence of T2D in PD and Predictors of T2D in LA

The Mexico City Diabetes Study (MCDS), a population-based survey of diabetes and cardiovascular risk factors initiated in 1989 in a low-income neighborhood of Mexico City,[17] has characterized for the first time the incidence of T2D and its risk factors in an LA population. The incidence of T2D has been estimated at 14-15 cases per 1,000 person-years. Apparently, this rate has been sustained over the past 20 years.[6] These findings characterize the Mexican population with a higher incidence of T2D compared with other ethnic groups. In this study, a population-based cohort of 1,963 participants without diabetes (mean age 47 years) was prospectively followed. An oral glucose tolerance test (OGTT) was performed at baseline and 7 years later. IGT was five times more prevalent (13.5%) than IFG. In both categories, participants were older, heavier, more hyperinsulinaemic, hyperproinsulinaemic, and dyslipidaemic compared with participants with normal glucose tolerance. The relative risk of incident diabetes were similar for IFG and IGT [3.73 (95% CI: 2.18–6.39) and 4.01 (95% CI: 3.12–5.14), respectively], but the population-attributable risk (PAR) was five-fold higher for IGT [29% (95% CI: 26–32)] than for IFG [6% (95% CI: 5–7)]. Isolated IFG carried no increase in risk. Lowering the threshold of fasting plasma glucose from 6.1 to 5.6 mmol/l (110 mg/dl to 100 mg/dl) raised the PAR of IFG to 23% (95% CI: 20–25); its contribution to diabetes progression, however, was largely due to co-existing IGT. In multivariate analysis adjusting for sex, age, familial diabetes and BMI, fasting and 2-hr glucose were found to be independent predictors of T2D. However, although T2D can be predicted using fasting plasma glucose, the 2-hr post-challenge glucose in the OGTT is more powerful for the prediction of diabetes. Also, lowering the diagnostic threshold increases the PAR of IFG four-fold, but performing an OGTT captures additional people at risk compared with the number identified by IFG.[18]

Another important issue, not commonly addressed by epidemiological studies, is the natural history of hyperglycaemia, i.e., the rate and pattern of progression from normal glycaemia (either fasting or postprandial) to impaired glucose status (IFG, IGT, or both). The MCDS offered a unique opportunity to explore the longitudinal changes ("tracking") of glycaemia over time. Over the first 8 years of follow-up, 140 individuals of 1,647 with both normal fasting and 2-hr glucose (NGT) at baseline developed prediabetes: 108 (6.6%) developed IGT; 18 (1.1%) IFG and 14 (0.9%) combined IGT and IFG. The 8-year incidence of prediabetes was 8.6%. If we accept the rate of glucose progression as a continuum, we can estimate the average annual risk of middle-aged adults from Mexico City developing prediabetes approximates 1%.

1.3. Prevalence of Cardiovascular Risk Factors and their Relationship with Diabetes in LA

Obesity is an independent risk factor for cardiovascular diseases (CVD) and plays a crucial role in the development of diabetes.[20] In the last two decades, the prevalence of being overweight and obesity combined in LA has increased by more than 20% and currently its prevalence in most of LA countries exceeds 40%.[21] The INTERHEART study demonstrated that AO is the most frequent risk factor for an acute myocardial infarction (AMI) in LA,[22] with a PAR of 48.5%, while in the rest of the world it was 30.2%.[22] Recently, the INTERSTROKE study also demonstrated that in the LA countries, AO has a high PAR to ischemic and hemorrhagic stroke.[23]

There are a number of physiologic and metabolic changes associated with obesity that may contribute to an increased risk of CVD. Increased visceral adipose tissue disturbs adipocytokine secretion and leads to a low-grade chronic inflammatory state by the infiltration of macrophages into adipose tissue.[24] It is noteworthy that the LA population seems to have a higher sensitivity for developing systemic low-degree inflammation as a response to AO.[25] This inflammatory state is found to be associated with peripheral resistance to insulin-mediated glucose uptake[26–28] and atherosclerosis.[24] These metabolic alterations might lead to vascular endothelial dysfunction, abnormal lipid profile, hypertension, and vascular inflammation, and all of these factors could favor the development of T2D and CVD.[26,29–31]

Various studies have assessed the prevalence of CVD risk factors in LA,[22,32–36] the situation being critical (Table 1). The risk factors

Table 1. Prevalence of cardiovascular risk factors in Latin America.

	INTERHEART (3)	CARMELA (13)	LASO (14)	PURE study (15)	PURE – Colombia (17)
ApoB/ApoA-1	42.0%				
Hypercholesterolemia		14 (6–20%)	8.9 (6.9–11.4%)		17.6 (16.7–18.6%)
HDL-C			53.3 (47.0–63.4%)		38.8 (37.7–39.9%)
hypertriglyceridemia			26.5 (19.0–35.7%)		49.7 (48.5–50.9%)
Current smoking	48.1%	30 (22–45%)	25.8 (18.1–35.3%)	20.8 (20.6–20.9%)	34.7 (33.6–35.7%)
Type 2 diabetes mellitus	9.5%	7 (4–9%)	5.0 (3.4–7.9%)	10.6 (10.5–10.8%)	5.8 (5.2–6.4%)
Hypertension	29.1%	18 (9–29%)	20.2 (12.5–31.0%)	41.6 (41.4–41.9%)	37.1 (35.9–38.2%)
Obesity					
WHR	48.6%				
BMI ≥ 30 kg/m^2		23 (18–27%)	16.1 (11.1–22.8%)	16.2 (15.9–16.3%)	18.8 (17.9–19.7%)
Waist circumference	33.3%		32.8 (25.4–47.8%)		58.9 (57.7–60.0%)

CARMELA Study: Hypertension: ≥140/≥90 mmHg or current antihypertensive drug treatment; Hypercholesterolemia: ≥240 mg/dL; Diabetes: fasting glucose ≥126 mg/dl or self-reported diabetes; Obesity: BMI ≥30 kg/m^2; Smoking: daily or occasional consumption of cigarettes, cigars, or pipe tobacco. **LASO**: Hypertension: ≥140/≥90 mmHg or self-reported current antihypertensive drug treatment; Diabetes: fasting glucose ≥126 mg/dl or self-reported diabetes; Hypercholesterolemia ≥240 mg/dL, Smoking. Current cigarette smokers were those who had smoked >100 cigarettes over their lifetime and smoked at the time of the interview; Obesity: BMI ≥30 kg/m2 and AO as WC ≥88 cm in women and ≥102 cm in men. **PURE study**: Hypertension ≥140/≥90 mmHg or self-reported current antihypertensive drug treatment; Diabetes: fasting glucose ≥126 mg/dl or self-reported diabetes; Smoking: Current cigarette smokers who smoked at least 1 tobacco product daily in the previous 12 month, including those who had stopped within the past year; Obesity: was defined as a BMI ≥30 kg/m^2. **PURE - Colombia**: The same as PURE study but AO as WC ≥80 cm in women and ≥94 cm in men.

associated with insulin resistance are very prevalent: 53.3% of LA populations have low levels of high-density lipoprotein cholesterol (HDL-C),[14] and 49.7% high levels of triglycerides (TG) in Colombia.[36] Smoking prevalence varies between 21.8% and 48%, and hypertension prevalence between 18% and 42%.[3,13–17] T2D prevalence in several LA countries is among the highest in the world, e.g., Mexico at 14.4%.[37,38] However, data are scanty and the percentage of patients without confirmation of the diagnosis is 30–50%, which may be even higher in rural areas.[39] Microvascular and macrovascular disease occurrence in people with T2D are also high.[40,41] The worldwide INTERHEART study identified nine potentially modifiable risk factors for a first AMI, and in LA T2D accounted for 12% of PAR for AMI.[22] However, this association between dysglycemia and CVD should not be considered from a specific cutoff point, but as a continuum. An increase in risk for CVD before the diagnosis of T2D has also been noted.[42] A Colombo-Ecuadorian study found that 37% of patients with a first AMI had prediabetes.[43] Moreover, hyperinsulinaemia has been established as an important factor associated with the occurrence of new CVD events in patients with a first AMI.[44]

2. INITIATIVES OF DIABETES SCREENING IN LA

Who should be screened for diabetes is an important question, since the benefits of diabetes prevention have been observed in people with prediabetes, although adopting a healthy lifestyle will benefit the entire population. Several LA countries have established, at least theoretically, institutional screening programs for early detection of T2D, the majority using opportunistic strategies with sporadic population-based campaigns. Despite this, diabetes is still undiagnosed in more than 45% of Central and South American adult populations.[1] In general, these screening strategies are not systematically implemented, the algorithms used are poorly adapted to the region-specific context, and without information as to their internal and external validation.

The first official institutional screening strategy was instituted in Mexico in 1998[45] based on a risk factor questionnaire that was literally translated from the questionnaire developed by Herman *et al.* in 1995, and adopted by the ADA.[46] Since the algorithm has undergone many changes without any validity assessment, and currently there is widespread heterogeneity in its components (WC cut-off values, use of casual capillary glucose) and how it is implemented across different regions of the country (the decision tree is poorly defined or the use of the 2-hr OGTT is totally absent in the strategy). Furthermore, the few studies that have evaluated its validity have shown that the specificity of the recommended cutoff to classify individuals as "high-risk" is very low (<50%).[47] Also, the specificity only increases to 59%, with a positive predictive value of 17%, when a casual capillary glucose determination is added to the screening strategy.[48] The issue of identifying individuals with intermediate hyperglycemia, i.e., prediabetes, is practically absent in most of these institutional screening strategies in LA.

Given the poor performance of these previous strategies for the early detection of T2D, the identification of prediabetes, which requires the addition of the 2-hr OGTT, will increase the costs considerably. Therefore, before implementing any strategy, it will be necessary to generate strong evidence about its cost-utility in the LA region. This would mean that well-designed and evaluated pilot studies are needed. The most recent systematic review of economic modeling[49] concluded that the strategies for early detection of diabetes and prediabetes are cost-effective, especially for detecting high-risk individuals who may derive benefit from not only glucose-lowering therapy but also other interventions to reduce cardiovascular risk such as statins or antihypertensive drugs. However, this analysis did not include any information for the LA region.

Recently, a new screening model *Instrumento para tamizaje de la Diabetes tipo 2* was developed in Mexico. It was designed as an external validation cohort study in 525 people, aged 20-65 years who were followed for 7 years. The components of the score included personal history, anthropometric and laboratory measurements. Its performance to detect incident diabetes was demonstrated by an area under the receiver operating characteristic curve (AUROC) value of 0.91 (sensitivity 92%, specificity 71%).[50] As there is a substantial deficiency of diabetes educators in most LA countries, opportunistic screening to identify people at high-risk and who can readily join existing primary-care lifestyle intervention programs should be initiated.

2.1. Local Validation of the Finnish Diabetes Risk Score (FINDRISC) for Screening

Recent long-term studies have demonstrated that diabetes can be prevented by early intervention in those with IGT, whether isolated or combined with IFG. These individuals can only be identified by screening and blood testing that may not always be available or accepted. Therefore, diabetes risk scores may become very useful to screen for impaired glucose regulation. The FINDRISC is one of the most efficient and certainly most commonly used screening tools to predict or detect new cases of T2D.[51] Several countries in LA have started to validate and use the FINDRISC for detecting those at high-risk for dysglycemic conditions. The FINDRISC score includes well-known metabolic risk factors such as AO, but it categorizes the latter using cutoffs for WC adopted for Europe and the USA. Recently, it was demonstrated that the cutoff for WC to identify AO were different in the LA population[10] and therefore was incorporated in a modified version of the FINDRISC where a WC $\geq$ 94 cm in men and $\geq$90 cm in women rendered 4 points and lower values rendered 0 points. This version has been validated in two LA cities: Bogotá (Colombia) and Barquisimeto (Venezuela).[52] In both places, the modified FINDRISC was able to discriminate so as to identify individuals with disorders of glucose metabolism (IFG, IGT, T2D) with an area under the curve (AUC) $\geq$ 0.77. The discriminative power of the modified FINDRISC for LA significantly improved in women when compared with the original version. There was no difference in men. A cutoff score >12 points had the best sensitivity/specificity ratio to screen subjects of both sexes and detect those with impaired glucose regulation who would be eligible for blood glucose testing. Nevertheless, there were differences in the best cutoff score in the two populations and therefore we recommend that local validation be conducted prior to its routine use.

2.1.1. *Current Experience with the FINDRISC in LA*

In early 2010, a first pilot study (IBERCARMEN) was conducted in four municipalities of Argentina (Mar del Plata), Colombia (Barranquilla), Peru (Lima), and Venezuela (Simón Planas) to evaluate the feasibility of implementing community screening programs for T2D and associated cardiovascular risk factors. Individuals aged 35-75 years were selected in Colombia, Peru, Venezuela, and Argentina. Using the aforementioned cutoff of WC for the LA region (≥94 cm in men and ≥90 cm in women), the modified FINDRISC classified as "high-risk for T2D" (FINDRISC score of 13 or higher) more women (28.9%) than men (12.5%). Prediabetes (IFG, IGT, or both) was also more frequent ($p < 0.05$) among women (15.5%) than men (13.9%). WC was similar in men and women (96.3 ± 9.3 cm vs. 93.0 ± 12.7 cm, respectively; p = NS). Significant differences between men and women were not observed for other cardiovascular risk factors such as systolic and diastolic blood pressures, total cholesterol, TG, but for HDL-cholesterol: 40.7 ± 9.29 mg/dl (1.05 ± 0.24 mmol/L) in men vs. 45.7 ± 11.9 mg/dl (1.18 ± 0.31 mmol/L) in women; $p<0.05$. This preliminary experience showed the feasibility of implementing diabetes screening programs in the community, and a possibly higher risk of T2D in women than men in LA.[53]

The initial report from DEMOJUAN, an IDF-Bridges Program funded project in Barranquilla, Colombia, regarding the implementation of FINDRISC in that country is very promising. DEMOJUAN is the first structured community-based program on screening and prevention of T2D that aims to improve the prevention and clinical management of T2D among communities living in the Caribbean coast region where poverty, obesity and lack of physical activity are exacerbating a dramatic rise in chronic non-communicable diseases.

The principal objective of DEMOJUAN is to investigate to what extent it is possible to reach normal glucose metabolism and optimal levels of risk factors for cardiovascular disease with early lifestyle interventions in those at high-risk of developing T2D, compared with those receiving standard therapy only. Since October, 2010 individuals between 34-60 years living in five primary health care areas of Barranquilla (El Pueblo, Simón Bolívar, El Bosque de María, COOSALUD, and Paso Juan Mina) are being systematically screened using FINDRISC. Those with a FINDRISC score >13 are offered a standard OGTT. Those diagnosed with IGT, IFG, or both are invited to participate in a lifestyle intervention program. In total, 14,193 participants completed the FINDRISC questionnaire. Thirty-five percent (n = 4915) had a score of 13 or higher (23%

men, 40% women) and were classified as "high-risk for T2D". Only 46% of men and 35% of women had a normal BMI (<25 kg/m^2). Similarly, central obesity using the WHO WC criteria (≥102 cm and ≥88 cm) was very frequent (70% women and 57% men). Only 33% of men and 20% of women reported at least 30 minutes of daily physical activity. The percentage of people reporting daily intake of fruits and vegetables was 32% among men and 34% in women. Approximately 40% of people reported a positive family history of T2D and 16% used antihypertensive drugs. Among "high-risk" people with the FINDRISC >13, the prevalence of screen-detected T2D was 18% in men and 12% in women. The prevalence of isolated IGT, isolated IFG, and IFG plus IGT, both sexes combined, were 8%, 11%, and 8%, respectively.[54]

Other countries such as Argentina, Chile, and Peru, are currently working on the validation and implementation of FINDRISC. For instance, CENEXA and the National University of La Plata have started a program this year to prevent T2D using the FINDRISC questionnaire to identify people at high-risk of T2D in three municipalities of the province of Buenos Aires in Argentina. The Peruvian Diabetes Association and the Ministry of Health of Chile are working on the validation of FINDRISC in their populations as well.

Carvalho and colleagues in Sao Paulo, Brazil evaluated whether FINDRISC can also be used to screen for the presence of hepatic steatosis due to non-alcoholic fatty liver disease.[55] The study sample consisted of 821 without diabetes or previous hepatic disease; 81% were men (mean age 45 ± 9 years) and 19% women (mean age 41 ± 10 years). The FINDRISC score was associated with liver steatosis and thus may also be a useful primary screening tool for its presence.

García-Alcalá and co-workers studied the frequency of T2D, IFG, and IGT in higher-risk groups using a FINDRISC survey in an urban Mexican population.[56] They concluded that the FINDRISC survey is a very useful tool for identifying individuals at high risk of developing diabetes and prediabetic states, especially in those older than 50 years.

It has been recommended to validate the FINDRISC in populations with characteristics different from those of the Finnish population before applying it in order to improve its sensitivity and specificity.[57] In subsequent years, more evidence will be available with regard to the validation and implementation of FINDRISC in primary health care systems of several LA countries.

New technology information systems offer interesting and useful e-health tools for screening chronic conditions. Web-based screening programs are now being developed by several organizations worldwide. The Spanish Foundation of Diabetes (www.fundaciondiabetes.org) recently successfully launched a web-based screening tool to detect high-risk individuals for developing diabetes using the Spanish version of e-FINDRISC. During the first year of the program, e-FINDRISC was completed by more than 26,000 people in the Spanish-speaking world. Nearly 6000 e-FINDRISC (23%) were completed by LA inhabitants (55% females, mean age 39 years), coming mainly from Mexico (33.6%), Argentina (25.6%), Venezuela (6.8%), Colombia (6.7%), Chile (6.1%), and Peru (5.8%). e-FINDRISC classified as high-risk 20.8% of individuals (28.5% of males and 20.3% of females). This pilot experience shows that websites are useful e-health tools for the dissemination of the awareness of T2D risk factors in the population, and for self-assessment of T2D risk in the Spanish-speaking world.[58]

3. PRIMARY PREVENTION PROGRAMS FOR DIABETES IN LA

Clinical trials have demonstrated that T2D can be prevented with lifestyle intervention but their translation to clinical practice may pose difficulties. In North America, several trials attempted to translate the Diabetes Prevention Program (DPP) lifestyle interventions into practice in primary-care settings, but in the rest of the Americas, real world examples are scarce. A few trials are on-going but are still insufficient. Strategies for primary prevention of T2D at the patient level include early identification individual at high-risk to implement interventions with both lifestyle modification and pharmacotherapy. As mentioned above, these strategies have been poorly implemented and limited to local experiences without a clear plan for scaling to national programs. However, at least two pilot projects, both funded by the BRIDGES-IDF Program, are ongoing in Venezuela and Colombia.

In a pilot clinical trial, 140 Latino subjects with prediabetes (63.6% women) 48.1 ± 11.8 years old, with BMI of 32.1 ± 5.5 kg/m² were randomly assigned to receive either standard of care (SC, $n = 70$) or group lifestyle (LS, $n = 70$) intervention for 2 years in the health care system of Maracaibo, Venezuela. Ideal cardiovascular health behaviors (non-smoking, achieving normal weight, enough physical activity, and a healthy diet) and ideal cardiovascular health factors [total cholesterol <200 mg/dl (5.2 mmol/l), blood pressure <120/80 mmHg, and fasting blood glucose <100 mg/dl (5.5 mmol/l)] were evaluated at baseline and every 6 months. The American Heart Association (AHA) global cardiovascular health score was calculated assigning 1 for each ideal behavior and factor (for a maximum of 7) and 0 for poor status to each one. The cardiovascular score at baseline was 3.9 ± 0.1 (84.3% in SC and 88.6% in LS had poor to intermediate cardiovascular scores). Larger improvements in cardiovascular scores from baseline were obtained in the LS vs SC ($p < 0.0001$) at 24 months (2.0 ± 0.9 vs. 0.8 ± 0.6) of intervention. At study end, only 4.3% of LS and 47.1% of SC participants had poor-intermediate cardiovascular scores ($p < 0.01$). The implementation of DPP-based lifestyle intervention leads to moderate improvements in overall CV health among Latinos with prediabetes in Venezuela.[59]

The Finnish DPS lifestyle program is also now being implemented in Barranquilla, Colombia.[54] This DEMOJUAN project is a primary prevention program aimed to improve the prevention and clinical management of T2D among communities living in the Caribbean coast region. The intervention program is based on the local culture and environment targeting a low socio-economic segment of the general population. The intervention comprises several individual appointments with nutritionists and physical activity coaches as well as monthly workshops with some local adaptations such as dancing as a main exercise or promotion of local fruits and vegetables. The first intervention cohort will complete one year of follow-up by the end of 2013 and initial results are expected in 2014. This project has been brought to the attention of the Ministry of Health of Colombia. Barranquilla is planned to be established as a national demonstration region for implementing prevention and health promotion strategies in diabetes. They have proposed to establish a training center in Barranquilla for health care staff from other provinces of the country for learning to screen those at high-risk of T2D and implementing lifestyle intervention strategies.

Other examples of this perspective of prevention at the patient level in the region is represented by recent initiatives of structural changes in the primary level of care, with the creation of specialized clinics to treat patients with diabetes and related conditions including obesity and the metabolic syndrome. A system of primary health clinics was recently launched in Mexico focused on treatment of obesity, diabetes, dyslipidemias, and high blood pressure (UNEMES *Crónicas*) with an interdisciplinary team (psychologist, social worker, dietician, nurse, and physician).[60]

Recently, a group of international experts developed a Transcultural Diabetes Nutrition Algorithm (tDNA) to facilitate and simplify the implementation of medical nutritional therapy and lifestyle changes in prediabetes and T2D.[61] Other countries have created their own versions based on specific epidemiological, physiological, nutritional, and pathological parameters, as well as body composition and lifestyle characteristics that are unique to each locale. A Venezuelan application of tDNA has been developed and the resultant algorithmic modifications include using the LA-modified version of FINDRISC (mentioned above) as a screening tool for prediabetes in order to initiate biochemical monitoring and lifestyle counseling.[62] The next step will be to design simple and practical tools to facilitate implementation and validation of tDNA in Venezuela, Mexico, Brazil, and other countries. While all these initiatives have been implemented and shown some benefit, none has been properly evaluated and so their effectiveness and impact remain to be proven.

A new proposal to reduce the burden of T2D by education and lifestyle interventions in people at high-risk is now under review (www.cyted.org) for LA. The LATIN-PLAN project will implement an intervention programmed at the primary health care level in Mexico, Panamá, Brazil, Colombia, Ecuador, Bolivia, and Venezuela. The project is based on current evidence and best practices in the prevention of T2D, especially those found in European diabetes prevention projects (DE-PLAN and IMAGE projects). It will also develop and implement a curriculum for training diabetes prevention managers in Latin America, which will provide a basis for long-term activities at the population level, and guarantee sustainability and continuity at the community level. Finally, the Latin American Diabetes Association or *Asociación Latinoamericana de*

Diabetes (ALAD) has developed a guideline for the prevention of diabetes that awaits implementation.[63]

4. PUBLIC POLICY AND DIABETES PREVENTION IN LA

In the last decade, many countries in the region have prioritized strategies at the population level especially focused on the prevention of obesity and consequently all related chronic diseases including diabetes. This has been motivated by several declarations from influential non-governmental professional societies such as the *Declaración de Acapulco*[64] and similar statements (*Consenso sobre Prediabetes)* from ALAD,[65] and the *The Salvador de Bahia Call for Action,*[66] a collaborative effort of the Pan American Health Organization (PAHO), Regional Office of the World Health Organization (PAHO-WHO), the Brazilian Ministry of Health, and the World Diabetes Foundation, clearly bolstered globally by the recent call for action from the UN in the *Political Declaration of the High-level Meeting of the General Assembly on the Prevention and Control of Non-communicable Diseases in 2011.*[67] All of these clearly addressed the urgent need for prevention and control of diabetes and recommended specific urgent action relevant for prevention to address and mitigate this threat. In general, these strategies seek to reduce the "obesigenic" environment through actions that necessarily involve the participation of multiple sectors and non-governmental stakeholders, such as private industry and civil society organizations. This strategy ranged from food regulatory measures to decrease access to products that increase the risk of these conditions (taxes, advertising regulation, nutritional labelling, etc.) to planning of urban environments and public spaces that encourage physical activity.

A good example of this is the National Agreement for Health Food (ANSA) (Acuerdo Nacional para la Salud Alimentaria Estrategia contra el sobrepeso y la obesidad. Primera edición, 2010. Secretaría de Salud. México, D.F) recently launched by the Mexican government that represented an effort of considerable value in public health, where several public and private sectors and civil society and academic organizations reached a series of agreements for a comprehensive multisectoral and multilevel strategy directed at controlling obesity and associated chronic diseases, setting clear goals for the coming years. This agreement initiated a series of initiatives that are currently in various stages of implementation:

1. Recommendations for drinks to promote a healthy life.
2. Tax on sugary drinks. This strategy has proven effective in reducing consumption of sugary drinks and currently Mexico, Brazil, and Chile have already proposed to include this tax which is still under discussion in the chambers of representatives.
3. Guidelines for food distribution and supply in the primary schools.
4. The "Five Steps Healthy Living" ("*Cinco pasos por tu salud*"): A massive communication program including recommendations to consume water (instead of soft drinks or other caloric beverages), increase physical activity, increase consumption of fruits and vegetables, and regular evaluation of health and weight.
5. Developing Front Labelling Systems for Food and Beverages to promote healthy choices in the population.

All of these strategies have proven to be cost-effective in several countries and most likely will be implemented across the LA region in the coming year.

5. NATIONAL INITIATIVES ON DIABETES PREVENTION: MEXICO

Statistics identify Mexico as the country with the highest burden of disease and risk of diabetes in LA. During the past six years, Mexico has been a pioneer among LA countries in proposing and developing public health policies on the prevention of diabetes. This section presents an overview of the status of preventive efforts directed to contain the T2D epidemic in Mexico that can be a model for other LA countries. Since the area is in constant change in all aspects: scientific, social, and political as well, it is important to recognize that a new federal government was elected on December 1, 2012. This will generate significant changes in all sectors including the health care arena. Efforts towards universal care as well as portability of health care insurance are the hallmark of expected transformations.

5.1. The Recent Past: 2006–2012

A significant change in the field of T2D prevention in Mexico took place during the last federal administration. The challenge that T2D represents for the country was recognized and a comprehensive list of actions was elaborated. A national program was identified to combat diabetes. The challenges for diabetes prevention and care in Mexico are listed below:

1. Availability of pharmacological agents throughout the country
2. Inadequate infrastructure for health care and prevention
3. Inadequate infrastructure of clinical laboratories
4. Detection and referral with inappropriate delays; policies/portability of health care insurance
5. Inadequate infrastructure for physical activity promotion
6. Insufficient nutritional/psychological social support

These are all situations and factors that are closely interrelated.[68] The actions listed by the federal health authorities in the health care sector to address these challenges during the six-year term that ended in 2012 were:

1. Promotion of the use of the preventive polypill. Low dose of agents (metformin, statin, aspirin, antihypertensive drugs) presumably reducing risk
2. Innovative health care models UNEMES. Specialized units dedicated to T2D care
3. Increase in health care training of the health care professional
4. Health care promotion. Incremental societal awareness
5. Joint efforts with various societal sectors: public/private, co-responsibility

Of these, some are particularly relevant to diabetes prevention. The administration successfully committed to the creation of a new model of health care provider specialized in the clinical management of T2D. This model was mostly focused towards the improvement of T2D care in order to promote better outcomes in metabolic control and by these means, achieve better prevention of acute and chronic complications associated with T2D. The program was implemented in several locations throughout the country; it is yet too early to assess its efficacy and sustainability although preliminary evaluations have yielded promising results. Another significant move was a national agreement regarding the nutritional quality of foods and drinks offered in elementary schools. The center of this agreement was to remove high-density caloric foods and drinks from the school environment, which took significant political negotiation involving educational authorities as well as several representatives of the economic sector. It was implemented with several amendments to the original proposal and needs to be reinforced and improved. The fundamental elements in the T2D prevention strategy identified by the previous administration are listed below:

1. Community-based awareness campaigns
2. Risk factors surveys
3. Training of health care professionals
4. Patient support groups (11,040 new groups created, 308,400 participants involved)
5. 23 million detection efforts
6. 40 million screens

These elements include not only the principal strategy but some of the results obtained during a six-year period during the previous administration. The magnitude of this impressive effort should be noted. The main objectives were:

- Decrease in consumption of food with high caloric density by 50%
- Increase in non-fat / low-fat offerings to school children
- Increase in physical activity in the general public to 150 min/week
- Increase in health literacy & nutrition information in the general population
- Promotion of adequate information for diabetes self-care in patients with T2D

Clearly, to achieve attainable goals, the program needs time and resources.

5.2. The Current Situation (2013–present)

The differential exposure to obesigenic environments in which lower levels of physical activity and increased caloric intake coexist, is the main cause of the incremental incidence of overweight, obesity, and T2D. These factors have important components of social and economic determinants. Although these are elements that need to be addressed by public health policy, many important actions are beyond the realm of the health care sector. All countries of the world are confronting these contradictory forces, mostly because the "development" driver has been interpreted as a "consumption" driver. It is possible that this is the reason why the epicenter of the T2D epidemic worldwide is mostly occurring in developing nations. Mexico is one of these countries. Profound socioeconomic changes are occurring, and the penetrations of pro-consumption forces are intensely and effectively manipulating a relatively docile market.[68] The program, to be announced in the near future by Mexican health care authorities, most likely will contain elements that will recognize the need for a comprehensive approach encompassing all sectors involved. In September 2013, the House of Representatives received a proposal in which a tax increment will be applied to carbonated sweetened beverages (one of the high caloric foods to be restricted in the elementary schools). This is a means to diminish consumption already extremely high in the entire country and a way to obtain urgently needed funds to finance health promotion initiatives. The debate around this bill has just begun regarding the many aspects of this problem. The conflict is centered on economic implications; it is too early to foresee the eventual destiny of this initiative. This is one example of the initiatives expected in the immediate future. Diabetes clearly meets the four criteria required by the WHO for consideration as a priority health problem:

1. The condition represents a large proportion of the total burden of disease.
2. It displays large disparities across and within populations.
3. It disproportionately effects certain groups within populations.
4. It is an emerging epidemic.

Health authorities know the importance of a comprehensive program. It is widely recognized that an effective intervention needs to have reliability, sustainability, scalability, political feasibility, and appropriate economic logic as well technical support. The complexity of the phenomenon must be recognized and the conflicting interests that arise need to be reconciled, with the benefit for the entire society acting as the guiding compass in this high road approach.

A recently completed survey exploring a sample of 31 websites sponsored by federal entities, all related to the health care or educational sector, such as the Ministry of Health and the Ministry of Social Development has yielded interesting results. The intention of the website visit was to explore accessibility, clarity, focus on diabetes prevention, and interactive potential and to estimate the number of visits and if possible a metric of impact. The conclusions, albeit preliminary, were that of the explored sites, only two specifically mentioned diabetes prevention, none indicated the number visiting the site and the absence of interactive encounter with the user.[69] This represents a potentially useful opportunity for intervention. The magnitude of the problem that T2D represents for Mexico should be approached as a top priority that will require immediate utilization of all potential resources in order to ameliorate their impact. Strategies that could use information technology to prevent T2D should be explored systematically since these means could be effective.[70] The approach should be in the form of "translational research" examples of which are beginning to emerge.[71,72]

It has become quite clear that T2D represents an important challenge for the country. Its prevalence, incidence, associated costs, and limited efficacy of the current model of care[73] will have devastating consequences for the nation even if an effective strategy is implemented soon. The example now seen in the United States health care system should serve as a "détente" for the trajectory of the health care sector in Mexico. The important influence that the United States has over many aspects of the country, health care included, is already showing its effects: escalating costs of care with managed care organizations, for-profit hospitals and clinics proliferating throughout the country, and insurance industry charging more without exercising social responsibility. Mexico has an opportunity to create a truly innovative model of care that could be sustained by evidence-based scientific findings, principles, and moral grounds capitalizing from and responding to the urgent need to serve its populace.

The recent approval of incremental taxes that will be applied to sugary beverages has resulted in several important moves. The industry has displayed a highly visible media campaign directed at public opinion regarding the drinks they produce. These advertisements are very well-crafted and show an industry aware of the role of a healthy nation. In addition, hired professional lobbyists are very intensively involved politically in both chambers of government. The challenge remains at the implementation level. As the community is not adequately informed, consequently, the level of consumption may not diminish as expected. In parallel, federal authorities have launched a campaign with the slogan "Chécate (check yourself), Mídete (measure-restrain yourself), Actívate (activate yourself)." This slogan appears with a title "Más vale prevenir" (It is better to prevent). Health promotion, shown in all official media (printed and electronic), though substantial, when compared with the space bought by industry, is significantly lower. There is no public data available yet regarding the impact of this important effort. The campaign is mostly targeted in urban settings though where electronic media coverage tends to be wider.

It is important to highlight the commitment of the president of Mexico in the efforts to combat obesity and diabetes. He attended a prestigious tertiary specialized medical center in Mexico City to witness the institution's new program to treat diabetes. The core of this program is focused on secondary and tertiary prevention. Regardless of the final outcome, it should be noted that diabetes remains on center stage in Mexican society.

ACKNOWLEDGMENTS

To Noël C. Barengo, University of Tolima, Ibague, Colombia, for providing information about current experiences of the validation and use of the FINDRISC questionnaire in Latin America.

To Hermes J Florez, University of Miami and Universidad de Zulia, Maracaibo, Venezuela, for providing data of the Lifestyle Intervention Program in Latinos with Prediabetes in Maracaibo, Venezuela.

To Programa CYTED (Ciencia y tecnología para el Desarrollo en Iberomerica). Funder of the Iberoamerican Cooperative Network IBERCARMEN (Red de Prevención de Enfermedades Cardio-metabólicas en Iberoamérica) Index.

REFERENCES

1. *IDF Atlas*, 5th ed., 2012 update, www.idf.org.
2. Encuesta Nacional de Salud y. Salud Publica de Mexico, **52**, 2010 Nutrición 2006.
3. Escobedo J, Buitro LV, Velasco MF *et al.* on behalf of the Carmela study investigators. (2009) High prevalence of diabetes and impaired fasting glucose in urban Latin America: the CARMELA Study. *Diabet Med* **26**: 864–871.
4. Seclen S, Rosas M, Arias A. Prevalence of type 2 Diabetes in Peru: First Wave prevalence report from PERUDiab, a Population-Based Three-Wave Longitudinal Study (in advance of publication).
5. Aschner P. (2010) Diabetes epidemiology in Colombia. *Avances Diabetología* **29**: 95–100.
6. Carrasco E, Pérez F, Angel B *et al.* (2004) Prevalence of type 2 diabetes and obesity in two Chilean aboriginal populations living in urban zones. *Rev Méd Chile* **132**: 1189–1197.
7. Dal Fabbro AL, Franco LJ, Da Silva AS *et al.* (2013) High prevalence of type 2 diabetes mellitus in Xavante Indians from Mato Grosso, Brazil. *Ethnicity Dis* (in press).
8. De Maio FG, Linetzky B, Ferrante D, Fleischer NL (2012) Extending the income inequality hypothesis: Ecological results from the 2005 and 2009 Argentine National Risk Factor Surveys. *Glob Public Health* **7**: 635–647.
9. Linetzky B, De Maio F, Ferrante D, Konfino J, Boissonnet C. (2013) Sex-stratified socio-economic gradients in physical inactivity, obesity, and diabetes: Evidence of short-term changes in Argentina. *Int J Public Health* **58**: 277–284.
10. Aschner P, Buendía R, Brajkovich I *et al.* (2011) Determination of the cutoff point for waist circumference that establishes the presence of abdominal obesity in Latin American men and women. *Diabetes Res Clin Pract* **93**: 243–247.
11. Aschner P, Ruiz A, Balkau B, Massien C, Haffner SM. (2009) On behalf of the Latin America and the Caribbean International Day for Evaluation of Abdominal Adiposity (IDEA) National Coordinators and Investigators: Association of abdominal adiposity with diabetes and cardiovascular disease in Latin America. *J Clin Hypertens (Greenwich)* **11**: 769–774.
12. González-Villalpando C, Stern M, Villalpando E. Hazuda H, Haffener S, Lisci E. (1992) Prevalencia de diabetes e intolerancia a la glucosa en una población urbana de nivel económico bajo. *Rev Invest Clínica* **44**: 321–327.

13. Lorenzo C, Martinez-Larrad MT, Serrano-Rios M *et al.* (2001) Was the Historic Contribution of Spain to the Mexican Gene Pool Partially Responsible for the Higher Prevalence of Type 2 Diabetes in Mexican-Origin Populations? The Spanish Insulin Resistance Study Group, the San Antonio Heart Study, and the Mexico City Diabetes Study. *Diabetes Care* **24**: 2059–2064.
14. Stern PM, González-Villalpando C, Mitchell BD, Villalpando E, Haffner SM, Hazuda HP. (1992) Genetic and Enviromental Determinants of type 2 diabetes in Mexico City and San Antonio. *Diabetes* **41**: 484–492.
15. Sigma Consortium: Sequence variants in SLC16A11 are a common risk factor for type 2 diabetes in Mexico. *Nature* 2013 (in press).
16. Jimenez-Corona A, Aguilar-Salinas CA, Rojas-Martínez R, Hernández-Ávila M. (2013) Diabetes mellitus tipo 2 y frecuencia de acciones para su prevención y control. *Salud Pública de México* **55**: s137–s143.
17. Nannipieri M, Gonzales C, Baldi S *et al.* (2005) Liver enzymes, the metabolic syndrome, and incident diabetes: the Mexico City diabetes study. *Diabetes Care* **28**: 1757–1762.
18. Ferrannini E, Massari M, Nannipieri M, Natali A, Ridaura RL, Gonzales-Villalpando C. (2009) Plasma glucose levels as predictors of diabetes: the Mexico City diabetes study. *Diabetologia* **52**: 818-2.
19. González-Villalpando C personal communication.
20. Türkoglu C, Duman BS, Günay D, Cagatay P, Ozcan R, Büyükdevrim AS. (2003) Effect of abdominal obesity on insulin resistance and the components of the metabolic syndrome: Evidence supporting obesity as the central feature. *Obes Surg* **13**: 699–705.
21. Rueda-Clausen CF, Silva FA, López-Jaramillo P. (2008) Epidemic of overweight and obesity in Latin America and the Caribbean. *Int J Cardiol* **125**: 111–112.
22. Lanas F, Avezum A, Bautista LE *et al.* INTERHEART Investigators in Latin America. (2007) Risk factors for acute myocardial infarction in Latin America: the INTERHEART Latin American study. *Circulation* **115**: 1067–1074.
23. O'Donnell MJ, Xavier D, Liu L *et al.* INTERSTROKE investigators. (2010) Risk factors for ischaemic and intracerebral haemorrhagic stroke in 22 countries (the INTERSTROKE study): A case-control study. *Lancet* **376**: 112–123.
24. Galic S, Oakhill JS, Steinberg GR. (2010) Adipose tissue as an endocrine organ. *Mol Cell Endocrinol* **316**: 129–139.
25. Lopez-Jaramillo P, Lahera V, Lopez-Lopez J. (2011) Epidemic of cardiometabolic diseases: A Latin American point of view. *Ther Adv Cardiovasc Dis* **5**: 119–131.

26. DeFronzo RA, Ferrannini E. (1991) Insulin resistance. A multifaceted syndrome responsible for NIDDM, obesity, hypertension, dyslipidemia, and atherosclerotic cardiovascular disease. *Diabetes Care* **14**: 173–194.
27. Friedman JE, Dohm GL, Leggett-Frazier N *et al.* (1992) Restoration of insulin responsiveness in skeletal muscle of morbidly obese patients after weight loss. Effect on muscle glucose transport and glucose transporter GLUT4. *J Clin Invest* **89**: 701–705.
28. Henry RR, Scheaffer L, Olefsky JM. (1985) Glycemic effects of intensive caloric restriction and isocaloric refeeding in noninsulin-dependent diabetes mellitus. *J Clin Endocrinol Metab* **61**: 917–925.
29. Reaven GM. (1988) Role of insulin resistance in human disease. *Diabetes* **37**: 1595–1607.
30. Ferrannini E, Haffner SM, Mitchell BD, Stern MP. (1991) Hyperinsulinaemia: the key feature of a cardiovascular and metabolic syndrome. *Diabetologia* **34**: 416–422.
31. Koh KK, Han SH, Quon MJ. (2005) Inflammatory markers and the metabolic syndrome: insights from therapeutic interventions. *J Am Coll Cardiol* **46**: 1978–1985.
32. Schargrodsky H, Hernández-Hernández R, Champagne BM *et al.* CARMELA Study Investigators. (2008) CARMELA: assessment of cardiovascular risk in seven Latin American cities. *Am J Med* **121**: 58–65.
33. Miranda JJ, Herrera VM, Chirinos JA *et al.* (2013) Major cardiovascular risk factors in Latin America: A comparison with the United States. The Latin American Consortium of Studies in Obesity (LASO). *PLoS One* **8**: e54056.
34. Chow CK, Teo KK, Rangarajan S *et al.* (2013) PURE (Prospective Urban Rural Epidemiology) Study investigators. Prevalence, awareness, treatment, and control of hypertension in rural and urban communities in high-, middle-, and low-income countries. *JAMA* **310**: 959–968.
35. Teo K, Lear S, Islam S *et al.* (2013) PURE Investigators. Prevalence of a healthy lifestyle among individuals with cardiovascular disease in high-, middle- and low-income countries: The Prospective Urban Rural Epidemiology (PURE) study. *JAMA* **309**: 1613–1621.
36. López-Jaramillo P, Gómez-Arbeláez D, Camacho F, Álvarez J, Cañon W, David T *et al.* (2013) Obesidad y Sobrepeso en Colombia: Análisis del estudio PURE. *Rev Colombiana Cardiol* (In press).
37. Guzmán JR, Lyra R, Aguilar-Salinas CA *et al.* (2010) ALAD Consensus Group. Treatment of type 2 diabetes in Latin America: a consensus statement

by the medical associations of 17 Latin American countries. Latin American Diabetes Association. *Rev Panam Salud Publica* **28**: 453–471.

38. Villalpando S, Shamah-Levy T, Rojas R, Aguilar-Salinas CA. Trends for type 2 diabetes and other cardiovascular risk factors in Mexico from 1993–2006. *Salud Pública Mex* **52**: S72–S79.
39. López-Jaramillo P, Sánchez RA, Diaz M *et al.* (2013) Latin America Expert Group. Latin American consensus on hypertension in patients with diabetes type 2 and metabolic syndrome. *J Hypertens* **31**: 223–238.
40. Klein R, Klein BE, Moss SE, Cruickshanks KJ. (1994) Relationship of hyperglycemia to the long-term incidence and progression of diabetic retinopathy. *Arch Intern Med* **154**: 2169–2178.
41. Selvin E, Coresh J, Golden SH, Boland LL, Brancati FL, Steffes MW. (2005) Atherosclerosis risk in communities study. Glycemic control, atherosclerosis, and risk factors for cardiovascular disease in individuals with diabetes: the atherosclerosis risk in communities study. *Diabetes Care* **28**: 1965–1973.
42. Hu FB, Stampfer MJ, Haffner SM, Solomon CG, Willett WC, Manson JE. (2002) Elevated risk of cardiovascular disease prior to clinical diagnosis of type 2 diabetes. *Diabetes Care* **25**: 1129–1134.
43. López-Jaramillo P, Sanchez G, Perez M *et al.* (2011) Colombo-Ecuadorian study to determinate the prevalence of pre-diabetes in patients with a first acute myocardial infarction. *J Diabetes* **3**: 73.
44. García RG, Rincón MY, Arenas WD *et al.* (2011) Hyperinsulinemia is a predictor of new cardiovascular events in Colombian patients with a first myocardial infarction. *Int J Cardiol* **148**: 85–89.
45. Secretaría de Salud. Guía para la detección integrada de diabetes e hipertensión arterial. In. México, DF.; 1998:4.
46. Herman WH, Smith PJ, Thompson TJ, Engelgau MM, Aubert RE. (1995) A new and simple questionnaire to identify people at increased risk for undiagnosed diabetes. *Diabetes Care* **18**: 382–387.
47. Lopez-Molina R, Lopez-Ridaura R, Parra-Cabrera S, Trejo-Valdivia B, González-Villalpando C. Validity of the risk prediction questionnaire for type 2 diabetes in the Mexican population: Mexico City Diabetes study. (Submitted to *Salud Pública de Mexico*).
48. Alvear-Galindo MG, Laurell AC. (2010) Analysis of the diabetes mellitus screening program in the Federal District, Mexico. *Cad Saude Publica* **26**: 299–310.

49. Waugh N, Scotland G, McNamee P *et al.* (2007) Screening for type 2 diabetes: Literature review and economic modelling. *Health Technol Assess* **11**: 1–236.
50. Guerrero-Romero F, Rodriguez-Morán M. (2010) Validation of an instrument for screening cases of type 2 diabetes and monitoring at-risk individuals in Mexico. *Rev Panam Salud Publica* **27**: 181–186.
51. Lindström J, Tuomilehto J. (2003) The diabetes risk score: A practical tool to predict type 2 diabetes risk. *Diabetes Care* **26**: 725–773.
52. Aschner P, Nieto R, Marin A, Rios M. (2012) Evaluation of the FINDRISC score as a screening tool for people with impaired glucose regulation in Latin America using modified score points for waist circumference according to the validated regional cutoff values for abdominal obesity. *Minerva Endocrinologica* **37**: 114.
53. Gabriel R. (2011) Informe final de actividades de la Red Temática Cooperativa de Investigación en Enfermedades Cardiometabólicas (IBERCARMEN). CYTED. Madrid.
54. Barengo NC, Acosta T, Arrieta A, Ricaurte C, Mayor D, Tuomilehto JO. (2013) The DEMOJUAN study group. Screening for people with glucose metabolism disorders within the framework of the DEMOJUAN project (DEMOnstration area for primary prevention of type 2 diabetes, JUAN Mina and Barranquilla, Colombia). *Diabetes Metab Res Rev* September 2. [Epub ahead of print]
55. Carvalho JA, Barengo NC, Tuomilehto J, Conceição RD, Santos RD. (2011) The Finnish Diabetes Risk Score (FINDRISC) as a screening tool for hepatic eatosis. *Ann Med* **43**: 487–494.
56. García-Alcalá H, Genestier-Tamborero CN, Hirales-Tamez O, Salinas-Palma J, Soto-Vega E. (2012) Frequency of diabetes, impaired fasting glucose, and glucose intolerance in high-risk groups identified by a FINDRISC survey in Puebla City, Mexico. *Diabetes Metab Syndr Obes* **5**: 403–406.
57. Alberti KG, Zimmet P, Shaw J. (2007) International Diabetes Federation: A consensus on Type 2 diabetes prevention. *Diabet Med* **24**: 451–463.
58. Salaverria V, Marín MC, Dueñas B *et al.* The website of the Spanish Foundation of Diabetes, an useful and friendly e-tool for information and prevention in the Spanish speaking countries.
59. Florez HJ, Stepenka V, Castillo-Florez S *et al.* (2012) Lifestyle intervention improves global cardiovascular health in Latinos with prediabetes in Maracaibo, Venezuela. *Circulation* **125**: AP162.

60. Córdova-Villalobos JA, Barriguete-Meléndez JA, Lara-Esqueda A *et al.* (2008) Chronic non-communicable diseases in Mexico: Epidemiologic synopsis and integral prevention. *Salud Publ Mex* **50**: 419–427.
61. Mechanick JI, Marchetti AE, Apovian C *et al.* (2012) Diabetes-specific nutrition algorithm: A transcultural program to optimize diabetes and prediabetes care. *Curr Diab Rep* **12**: 180–194.
62. Nieto-Martínez R, Hamdy O, Marante D *et al.* Transcultural diabetes nutrition algorithm: The Venezuelan application. (Submitted article to *Nutrients*).
63. Rosas Guzmán J, Mesa JA, Alexanderson G *et al.* (2008) Recomendaciones para prevenir, detectar y tratar la prediabetes en América Latina. *Rev Asoc Latino Diabetes* **16**: 48–49.
64. Aguilar-Salinas CA, Gómez-Pérez FJ. (2006) The Acapulco Declaration: A proposal to reduce incidence of diabetes in México. *Rev Invest Clin* **58**: 71–77.
65. Rosas J, Calles J. On behalf of the ALAD working group: Prediabetes consensus: Position statement of the Latin American Diabetes Association (ALAD), www.alad-latinoamerica.org.
65. A Report From The Diabetes Summit for Latin America, Bahia, Brazil (30 June–2 July, 2010). *Pract Diab Int*, Copyright © 2010 John Wiley & Sons.
66. Political Declaration of the High-level Meeting of the General Assembly on the Prevention and Control of Non-communicable Diseases in 2011.
67. Secretaría de Salud, Subsecretaría de Prevención y Promoción de la Salud, Programa de acción específico 2007–2012. Diabetes Mellitus, Primera edición 2008, [Accessed septiembre 26, 2013] http://www.cenavece.salud.gob.mx/descargas/pdf/programa_dm.pdf.
68. Chen L, Magliano DJ, Zimmet PZ. (2012) The worldwide epidemiology of type 2 diabetes mellitus, present and future perspectives. *Nature* **8**: 229–236.
69. Jimenez-Corona A, Aguilar-Salinas CA, Rojas-Martínez R, Hernández-Ávila M. (2013) Diabetes mellitus tipo 2 y frecuencia de acciones para su prevención y control. *Salud Públ Méx* **55**: S137–S143.
70. Ramachandran A, Snehalatha C, Ram J *et al.* (2013) Effectiveness of mobile phone messaging in prevention of type 2 diabetes by lifestyle modification in men in India: A prospective, parallel-group, randomised controlled trial. *Lancet* **1**: 191–198.
71. García-Alcalá C, Genestier-Tamborero N, Hirales-Tamez O, Salinas-Palama J, Soto-Vega E. (2012) Frequency of diabetes, impaired fasting glucose, and glucose intolerance in high-risk groups identified by a FINDRISC survey in Puebla City, Mexico. *Diabetes Metab Syndr Obes* **5**: 403–406.

72. Pérez de Célis Herrero MC, Somodevilla-Garcia MJ, Gutiérrez Martínez MT *et al.* Prevención en diabetes (DM) una experiencia piloto usando TICs: Identificación de necesidades en la estrategia. 1 Proceeding of 5°. Congreso de Investigación en Salud Pública. Instituto Nacional de Salud Pública. Cuernavaca, Mor.
73. González-Villalpando C, López-Ridaura R, Campuzano JC, González Villalpando ME. (2010) The status of diabetes care in Mexican population: Are we making a difference? Results of the National Health and Nutrition Survey 2006. *Salud Publ Mex* **2010**: 5.

Index